Cognitive and Cultural Influences on Eye Movements

认知与文化的眼动研究

Edited by

Keith Rayner 凯斯 · 瑞纳
Deli Shen 沈德立
Xuejun Bai 白学军
Guoli Yan 阎国利

CRC Press
Taylor & Francis Group
Boca Raton London New York

CRC Press is an imprint of the
Taylor & Francis Group, an **informa** business

First published 2008 by Tianjin People Publishing House

First edition 2008

Published 2018 by CRC Press
Taylor & Francis Group
6000 Broken Sound Parkway NW, Suite 300
Boca Raton, FL 33487-2742

First issued in paperback 2018

ISBN-13: 978-1-138-96944-5 (pbk)
ISBN-13: 978-7-201-06107-8 (hbk)

Visit the Taylor & Francis Web site at
http://www.taylorandfrancis.com

and the CRC Press Web site at
http://www.crcpress.com

图书在版编目（CIP）数据

认知与文化的眼动研究=Cognitive and Culture Influence on Eye Movement:英文/白学军主编. — 天津：天津人民出版社，2008.11
ISBN 978-7-201-06107-8

I. 认… II. 白… III. 眼动 — 国际学术会议 — 文集 — 英文 IV. B842.2-53

中国版本图书馆CIP数据核字（2008）第174543号

Contents

Preface and overview of chapters

Over the past few years, researchers interested in various aspects of cognitive processes in reading, scene perception, and visual search have increasingly turned to eye movement data to investigate these topics. The present volume presents chapters on these topics, with special emphasis on cognitive and cultural influences on eye movements. The volume is largely based on talks presented at the Second China International Conference on Eye Movements in June, 2006 at Tianjin Normal University. This meeting was very successful in bringing a number of established eye movement researchers from the US and Europe to China. In addition, a large number of Chinese researchers attended the meeting (with many of them presenting talks or posters). The conference itself was very stimulating and followed an earlier meeting (in 2004) where the invited talks were published in the journal *Studies in Psychology and Behavior* published by the Academy of Psychology and Behavior at Tianjin Normal University. However, given that the second meeting was considerably larger, it was decided to publish the invited presentations and other selected presentations in the present volume. Fortunately, all invited speakers agreed to write chapters, as did all of those who were invited to contribute chapters. The resulting volume provides a good overview of research on many topics typically studied via eye movement data.

The volume begins with an overview chapter by Castelhano and Rayner in which eye movements during reading, visual search, and scene perception are reviewed. In Section 2, descriptions of the E-Z Reader model of eye movement control in reading by Pollatsek, Rayner, and Reichle and the SWIFT model by Risse, Engbert, and Kliegl are presented. Recently, there has been considerable research activity associated with the development of computational models that successfully predict both where readers look and when they move their eyes during reading and these two chapters provide descriptions of the two best known and successful models. In keeping with the theme of cultural influences on eye movements, Chapter 4 by Rayner, Li, and Pollatsek deals with an initial attempt to extend the E-Z Reader model to Chinese readers. In Section 3, Liversedge discusses recent research dealing with binocular eye movements in reading. Until recently, it was assumed that the two eyes were in the same place in reading and other information processing tasks. However, the work of Liversedge and colleagues demonstrates that this is not always the case. In Chapter 6, Benson discusses some very interesting research documenting characteristics of saccade orienting in special populations. The final two chapters in this section deal with using eye movements to understand complex visual comparisons by Cave et al. (Chapter 7) and in driving situations by Pollatsek, Fisher, and Pradham (Chapter 8). In Section 4, Nummenmaa, Hyönä, and Calvo (Chapter 9) discuss research on the extent to which emotional stimuli catch the eye, Menneer et al. (Chapter 10) discuss eye movements during visual search, and Hakki et al. (Chapter 11) discuss eye movements and individual differences in mental rotation.

With the exception of Rayner et al.'s chapter on the E-Z Reader model and Chinese, the other chapters in the first four sections focus pretty much exclusively with cognitive influences on eye movements in different tasks. The chapters in the last two sections of the volume deal exclusively with cultural influences on eye movements. All of the chapters in Section 5 deal with the eye movements of Chinese readers. In Chapter 12, Tsang and Chen provide an overview of eye movements when reading Chinese. The perceptual span in reading Chinese is the focus of Chapter 13 by Shen et al. and lexical processing is the focus of Chapter 14 by Gao, Zhang, and Chen. In Chapter 15, Wu et al. discuss word segmentation in reading. The penultimate chapter in the section, Chapter 16 by Wang, Yang, and Chen deals with eye movements and higher order processes in reading Chinese. The final chapter, Chapter 17, by Yan et al. deals with beginning Chinese reading. In Section 6, the theme of cultural influences continues with chapters by Boland, Chua, and Nisbett (Chapter 18) on cultural influences on scene perception and Li et al. (Chapter 19) examine individual differences in eye movements in different information processing tasks, while also considering cultural effects. The final chapter, Chapter 20, by Feng deals with what he calls the "paraorthographic linkage hypothesis" and the extent to which differences in writing systems influence eye movements.

As editors of this volume, we greatly appreciate the punctuality of the authors in providing chapters for this volume. We hope that readers of the volume will appreciate the insights contained in the chapters. We also thank Tianjin People's Pubilshing House for their efforts in publishing the book and Lucy Kennedy and Mike Forster of Psychology Press for their assistance in publishing the book outside of China. We also thank Abby Rothschild for her excellent copy-editing of the chapters. Finally, we note that the conference and the production of the book were supported financially by the Academy of Psychology and Behavior at Tianjin Normal University.

Keith Rayner
Deli Shen
Xuejun Bai
Guoli Yan

List of contributors

Xuejun Bai, Academy of Psychology and Behavior, Tianjin Normal University, Tianjin, 300074, China.

E-mail: psy-bxj@mail.tjnu.edu.cn

Valerie Benson, School of Psychology, University of Southampton, Southampton, S017 1BJ, UK.

E-mail: vb1@soton.ack.uk

Julie E. Boland, Department of Psychology, University of Michigan, Ann Arbor, MI 48109, USA.

E-mail: jeboland@umich.edu

Manuel G. Calvo, Department of Psychology, University of La Laguna, La Laguna, 38207, Spain.

E-mail: mgcalvo@ull.es

Kyle R. Cave, Department of Psychology, University of Massachusetts, Amherst, MA 01003, USA.

E-mail: kcave@psych.umass.edu

Monica S. Castelhano, Department of Psychology, Queen's University, Kingston, Ontario, K7L 3N6, Canada.

E-mail: castelm@queensu.ca

Hsuan-Chih Chen, Department of Psychology, The Chinese University of Hong Kong, Shatin, NT, Hong Kong.

E-mail: hcchen@psy.cuhk.edu.hk

Ju Chen, Department of Psychology, Sun-Yat Sen University, Guangzhou, 510275, China.

E-mail: qiqi05@gmail.com

Hannah Faye Chua, Department of Psychology, University of Michigan, Ann Arbor, MI 48109, USA.

E-mail: hchua@umich.edu

Andrew L. Cohen, Department of Psychology, University of Massachusetts, Amherst, MA 01002, USA.

E-mail: acohen@psych.umass.edu

Ibrahim Dahlstrom-Hakki, Department of Psychology, University of Massachusetts, Amherst, MA 01002, USA.

E-mail: ihakki@psych.umass.edu

Nick Donnelly, School of Psychology, University of Southampton, Southampton, SO17 1BJ, UK.

E-mail: n.donnelly@soton.ac.uk

Ralf Engbert, Department of Psychology, University of Potsdam, Potsdam, 14476, Germany.

E-mail: engbert@rz.uni-potsdam.de

Kris Evans, Department of Psychology, University of Massachusetts, Amherst, MA 01003, USA.

E-mail: hsiaochu@psych.umass.edu

Gary Feng, Department of Psychology and Neuroscience, Duke University, Durham, NC 27708, USA.

E-mail: garyfeng@duke.edu

Donald L. Fisher, Department of Engineering, University of Massachusetts, Amherst, MA 01003, USA.

E-mail: fisher@ecs.umass.edu

Dingguo Gao, Department of Psychology, Sun-Yat Sen University, Guangzhou, 510275, China.

E-mail: edsgao@mail.sysu.edu.cn

Hua Shu, School of Psychology, Beijing Normal University, Beijing, 100875, China.

E-mail: shuh@bnu.edu.cn

Jukka Hyönä, Department of Psychology, University of Turku, Turku, 20014, Finland.

E-mail: hyona@utu.fi

Reinhold Kliegl, Department of Psychology, University of Potsdam, Potsdam, 14476, Germany.

E-mail: kliegl@uni-potsdam.de

Hong Li, School of Psychology, Beijing Normal University, Beijing, 100875, China.

E-mail: psy.lihong@gmail.com

Xingshan Li, Department of Psychology, Vanderbilt University, Nashville, TN 37203, USA.

E-mail: xingshan@gmail.com

Simon P. Liversedge, School of Psychology, University of Southampton, Southampton, S017 1BJ, UK.

E-mail: s.p.liversedge@soton.ac.uk

Anthony McCaffrey, Department of Psychology, University of Massachusetts, Amherst, MA 01003, USA.

E-mail: amccaffr@psych.umass.edu

Tamaryn Menneer, School of Psychology, University of Southampton, Southampton, S017 1BJ, UK.

E-mail: t.menneer@soton.ac.uk

Brett Miller, National Institute of Child Health and Development, Bethesda, MD 20892, USA.

E-mail: millerbre@mail.nih.gov

Kevin F. Miller, Department of Psychology, University of Michigan, Ann Arbor, MI 48109, USA.

E-mail: kevinmil@umich.edu

Richard E. Nisbett, Department of Psychology, University of Michigan, Ann Arbor, MI 48109, USA.

E-mail: nisbett@umich.edu

Lauri Nummenmaa, MRC Cognition and Brain Sciences Unit, Cambridge, CB2 2EF UK.

E-mail: Lauri.Nummenmaa@mrc-cbu.cam.ac.uk

and Department of Psychology, University of Turku, Turku, 20014, Finland.

E-mail: lauri.nummenmaa@utu.fi

Alexander Pollatsek, Department of Psychology, University of Massachusetts, Amherst, MA 01003, USA.

E-mail: pollatsek@psych.umass.edu

Anuj Pradhan, UMass Transportation Center, University of Massachusetts, Amherst, MA 01003, USA.

E-mail: anujkp@acad.umass.edu

Keith Rayner, Department of Psychology, University of Massachusetts, Amherst, MA 01003, USA.

E-mail: rayner@psych.umass.edu

and Department of Psychology, University of California, San Diego, 92093, USA.

E-mail: krayner@ucsd.edu

Erik D. Reichle, Department of Psychology, University of Pittsburgh, Pittsburgh, PA 15260, USA.

E-mail: reichle@pitt.edu

Sarah Risse, Department of Psychology, University of Potsdam, Potsdam, 14476, Germany.

E-mail: srisse@rz.uni-potsdam.de

Michael G. Ross, Department of Psychology, University of Massachusetts, Amherst, MA 01003, USA.

E-mail: mgross@psych.umass.edu

Caren M. Rotello, Department of Psychology, University of Massachusetts, Amherst, MA 01003, USA.

E-mail: caren@psych.umass.edu

Deli Shen, Academy of Psychology and Behavior, Tianjin Normal University, Tianjin, 300074, China.

E-mail: b126@eyou.com

Timothy J. Slattery, Department of Psychology, University of California, San Diego, 92093.

E-mail: tslattery@ucsd.edu

Michael J. Stroud, Department of Psychology, University of Massachusetts, Amherst, MA 01003, USA.

E-mail: mtroud@psych.umass.edu

Yiu-Kei Tsang, Department of Psychology, The Chinese University of Hong Kong, Shatin, NT, Hong Kong.
E-mail: yktsang@psy.cuhk.edu.hk

Suiping Wang, Department of Psychology, South China Normal University, Guangzhou, 510631, China.
E-mail: suipingscnu@263.net

Arnold D. Well, Department of Psychology, University of Massachusetts, Amherst, MA 01003, USA.
E-mail: well@psych.umass.edu

Carrick C. Williams, Department of Psychology, Mississippi State University, Mississippi State, MS 39762, USA.
E-mail: cwilliams@psychology.msstate.edu

Jun Wu, Department of Psychology, South China Normal University, Guangzhou, 510631, China.
E-mail: junwupsy@gmail.com

Guoli Yan, Academy of Psychology and Behavior, Tianjin Normal University, Tianjin, 300074, China.
E-mail: psyygl@yahoo.com

Ming Yan, School of Psychology, Beijing Normal University, Beijing, 100875, China.
E-mail: mingyan1981@gmail.com

Jinmian Yang, Department of Psychology, University of Massachusetts, Amherst, MA 01003, USA.
E-mail: jinmian@psych.umass.edu

Min Zeng, Department of Psychology, University of Massachusetts, Amherst, MA 01003, USA.
E-mail: zeng@psych.umass.edu

Ruijian Zhang, Department of Psychology, Sun-Yat Sen University, Guangzhou, 510275, China.
E-mail: the only moon@126.com

Matthew Zivot, Department of Psychology, University of Massachusetts, Amherst, MA 01003, USA.
E-mail: mzivot@psych.umass.edu

Section 1
Introduction

Chapter 1

Eye movements during reading, visual search, and scene perception: An overview

Monica S. Castelhano and Keith Rayner

In this chapter, we provide an overview of research on eye movements during reading, visual search, and scene perception. Our overview of reading will be more complete than our overview of visual search or scene perception. The reason for this is quite simple. We know more about the nature of eye movements in reading than in the other two tasks. And, the reason for this is also quite apparent. In reading, there is a well-defined task for the viewer: People generally read to understand or comprehend the text. This involves a sequence of eye movements that typically move from left-to-right across the page and then down the page. Of course, the task can be varied somewhat so that, for example, readers are asked to skim the text, and this will result in different eye movement characteristics. Yet, the vast bulk of the research on eye movements during reading has utilized comprehension as the goal of the reader. On the other hand, in scene perception, the nature of the task is inherently much vaguer. Viewers may be asked to look at a scene to remember it, but the sequence in which they examine the scene may be highly idiosyncratic and variable. In visual search, there are many different types of search tasks (search for a letter, search for a colored object, search for a person in a large group picture, search for Waldo in a "Where's Waldo" children's book, and so on), and viewers can use idiosyncratic strategies in dealing with the task. Despite these differences, a fair amount of information on the nature of eye movements in each task is available. In this chapter, we will review some of the main findings concerning eye movements in these tasks as background information for the other chapters in the volume, which deal with these issues and also with the influence of cultural variables on eye movements.

Basic characteristics of eye movements

While we are reading or searching a visual array for a target or simply looking at a new scene, our eyes move every 250-350 ms. These eye movements serve to move the fovea (the high resolution part of the retina encompassing 2 degrees at the center of the visual field) to an area of interest in order to process it in greater detail. Because of acuity limitations in the retina, eye movements are necessary for processing the details of the array. Our ability to discriminate fine detail drops off markedly outside of the fovea in the parafovea (extending out to about 5 degrees on either side of fixation) and in the periphery (everything beyond the parafovea). During the actual eye movement (or saccade), vision is suppressed[1] and new information is acquired only during the fixation (the period of time when the eyes remain still for about 250-350 ms). Although we have the impression that we can process the entire visual array in a single fixation and while we can rapidly obtain the gist of the scene from a single fixation, in reality we would be unable to fully process the information outside of foveal vision if we were unable to move our eyes (Rayner, 1978, 1998).

While it is true that we can move our attention independently of where the eyes are fixated, it does not seem to be the case in everyday viewing. The separation between attention and fixation is often attained in very simple tasks (Posner, 1980); however, in tasks like reading, visual search, and scene perception, covert attention and overt attention (the exact eye location) are tightly linked. Although when we look at a complicated scene, we can dissociate covert and overt attention, generally speaking it takes either a certain amount of effort to maintain it (as when we hold fixation and move our attention elsewhere) or it is a natural consequence of programming eye movements. There is considerable evidence that before an eye movement is made, attention typically

1 It is important to note that although vision is suppressed, mental processes continue during the saccade for many cognitive tasks (see Irwin, 2004 for a review of when cognition is also suppressed during saccades).

precedes it to the intended target (Deubel & Schneider, 1996; Hoffman & Subramaniam, 1995; Kowler, Anderson, Dosher, & Blaser, 1995; Rayner, McConkie, & Ehrlich 1978).

Because eye movements are essentially motor movements, it takes time to plan and execute a saccade. In simple reaction time experiments, where there is no necessity of cognitive processing of the fixated material and participants merely need to monitor when a simple fixation target moves from one location to another (and move their eyes accordingly), it takes on the order of 175 ms to move the eyes under the best of circumstances (Becker & Jürgens, 1979; McPeek, Skavenski, & Nakayama, 2000; Rayner, Slowiaczek, Clifton, & Bertera, 1983). In addition, it is important to note that eye movements are more or less ballistic movements. Once initiated, it is difficult (though not impossible) to change their trajectory. While it has generally been assumed that the two eyes move in synchrony and that they fixate the same point in space, recent research summarized by Liversedge (this volume) clearly demonstrates that this is not the case and the two eyes are frequently deviated from each other.

Table 1.1 Eye movement characteristics in reading, scene perception, and visual search

Task	Mean fixation duration (ms)	Mean saccade size (degrees)
Silent reading	225-250	2 (7-9 letter spaces)
Oral reading	275-325	1.5 (6-7 letter spaces)
Scene perception	260-330	4
Visual search	180-275	3

There is considerable evidence that the nature of the task influences eye movements. A summary of the average amount of time spent on each fixation and the average distance the eyes move in reading, visual search, and scene perception are shown in Table 1.1. From this table, it is immediately apparent that while the values presented in the table are quite representative of the different tasks, they show a range of average fixation durations and for each of the tasks there is considerable variability both in terms of fixation durations and saccade lengths. This is also clearly illustrated in Figure 1.1, which shows frequency distributions of fixation durations in the three tasks. From these graphs, it is very evident that there is a great amount of variability in fixation time measures.

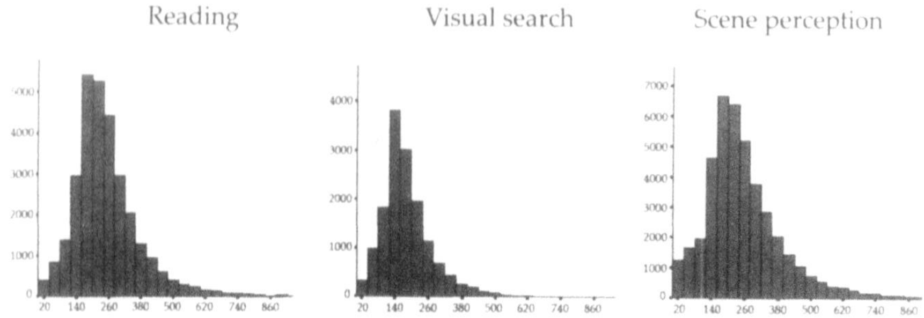

Figure 1.1 Fixation duration frequency distributions for reading, visual search, and scene perception. The data are from the same 24 observers engaged in the three different tasks. No lower cutoffs of fixation duration were used in these distributions while an upper cutoff of 1000 ms was used.

At one time, researchers believed that the eyes and the mind were not tightly linked during information processing tasks like reading, visual search, and scene perception. This conclusion was based on the relatively long latencies of eye movements (or reaction time of the eyes) and the large variability in the fixation time measures. They questioned the influence of cognitive factors on fixations given that eye movement latency was so long and the fixation times were so variable. It seemed unlikely that cognitive factors could influence fixation times from fixation to fixation. Actually, an underlying assumption was that everything proceeded in a serial fashion and that cognitive processes could not influence anything until very late in a fixation, if at all. However, a great deal of research since has established a tight link between the eye and the mind, and it is now clear that saccades can be programmed in parallel (Becker & Jürgens, 1979) and, furthermore, that information processing continues in parallel with saccade programming.

With this preamble (and basic information) out of the way, let's now turn to a brief overview of eye movements in each of the three tasks. We'll begin with reading (which will receive the most attention given that there is more research on eye movements in this task than the other two), and then move to visual search and scene perception.

Eye movements in reading

During reading, the average fixation duration in reading is about 225-250 ms and the average saccade size is 7-9 character spaces. In reading, unlike the other tasks, character spaces are used as the metric for how far the eyes move rather than visual angle. This is because it has been demonstrated that character spaces are the more appropriate unit than visual angle. So, if the size of the print is held constant and the viewing distance varied (so that there are either more or fewer characters per degree of visual angle), how far the eyes travel is determined by character spaces, not visual angle (Morrison & Rayner, 1981). Another important characteristic of eye movements while reading is that about 10%~15% of the time readers move their eyes back (regress) to previously read material in the text. These regressions, as they are called, tend to depend on the difficulty of the text. As would be expected, saccade size and fixation duration are also both modulated by text difficulty: As the text becomes more difficult, saccade size decreases, fixation durations increase, and regressions increase. From these measures alone, it is very clear that global properties of the text influence eye movements greatly. In addition, these three main global measures (saccade size, fixation duration, and number of regressions) are also influenced by the type of material being read and the reader's goals in reading (Rayner & Pollatsek, 1989). For instance, reading a text for understanding produces a very different pattern of eye movement measures when compared to skimming a text while proofreading.

In addition to global effects, studies have shown clear local effects on words. Measures in these studies focus on the processing of a target word (versus looking at an average measure that is pooled from all words in a sentence, such as the average fixation duration). Local measures include: first fixation duration (the duration of the first fixation on a word), single fixation duration (those cases where only a single fixation is made on a word), and gaze duration (the sum of all fixations on a word prior to moving to another word). Global measures would be more useful if every word was fixated in a sentence and fixated only once. However, reading patterns are not so: Many words are skipped during reading (i.e., never receive a direct eye fixation) and some words are fixated more than once. There is good reason to think that words that are skipped are processed on the fixation prior to the skip. There is also good reason to believe that when words are re-fixated (before moving on in the text), it is because more time is needed to process these words' meaning. The solution then is to use eye movement measures that are more local (as described above) and so, are able to provide a reasonable estimate of the processing of a particular word (Rayner, 1998).

The perceptual span

A very important issue in reading is how much information the reader is able to process and use during a single fixation, which, as we've noted above, typically lasts for 200-250 ms. This measure is referred to as the perceptual span (also called the functional field of view or, to a lesser degree, the region of effective vision). Although we have the impression that we can see an entire line of text or even an entire page of text, this is an illusion. This fact has been clearly demonstrated in a number of studies over the years that use a gaze-contingent moving window paradigm (see Figure 1.2), introduced by McConkie and Rayner (1975; Rayner & Bertera, 1979).

The logic behind the gaze-contingent moving window paradigm is that we can determine how much of the text is being processed by varying the window size in which the text appears normal. Therefore, how much information is available to a reader is determined by how large the window (showing the normal text) has to be for readers to read normally. Or conversely, how small the window can get before there is disruption to reading. In this paradigm, the text within the window is normally presented, but the text outside the window is manipulated by either replacing the correct letters with other letters or replacing them all with Xs. Studies using this paradigm have demonstrated that English readers acquire useful information from an asymmetrical region around the fixation point (extending 3-4 character spaces to the left of fixation and about 14-15 character spaces to the right)[2]. So, if the fixated word and the word to the right of fixation are normal and all other letters are replaced with visually similar letters, we find that readers are not aware that the words outside of the window have been changed, and their reading speed only decreases by about 10%. If two words to the right of fixation are normally displayed, then we see little slowdown in reading. Research has also found that readers do not utilize information from the words on the line below the currently fixated line (Rayner, 1998). Finally, the moving window paradigm can be reversed to produce a moving mask paradigm (Rayner & Bertera, 1979; Rayner, Inhoff, Morrison, Slowiaczek, & Bertera, 1981). In this case, a mask moves with the eyes on each fixation covering the letters in the center

2 The size of the perceptual span is also influenced by the nature of the writing system, but a description of this influence is beyond the scope of this chapter (a review; see also the chapter by Shen et al., this volume).

of vision (see Figure 1.2). From this paradigm, results demonstrate that reading is almost impossible when only letters in parafoveal vision are presented normally, while the central region is masked.

```
Normal Line:
Studying people while reading versus looking at

Moving Window Paradigm (13 character window):
Xxxxxxxx xeople while rxxxxxx xxxxxx xxxxxxx xx
                *

Xxxxxxxx xxxxxx xxile reading vxxxxx xxxxxxx xx
                        *


Moving Mask Paradigm (7 character mask):
Studying people wxxxxxxxading versus looking at
                    *

Studying people while rexxxxxxxersus looking at
                           *


Boundary Paradigm:
Studying people while feeding versus looking at
                  *

Studying people while reading versus looking at
                          *
```

Figure 1.2 Examples of a moving window (with a thirteen character window), a moving mask (with a 7 character mask), and the boundary paradigm. When the reader's eye movement crosses an invisible boundary location (the letter *e*), the preview word *feeding* changes to the target word *reading*. The asterisk represents the location of the eyes in each example.

Another gaze-contingent display change paradigm (see Figure 1.2), called the boundary paradigm (Rayner, 1975), has been used to investigate the degree to which information outside the fixated region is processed. In this paradigm, the word to the right of fixation can be the target word (i.e., a valid preview), or it may be replaced with another word, a non-word, or random string of letters (i.e., an invalid preview). When the reader's eye movement crosses an invisible boundary location, the preview (either the valid preview or an invalid preview) changes to the target word; since vision is suppressed during the eye movement, readers are not aware of the change. Researchers have found that when a reader has a invalid preview of the word to the right of fixation, they spend about 30-50 ms more fixating that word (following a saccade to it) than when they have a valid preview. It is also interesting to note that using this technique, studies have revealed that readers don't combine a literal representation of the visual information across saccades, but rather combine abstract (and phonological) information across eye fixations (McConkie & Zola, 1979; Rayner, McConkie, & Zola, 1980).

Linguistic influences on fixation time

As briefly mentioned above, the difficulty of the text being read has an impact on eye movement patterns (fixation duration, saccade length, and frequency of regressing to previously read text). Over the past few years, it has become very clear that how long the eyes remain in place is influenced by a host of linguistic factors. These factors include the frequency of the fixated word (Inhoff & Rayner, 1986; Rayner & Duffy, 1986), how predictable the fixated word is (Ehrlich & Rayner, 1981; Rayner & Well, 1996), how many meanings the fixated word has (Duffy, Morris, & Rayner, 1988; Sereno, O'Donnell, & Rayner, 2006), when the meaning of the word was acquired (Juhasz & Rayner, 2003, 2006), semantic relations between the word and prior words (Carroll & Slowiaczek, 1986; Morris, 1994), and how familiar the word is (Williams & Morris, 2004). For a more in-depth review of these factors and others (see Rayner 1998).

The most compelling evidence that cognitive processing drive the eyes through the text perhaps comes from experiments in which the fixated word either disappears or is masked after 50-60 ms (Ishida & Ikeda, 1989; Liversedge, Rayner, White, Vergilino-Perez, Findlay, & Kentridge, 2004; Rayner et al., 1981; Rayner, Liversedge, & White, 2006; Rayner, Liversedge, White, & Vergilino-Perez, 2003). In these studies, readers are allowed to see the fixated word for 50-60 ms before it disappears. Under these conditions, they read quite normally; however, if the word to the right of fixation also disappears or is masked, then reading is disrupted (Rayner et al., 2006). This result indicates quite strongly that the word to the right of fixation is very important in reading. For the present purposes, it is important to note that when the fixated word disappears after 60 ms, fixation duration on that word is determined by the frequency of the word: If it is a low frequency word, the eyes remain in place longer (Rayner et al., 2003, 2006). So, even though the word is no longer visible, how long the eyes remain fixated is determined by that words' frequency. This evidence is very compelling and supports the notion that the cognitive processes associated with a fixated word are what drive eye movements through the text.

To summarize, it is clear that readers obtain information from a limited region during a fixation (extending to about 14-15 character spaces to the right of fixation). Information used for word identification is obtained from an even smaller region (extending to about 7-8 character spaces to the right of fixation). Furthermore, the word to the right of fixation is important and some information about that word is processed, as shown by preview benefit from that word. On some fixations, readers process the meaning of the fixated word and the word to the right of fixation, and will subsequently skip the word to the right of fixation. Finally, the ease or difficulty associated with processing the fixated word strongly has an effect on how long readers look at that word.

Models of eye movements in reading

Based on the vast amount of information about eye movements during reading learned in the past 25-30 years, a number of models of eye movements in reading have recently appeared. The E-Z Reader model (Pollatsek, Reichle, & Rayner, 2006; Rayner, Ashby, Pollatsek, & Reichle, 2004; Rayner, Reichle, & Pollatsek, 1998; Reichle, Pollatsek, Fisher, & Rayner, 1998; Reichle, Pollatsek, & Rayner, 2006; Reichle, Rayner, & Pollatsek, 2003) is typically regarded as the most influential of these models. Due to space limitations, other models will not be discussed here.[3] The E-Z Reader model can account for all of the results discussed above, and also does a good job of predicting how long readers look at words, which words they skip, and which words will most likely be refixated. Importantly, it can account for global aspects of eye movements in reading, as well as more local processing characteristics; competitor models also account for similar amounts of data (see the chapter by Risse et al.). In many ways, these models share many similarities, though they differ on some precise processing details and on how certain effects are explained. As a computational model, E-Z Reader has the virtue of being highly transparent, so it makes very clear predictions and when it can't account for certain data, it is very clear why it can't (thus enabling one to change parameter values in the model). The model has also enabled us to account for data patterns that in the past may have been difficult to explain. However, this model isn't perfect and it has some limitations. For example, in this model, higher order processes due to sentence parsing and discourse variables currently have no influence. The model primarily assumes that lexical processing is driving

3 For a comprehensive overview of these models, see the special issue of *Cognitive Systems Research*, 2006 (vol. 7). In addition, Risse, Engbert, and Kliegl (this volume) discuss the other major model, SWIFT.

the eyes through the text, and we believe that this is a reasonable assumption.[4]

With careful experimentation and with the implementation of computational models that simulate eye movements during reading, we see from the foregoing that great advances have been made in understanding eye movements in reading (and inferring the mental processes associated with reading). In the next two sections, eye movements during visual search and scene perception will be discussed, in turn. Although there hasn't been as much research on these areas as on reading, it is still the case that some clear conclusions emerge from the work that has been done.

Eye movements and visual search

Visual search is a research area that has received considerable effort over the past 40 years. However, the vast majority of this research has been done in the absence of considering eye movements (Findlay & Gilchrist, 1998), because it was largely assumed that eye movements are not particularly important in understanding search. With more recent research, this attitude seems to be changing, as there are now many more experiments examining aspects of visual search which report eye movement measures (see Benson, this volume; Menneer, Stroud, Cave, Donnelly, & Rayner, this volume). Though, many of these studies are often focused on using the search task to uncover properties of the saccadic eye movement system itself (see Findlay, 2004; Findlay & Gilchrist, 2003), many also use eye movements to learn about search behavior.

In this chapter, we'll focus primarily on research that has some implications for how viewers search through arrays to find specific targets. Fixation durations in search tend to be highly variable. Some studies report average fixation times as short as 180 ms while others report averages on the order of 275 ms. This is undoubtedly due to the fact that the level difficulty of a search (i.e., how dense or cluttered the array is) and the exact nature of the search task will strongly influence how long viewers pause on each item. Typically, saccade size is a bit larger than in reading (though saccades can be quite short with very

4 Our primary argument is that lexical processing drives the eyes through the text and higher order processes primarily serve to intervene when something doesn't compute (see Rayner, Warren, Juhasz, & Liversedge, 2004).

dense arrays).

The search array matters

Perhaps the most obvious thing about visual search is that the properties of the search array have an enormous influence on the ease with which a target is found. When an array is very cluttered (with many objects and distractors), the search becomes more demanding than when the array is simple. The eye movements on each of these types of arrays typically reflect this property of an array (Bertera & Rayner, 2000; Greene & Rayner, 2001a. 2001b). As the array becomes more complicated, we see an increase in the fixation duration and the number of fixations, as well as a decrease in the average saccade length (Vlaskamp & Hooge, 2006). Another influential property on the pattern of eye movements is the configuration of the search array. An array of objects arranged in an arc tends to have more fixations that fall in-between objects, progressively getting closer to the area where viewers think the target is located (Zelinsky, 2005; Zelinsky, Rao, Hayhoe, & Ballard, 1997). On the other hand, in randomly placed arrays, fixations tend to fall directly on an item within an array and other factors such as color of the items and shape similarity to the target object preferentially attract fixations (Williams, Henderson, & Zacks, 2005).

Does visual search have a memory?

Horowitz and Wolfe (1998) initially proposed that visual search doesn't have a good memory and that the same item will be re-sampled during multiple encounters with the same search array. However, this assertion was based on reaction time functions. Ideally, eye movement data would better address this question, because one can directly examine how often the eyes return to a previously sampled part of the array. Studies using eye movement measures have made it clear that while searching, viewers generally do not return to previously searched items (Beck, Peterson, Boot, Vomela, & Kramer, 2006; Beck, Peterson, & Vomela, 2006; Peterson, Kramer, Wang, Irwin, & McCarley, 2001).

The perceptual span

As discussed in the reading section of this chapter, how much information is processed on each fixation is an important factor in determining eye movement patterns. Using the moving window paradigm, Rayner and Fisher (1987a, 1987b) asked viewers to search through horizontally arranged letter strings for a specified target letter. They found that the size of the perceptual span varied as a function of the difficulty of the distractor letter. That is, the perceptual span was smaller when distractor letters were visually similar to the target letter than when the distractor letters were distinctly different. This suggested that there were two qualitatively different regions within the span: a decision region (where information about the presence or absence of a target is available), and a preview region where some letter information is available, but where information on the absence of a target is not yet available.

In another study, Bertera and Rayner (2000) asked viewers to search though a randomly arranged array of letters and digits for the presence of a target letter. They used both the moving window and moving mask techniques. They varied the density of the array by changing the size of the array (so that it was 13 degrees by 10 degrees, 6 degrees by 6 degrees, or 5 degrees by 3.5 degrees), while holding the number of items constant. The size of the moving mask was directly related to the accuracy and the time it took to complete the search: Increasing the mask size, increased search time and decreased accuracy. When given a moving window, viewers' search performance reached asymptote when the window was approximately 5 degrees. That is, all letters/digits falling within 2.5 degrees from the fixation point were visible, while all other items were masked.

Where and when to move the eyes

Many studies have tried to determine the factors involved in deciding where and when to move the eyes during search (Greene, 2006; Greene & Rayner, 2001a, 2001b; Hooge & Erkelens, 1996, 1998; Jacobs, 1986; Vaughan, 1982). However, despite this effort, no clear answers have emerged. In some cases, researchers concluded that fixation durations in visual search are the result of both preprogramming saccades and processing currently fixated information (Vaughan, 1982). In other cases, some researchers suggested that the completion of foveal analysis is not necessary to trigger an eye movement (Hooge & Erkelens, 1996, 1998), while others have suggested that it is (Greene & Rayner, 2001b). Rayner (1995) suggested that the trigger to move the eyes in a search task is determined by a check processes that determines whether the target is present in the decision area of the perceptual span. If not, a new saccade is programmed to move the eyes to a location that has not been examined. As with reading, attention would first move to the region targeted for the next saccade (and as described above, would favor items that shared a similar shape or color with the target, Williams et al., 2005).

As a final point, the decision about where to fixate next and when to move the eyes will undoubtedly be influenced by characteristics of the specific search task and the density of the array. In a recent study, van Zoest, Donk, and Theeuwes (2004) investigated what type of information had more influence over the placement of fixations: goal-driven information (i.e., target knowledge) or distractor saliency. Results indicated that the timing of the fixations was linked to where the eyes would land. When fixations were made quickly, viewers tended to fixate the target and distractor equally. However, when the fixation latency was longer, the target was more likely fixated. So, the longer viewers took to choose a location and execute the saccade, the more likely it would be influenced by goal-driven control. Consequently, it seems that for fixations made early on, visual saliency may play a greater role in directing fixations.

Eye movements and scene perception

The eye movement pattern of a viewer on a scene is shown in Figure 1.3 (A). As is very evident in this figure, not every part of the scene is fixated. This is largely because in scene perception information can be obtained over a wider region than is found in reading and possibly, visual search arrays. However, it is clear that the important aspects of the scene are typically fixated (and generally looked at for longer periods than less important parts of the scene). In Figure 1.3 (B), the fixations from multiple viewers have been compiled and show that most fixations are on the informative parts of the scene. That is, viewers do not tend to fixate on the sky or the road in front of the houses. As noted at the outset, the average fixation duration in scene perception tends to be longer than that in reading, and likewise the average saccade size tends to be longer. In this section, we will briefly summarize where people tend to look in scenes, the perceptual span region for scenes, and the nature of eye movement control when looking at scenes.

Getting the gist of a scene

The gist of a scene has been defined as the general scene concept (Potter, 1999), and is most often referring to a scene's basic-level category when investigated in the literature (Oliva, 2005). One very important general finding is that viewers are able to acquire scene gist in a single glance. That is, the gist of the scene is understood so quickly, it is thought to be processed even before the eyes begin to move (De Graef,

A.

B.

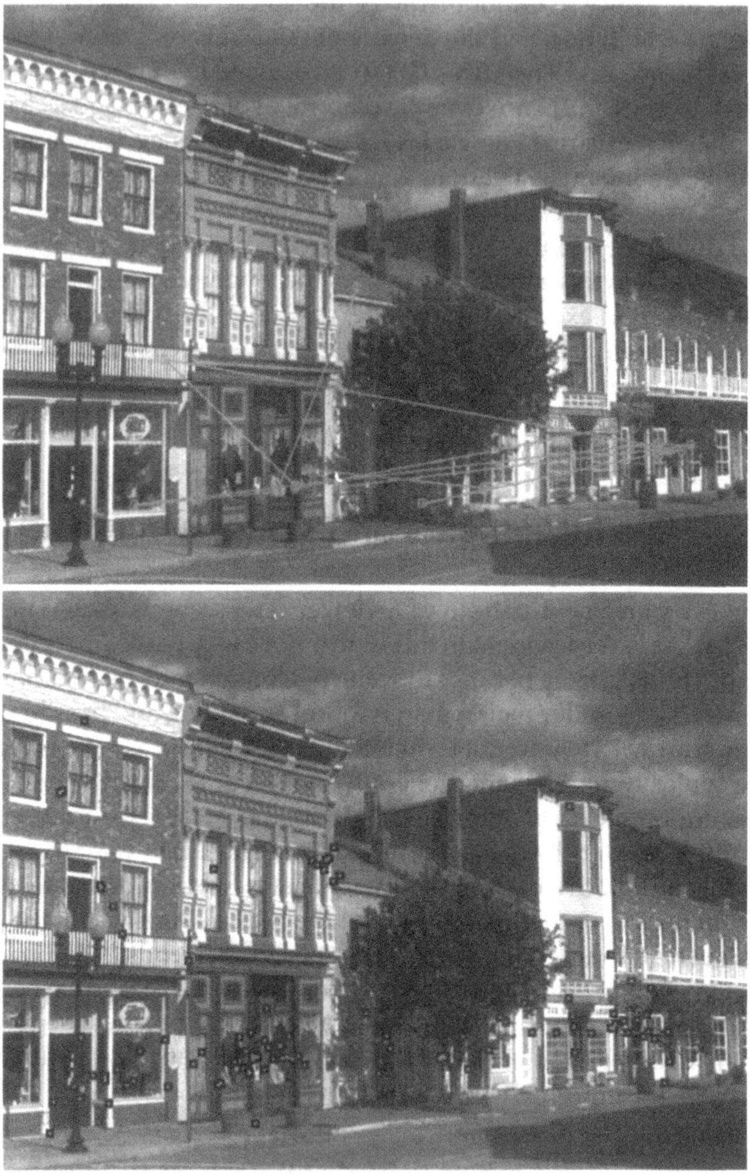

Figure 1.3 Examples of where viewers look in scenes. The top portion of the figure shows where one viewer fixates in the scene (the dots represent fixation points and the lines represent the sequence). The bottom portion shows where a number of different viewers fixate (with the dots representing fixation locations across a number of viewers).(*See Plate 1.*)

2005). In a recent study, Castelhano and Henderson (2008) showed that when viewers were shown a scene for as little as 40 ms, they were able to extract enough information to understand the scene gist. Typically, the scene gist is thought to be acquired within the first fixation in order to orient subsequent fixations to appropriate or interesting regions within the scene. We will turn to this question in the next section.

Where do viewers look in scenes?

Pioneering works of Buswell (1935) and Yarbus (1967) first documented how a viewer's gaze is drawn to important aspects of a visual scene and that task goal very much influences eye movements. Much of the research that followed illustrated that the eyes are drawn to informative areas in a scene quickly (Antes, 1974; Mackworth & Morandi, 1967), and an object that is out-of-place in a scene tends to attract a lot of early fixations (Friedman, 1979; Loftus & Mackworth, 1978). It is important to note however, that the out-of-place objects in these studies tended to differ from the appropriate objects on a number of dimensions (Rayner & Pollatsek, 1992). For example, an octopus in a farm scene is not only semantically out-of-place, but it also tends to have more rounded features than the objects typically in a farm scene. So, these early studies confounded visual saliency and semantic saliency. Recent experiments that control for visual saliency of the out-of-place objects raise some uncertainty about the earlier findings, and suggest that the eyes are not immediately drawn to out-of-place objects that differ in semantics alone (De Graef, Christiaens, & d'Ydewalle, 1990; Henderson, Weeks, & Hollingworth, 1999), though see Becker, Pashler, and Lubin (2007) for conflicting evidence.

Nonetheless, it has become clear that the eyes can quickly go to parts of a scene that are relevant and important. A recent study investigated the influence of scene context on the placement of eye movements while viewers searched for certain objects within pseudo-realistic scenes (Neider & Zelinsky, 2006). Viewers were asked to look for a target object that was typically constrained to a certain part of the scene (i.e., a jeep on the ground or a blimp in the sky). When a target was present, fixations were largely limited to the area where one would expect to find the target object (i.e., ground or sky); whereas, when the target was absent, eventually there was less of an inclination to restrict search to these areas. In addition, when the target was in its expected area, search times were about 19% faster. From these results, they concluded that not only do viewers immediately focus fixations in the target's expected area, but also that the visual system is flexible enough to quickly switch to a "look everywhere" strategy when the first proves fruitless. Thus, it seems that although likely target context can serve as a good search strategy, it is not generally with strict adherence.

Other studies have also made it clear that saliency of different parts of the scene greatly influences where viewers tend to fixate (Parkhurst & Niebur, 2003; Mannan, Ruddock, & Wooding, 1995, 1996). As discussed with visual search, saliency is typically defined in terms of low-level components of the scene (such as contrast, color, intensity, brightness, spatial frequency, etc.). There are a number of computational models (Baddeley & Tatler, 2006; Itti & Koch, 2000, 2001; Parkhurst, Law, & Niebur, 2002) that use the concept of a saliency map to model eye fixation locations in scenes. With this approach, the bottom-up properties of a scene (i.e., saliency map) make explicit predictions about the most visually prominent regions of the scene. The models are basically used to derive predictions about the distribution of fixations on a given scene based on these prominent regions.

While these models can account for some of the variability in the distribution of fixations across a scene, they are limited by the assumption that fixations are primarily driven by bottom-up factors. Research has shown that higher-level factors also have a strong influence on where viewers direct their gaze in a scene (Castelhano & Henderson, 2007; Henderson & Castelhano, 2005; Henderson & Ferreira, 2004). Recently, Torralba, Oliva, Castelhano, and Henderson (2006) presented a model that incorporates the influence of top-down and cognitive strategies. Although there is considerable research on localizing *where* viewers move their eyes while looking at scenes, very few studies have investigated what controls *when* the eyes move. In contrast, reading research has focused on both *where* to move the eyes and *when* to move the eyes. A recent study (that attempted to investigate when the eye move) examined the effect of repeated exposure to a scene on fixation durations (Hidalgo-Sotelo, Oliva & Torralba, 2005). In this study, the viewers' task was to search for a target (i.e., a person) in the scene while their eye movements were tracked. Unbeknownst to them, there were certain scene-target combinations that repeated throughout the experiment twenty times. As expected, these repeated searches showed a large decrease in response time. Interestingly, although the number of fixations did not decrease, the average fixation duration prior to fixating the target object did. Furthermore, the results showed that the proportion of target objects that were fixated before a response was made did not change with increased repetitions (85%). Furthermore, average gaze durations on the target dropped from 450 ms during the first exposure to 310 ms in the twentieth. Despite the fact that the target presence was highly correlated with the scene, it seems that observers chose to verify the target object presence before making their response. These results demonstrated that with repeated exposure, the reduced response time is primarily due to a decrease in the average duration of fixations during the search, as well as in the time taken to verify the target object. Thus, performance improvements on a repeated search stemmed from a facilitation of identifying the fixated regions as non-targets and targets, but not from a reducing the number of fixations made overall.

Another difference between scenes and reading is the question of how recently acquired information is used to guide eye movements. We know that in reading, prior context provided by the material read up until that point plays a large role in determining the directing of subsequent fixations (such as deciding between a forward-going saccade or a regressive saccade). In scenes, the role that previously viewed information plays in directing fixations is not as clear. Many of the models that use saliency as the primary driving force of the eyes do not consider how information gathered initially may influence subsequent fixations. In a recent study, Castelhano and Henderson (2007) investigated whether the initial representation of a scene can be used to guide eye movements on a real-world scene. After a brief preview of the search scene, viewers were asked to find the target object. In the experiment, the moving window technique was used and it blocked out all scene information, with the exception of the scene at the point of fixation; thus, immediately available visual information from the surrounding scene could not be used to plan fixations. Instead, viewers had to rely on the information that was gathered during the preview. When the preview was of the search scene itself, performance was much more efficient than when the preview was a meaningless control. Using a preview of another scene within the same semantic category (thereby providing general semantic information without the same visual details) resulted in no improvement in search efficiency; this suggests that the information used to guide the eyes was not based on general semantics. With a reduced scale preview of the search scene, performance was just as high as when the full-scale preview was shown. Taken together, this study suggests that to guide the eyes, the visual system relied on abstract visual information. Thus, the information used to guide eye movements in scenes is said to have multiple sources, such as the saliency of the regions, abstract visual information previously extracted from the scene, and top-down knowledge about the context and scene type.

The perceptual span

How much information is extracted from a single fixation on a scene? As noted at the beginning of this section, it is known that the extent of the visual field used to extract useful information is much larger in scene viewing than it is in reading. Using a moving mask paradigm (to cover the part of the scene around the fixation point) during scene exploration, Henderson, McClure, Pierce, and Shrock (1997) found that although the foveal mask had an influence on looking time, it did not have nearly as deleterious effects for object identification as was found for word identification in reading.

In an early study, Nelson and Loftus (1980) examined object recognition as a function of the closest fixation to that object. Results showed that objects located within about 2.6 degrees from fixation were generally recognized. The results also suggested that information acquired from the region 1.5 degrees around fixation is qualitatively different from regions farther away (see also Nodine, Carmody, & Herman, 1979). A study by Parker (1978) found that the functional field of view for specific objects in a scene is quite large: with a radius of at least 10° around fixation resulting in a perceptual span of up to 20° (see Henderson & Ferreira, 2004 for discussion). However, more recent studies using more natural images suggest that the functional field of view extends about 4° away from fixation (Henderson & Hollingworth, 1999; Henderson, Williams, Castelhano, & Falk, 2003).

In an early study, Saida and Ikeda (1979) used the moving window paradigm and found that the functional field of view is quite large, and can consist of about half of the total scene regardless of the absolute size of the scene (at least for scenes that are up to 14.4 degrees by 18.8 degrees). In this and other studies using the moving window paradigm (van Diepen & d'Ydewalle, 2003; van Diepen, Wampers, & d'Ydewalle, 1998) normal scene information within the window area around a fixation point is presented normally, but the information outside of the window is degraded in some systematic way. Saida and Ikeda (1979) found a serious deterioration in recognition of a scene when the window was limited to a small area (about 3.3 degrees × 3.3 degrees) on each fixation. Performance gradually improved as the window size became larger, as noted, up to about 50% of the entire scene. Saida and Ikeda noted that there was considerable overlap of information across fixations.

Based on the studies reviewed above, it should now be clear that the question of how large the perceptual span during scene viewing hasn't been answered as conclusively as it has in reading or visual search. And yet, it does appear that viewers typically gain useful information from a fairly wide region of the scene and that it probably varies as a function of the scene and the task of the viewer. For example, the ease with which an object is identified within a scene is influenced by its orientation (Boutsen, Lamberts, & Verfaillie, 1998), how well camouflaged it is (De Graef, et al., 1990), and the frequency with which it is typically encountered within a scene context (Hollingworth & Henderson, 1998). As shown for the perceptual span in reading (Henderson & Ferreira, 1990), it is highly probable that identification of the fixated object has an effect on the extent to which information in the periphery is processed.

Preview benefit

Just as with reading, before fixating an object, viewers obtain preview benefit from it (Henderson, 1992; Henderson, Pollatsek, & Rayner, 1987, 1989; Pollatsek, Rayner, & Collins, 1984; Pollatsek, Rayner, & Henderson, 1990). Further, the preview benefit for objects is about 100 ms, making it much larger than the effects found for words in reading. Interestingly, viewers are rather insensitive to large changes in a scene. In a series of experiments by McConkie and Grimes (McConkie, 1991; Grimes & McConkie, 1995; Grimes, 1996) viewers were asked to try to memorize scenes that were shown for a predetermined amount of time. In addition, they were informed that it was possible that some changes to the image could be made while they were studying it, and they were instructed to press a button when one of those changes was detected. During this study phase, changes to the scene were made when the viewer launched a saccade. As discussed earlier, vision is suppressed during saccades so that these changes would not have been visible as they were occurring. Surprisingly, observers were unaware of most changes, which included the appearance and disappearance of large objects and the changing of colors of large regions of the scene. All of these changes occurred while the scene was being viewed. Although later studies found that any disruption served to induce an inability to detect changes, such as inserting a blank screen in between two changing images (Rensink, O'Regan, & Clark, 1997), movie cuts (Levin & Simons, 1997), or the simultaneous onset of patches or 'mudsplashes' which covered portions of the scene (O'Regan, Rensink, & Clark, 1999). These experiments highlighted the relation between what is viewed during the initial exploration of a scene and what is remembered about that scene. Further studies have shown that this lack of awareness does not mean that there is no recollection of any visual details, but rather that the likelihood of remembering visual information is highly dependent on the processing of that information (Hollingworth & Henderson, 2002; Hollingworth, 2003). Thus, knowing something about the processes that go on during a fixation on a scene is extremely important if one would want to predict how well visual information will be remembered later on, or even while the scene is being explored further.

When do viewers move their eyes when looking at scenes?

Past studies have shown that attention precedes an eye movement to a new location within a scene (Henderson, 1992; van Diepen & d'Ydewalle, 2003). So, it would follow that the eyes will move once the visual information at the center of vision has been processed and a new fixation location has been selected and programmed. In a recent study, van Diepen and d'Ydewalle (2003) investigated when this shift in attention (from the center of fixation to the periphery) took place in the course of a fixation. They had observers view scenes whose information at the center of fixation was masked during the initial part of fixations (from 20- 90 ms). In another case, the periphery was masked at the beginning of each fixation (for 10-85 ms). As expected, this study demonstrated that when the center of fixation was masked initially, fixation durations increased with longer mask durations (a 61% increase). When the periphery was masked, they found a slight increase in fixation durations, but not as much as with a central mask (a 15% increase). Interestingly, their results also showed that as mask durations in the periphery were increased, the average distance of saccades decreased and the number of fixations increased. They surmised that increasing the duration of the peripheral mask does not prevent the visual system from making a saccade, but instead information that is immediately available is often chosen for the next fixation. Taken together, these results suggest that at the fovea information is extracted very rapidly, and attention is directed to the periphery almost immediately following the extraction of information (70-120 ms) to choose a viable saccade target. The general timing of the switch between central and peripheral information processing is currently being investigated; however, the inherent variability across scenes makes it difficult to find as specific a time frame as in reading.

Finally, a very interesting issue that has received attention lately is the extent to which emotional aspects of a scene influence eye movements. Do emotional aspects of a scene lead viewers to quickly look at that part of the scene conveying strong emotional content? Nummenmaa, Hyönä, and Calvo (this volume) review this issue. It seems quite clear that emotional aspects of scenes do have an immediate impact on eye movements.

General comments on eye movements

In the preceding sections, we have reviewed research on eye movements in three tasks: reading, visual search and scene perception. Although there are obviously many differences between these tasks, there are some general principles that are likely to hold across them. First, how much information is processed on any fixation (the perceptual span or functional field of view) varies as a function of the task. The perceptual span is clearly smaller in reading than in either scene perception or visual search. Hence, for example, fixations in scene perception tend to be longer and saccades are longer because more information is being processed in a single fixation. Second, the difficulty of the stimulus influences eye movements: In reading, when the text becomes more difficult, eye fixations get longer and saccades get shorter; likewise in scene perception and visual search, when the stimulus is more crowded, cluttered, or dense, fixations get longer and saccades get shorter. Fourth, the difficulty of the specific task (reading for comprehension versus reading for gist, searching for a person in a scene versus looking at the scene for a memory test, and so on) obviously influences how the eyes move. Finally, in all three tasks there is some evidence (Najemnik & Geisler, 2005; Rayner, 1998) that viewers integrate information poorly across fixations and it is more critical that information is processed efficiently on each fixation.

Cultural influences on eye movements

In the prior sections of this chapter, we have not commented on cultural influences on eye movements. However, there is currently a great deal of interest in this issue and many chapters in the present volume deal specifically with this issue. The chapter by Rayner, Li, and Pollatsek (this volume) provides a discussion of the extension of the E-Z Reader model to Chinese and a number of the chapters in the volume deal specifically with eye movements when reading Chinese text. The other recent development receiving attention is the extent to which cultural differences can influence how people look at a scene. The chapter by Boland, Chua, and Nisbett (this volume) reviews their interesting finding that culture can influence what people look at (and how early they look at) certain aspects of a scene. The chapter by Li, Williams, Cave, Well, and Rayner (this volume) raises some qualifications concerning the cultural effect. Clearly, more research is needed on this issue.

Summary

In this chapter, we have reviewed the basic findings concerning eye movements when (1) reading, (2) looking at a scene, and (3) searching through a visual array. Although there is no question that these tasks differ considerably, and that eye movements also differ considerably as a function of the task, it is the case that eye movements can be very informative about what exactly viewers do in each type of task. Each of these points has been discussed in the preceding sections. It will also be interesting to see how well the findings we have described above will hold up when viewers look at dynamically changing scenes (virtually all of the work that we described has dealt with static scenes).

We also suspect, as is clearly evident in the present volume, that there will be more and more research examining cultural influences on eye movements. It is also worth noting that eye movement data are now widely used to examine cognitive processing in a number of real world tasks such as driving (see Pollatsek, Fisher, and Pradhan, this volume), mental problem solving and visual comparisons (Cave et al.; Hakki et al., this volume), making tea and sandwiches (Land & Hayhoe, 2001), and so on. They are also increasingly used to study various types of special populations (see Benson, this volume). And, eye movement data are now also widely used in the so-called "visual world" paradigm (see Tanenhaus, Chambers, & Hanna, 2004) in which people listen to speech while simultaneously looking at a visual array. This research shows quite clearly that people tend to look at that part of the array that is being discussed in the narrative. Finally, as should be apparent from the foregoing discussion, our expectation is that eye movements will continue to play a valuable role for those interested in visual cognitive processing.

Acknowledgments

Preparation of this chapter was supported by a Grant from the Microsoft Corporation and by Grant HD26765 from the National Institute of Health.

References

Antes, J. R. (1974). The time course of picture viewing. *Journal of Experimental Psychology, 103,* 62-70.

Baddeley, R. J., & Tatler, B. W. (2006). High frequency edges (but not contrast) predict where we fixate: A Bayesian system identification analysis. *Vision Research, 46,* 2824-2833.

Beck, M. R., Peterson, M.S., Boot, W.R., Vomela, M., & Kramer, A.F. (2006). Explicit memory for rejected distractors during visual search. *Visual Cognition, 14,* 150-174.

Beck, M. R., Peterson, M. S., & Vomela, M. (2006). Memory for where, but not what, is used during visual search. *Journal of Experimental Psychology: Human Perception and Performance, 32,* 235-250.

Becker, M. W., Pashler, H., & Lubin, J. (2007). Object-intrinsic oddities draw early saccades. *Journal of Experimental Psychology: Human Perception and Performance, 33,* 20-30.

Becker, W., & Jürgens, R. (1979). Analysis of the saccadic system by means of double step stimuli. *Vision Research, 19,* 967-983.

Bertera, J. H., & Rayner, K. (2000). Eye movements and the span of effective stimulus in visual search. *Perception & Psychophysics, 62,* 576-585.

Boutsen, L., Lamberts, K., & Verfaillie, K. (1998). Recognition times of different views of 56 depth-rotated objects: A note concerning Verfaillie and Boutsen (1995). *Perception & Psychophysics, 60,* 900-907.

Buswell, G. T. (1935). *How people look at pictures.* Chicago: University of Chicago Press.

Carroll, P. J., & Slowiaczek, M. L. (1986). Constraints on semantic priming in reading: A fixation time analysis. *Memory & Cognition, 14,* 509-522.

Castelhano, M. S., & Henderson, J. M. (2007). Initial scene representations facilitate eye movement guidance in visual search. *Journal of Experimental Psychology: Human Perception and Performance, 33*, 753-763.

Castelhano, M. S., & Henderson, J. M. (2008). The influence of color on perception of scene gist. *Journal of Experimental Psychology: Human Perception and Performance, 34*, 660-675.

De Graef, P. (2005). Semantic effects on object selection in real-world scene perception. In G. Underwood (Ed.), *Cognitive processes in eye guidance*. Oxford: Oxford University Press.

De Graef, P., Christiaens, D., & d'Ydewalle, G. (1990). Perceptual effects of scene context on object identification. *Psychological Research, 52*, 317-329.

Deubel, H., & Schneider, W. X. (1996). Saccade target selection and object recognition: Evidence for a common attentional mechanism. *Vision Research, 36*, 1827-1837.

Duffy, S. A., Morris, R. K., & Rayner, K. (1988). Lexical ambiguity and fixation times in reading. *Journal of Memory and Language, 27*, 429-446.

Ehrlich, S. E., & Rayner, K. (1981). Contextual effects on word perception and eye movements during reading. *Journal of Verbal Learning and Verbal Behavior, 20*, 641-655.

Findlay, J. M. (2004). Eye scanning and visual search. In J. M. Henderson, & F. Ferreira (Eds.), *The interface of language, vision, and action: Eye movements and the visual world* (pp.135-160). New York: Psychology Press.

Findlay, J. M., & Gilchrist, I. D. (1998). Eye guidance and visual search. In G. Underwood (Ed.), *Eye guidance in reading and scene perception* (pp. 295-312). Oxford, England: Elsevier.

Findlay, J. M., & Gilchrist, I. D. (2003). *Active vision: The psychology of looking and seeing*. Oxford: Oxford University Press.

Friedman, A. (1979). Framing pictures: The role of knowledge in automatized encoding and memory for gist. *Journal of Experimental Psychology: General, 108*, 316-355.

Greene, H. (2006). The control of fixation duration in visual search. *Perception, 35*, 303-315.

Greene, H., & Rayner, K. (2001a). Eye movements and familiarity effects in visual search. *Vision Research, 41*, 3763-3773.

Greene, H., & Rayner, K. (2001b). Eye-movement control in direction-coded visual search. *Perception, 29*, 363-372.

Grimes, J. (1996). On the failure to detect changes in scenes across saccades. In K. Akins (Ed.), *Vancouver studies in cognitive science: Vol. 5. Perception* (pp.89-110). New York: Oxford University Press.

Grimes, J., & McConkie, G. (1995). On the insensitivity of the human visual system to image changes made during saccades. In K. Akins, (Ed.), *Problems in perception.* Oxford, UK: Oxford University Press.

Henderson, J. M. (1992). Identifying objects across saccades: Effects of extrafoveal preview and flanker object context. *Journal of Experimental Psychology: Learning, Memory, and Cognition, 18,* 521-530.

Henderson, J. M., & Castelhano, M. S. (2005). Eye movements and visual memory for scenes. In G. Underwood (Ed.), *Cognitive processes in eye guidance* (pp. 213-235). Oxford University Press.

Henderson, J. M., & Ferreira, F. (1990). Effects of foveal processing difficulty on the perceptual span in reading: Implications for attention and eye movement control. *Journal of Experimental Psychology: Learning, Memory, and Cognition, 16*(3), 417-429.

Henderson, J. M., & Ferreira, F. (2004). Scene perception for psycholinguists. In J. M. Henderson, & F. Ferreira (Eds.), *The interface of language, vision, and action: Eye movements and the visual world* (pp. 1-58). New York: Psychology Press.

Henderson, J. M., & Hollingworth, A. (1999). High-level scene perception. *Annual Review of Psychology, 50,* 243-271.

Henderson, J. M., McClure, K. K., Pierce, S., & Schrock, G. (1997). Object identification without foveal vision: Evidence from an artificial scotoma paradigm. *Perception & Psychophysics, 59,* 323-346.

Henderson, J. M., Pollatsek, A., & Rayner, K. (1987). The effects of foveal priming and extrafoveal preview on object identification. *Journal of Experimental Psychology: Human Perception and Performance, 13,* 449-463.

Henderson, J. M., Pollatsek, A., & Rayner, K. (1989). Covert visual attention and extrafoveal information use during object identification. *Perception & Psychophysics, 45,* 196-208.

Henderson, J. M., Weeks, P. A. Jr., & Hollingworth, A. (1999). Effects of semantic consistency on eye movements during scene viewing. *Journal of Experimental Psychology: Human Perception and Performance, 25,* 210-228.

Henderson, J. M., Williams, C. C., Castelhano, M. S., & Falk, R. J. (2003). Eye movements and picture processing during recognition. *Perception & Psychophysics, 65,* 725-734.

Hidalgo-Sotelo, B., Oliva, A., & Torralba, A. (2005). *Human learning of contextual priors for object search: Where does the time go?* Proceedings of 3rd Workshop on Attention and Performance at the International Conference in Computer Vision and Pattern Recognition (CVPR), San Diego CA.

Hoffman, J. E., & Subramaniam, B. (1995). The role of visual attention in saccadic eye movements. *Perception & Psychophysics, 57,* 787-795.

Hollingworth, A. (2003). Failures of retrieval and comparison constrain change detection in natural scenes. *Journal of Experimental Psychology: Human Perception and Performance, 29,* 388-403.

Hollingworth, A., & Henderson, J. M. (1998). Does consistent scene context facilitate object perception? *Journal of Experimental Psychology: General, 127,* 398-415.

Hollingworth, A., & Henderson, J. M. (2002). Accurate visual memory for previously attended objects in natural scenes. *Journal of Experimental Psychology: Human Perception and Performance, 28,* 113-136.

Hooge, I. T. C., & Erkelens, C. J. (1996). Control of fixation duration during a simple search task. *Perception & Psychophysics, 58,* 969-976.

Hooge, I. T. C., & Erkelens, C. J. (1998). Adjustment of fixation duration during visual search. *Vision Research, 38,* 1295-1302.

Horowitz, T. S., & Wolfe, J. M. (1998). Visual search has no memory. *Nature, 94,* 575-577.

Inhoff, A. W., & Rayner, K. (1986). Parafoveal word processing during eye fixations in reading: Effects of word frequency. *Perception & Psychophysics, 40,* 431-439.

Irwin, D. E. (2004). Fixation location and fixation duration as indices of cognitive processing. In J.M. Henderson, & F. Ferreira (Eds.), *The interface of language, vision, and action: Eye movements and the visual world* (pp. 105-134). New York: Psychology Press.

Ishida, T., & Ikeda, M. (1989). Temporal properties of information extraction in reading studied by a text-mask replacement technique. *Journal of the Optical Society A: Optics and Image Science, 6,* 1624-1632.

Itti., L., & Koch, C. (2000). A saliency-based search mechanism for overt and covert shifts of visual attention. *Vision Research, 40,* 1489-1506.

Itti, L., & Koch, C. (2001). Computational modeling of visual attention. *Nature Reviews: Neuroscience, 2,* 194-203.

Jacobs, A. M. (1986). Eye movement control in visual search: How direct is visual span control? *Perception & Psychophysics, 39,* 47-58.

Juhasz, B. J., & Rayner, K. (2003). Investigating the effects of a set of intercorrelated variables on eye fixation durations in reading. *Journal of Experimental Psychology: Learning, Memory, and Cognition, 29,* 1312-1318.

Juhasz, B. J., & Rayner, K (2006). The role of age-of-acquisition and word frequency in reading: Evidence from eye fixation durations. *Visual Cognition, 13,* 846-863.

Kowler, E., Anderson, E., Dosher, B., & Blaser, E. (1995). The role of attention in programming saccades. *Vision Research, 35,* 1897-1916.

Land, M. F., & Hayhoe, M. (2001). In what ways do eye movements contribute to everyday activities? *Vision Research, 41,* 3559-3565.

Levin, D. T., & Simons, D. J. (1997). Failure to detect changes to attended objects in morion pictures. *Psychonomic Bulletin & Review,* 4 (4), 501-506.

Liversedge, S. P., Rayner, K., White, S. J., Vergilino-Perez, D., Findlay, J. M., & Kentridge, R.W. (2004). Eye movements while reading disappearing text: Is there a gap effect in reading? *Vision Research, 44,* 1013-1024.

Loftus, G. R., & Mackworth, N. H. (1978). Cognitive determinants of fixation location during picture viewing. *Journal of Experimental Psychology: Human Perception and Performance, 4,* 565-572.

Mackworth, N. H., & Morandi, A. J. (1967). The gaze selects informative details within pictures. *Perception & Psychophysics, 2,* 547-552.

Mannan, S. K., Ruddock, K. H., & Wooding, D. S. (1995). Automatic control of saccadic eye movements made in visual inspection of briefly presented 2-D images. *Spatial Vision, 9,* 363-386.

Mannan, S. K., Ruddock, K. H., & Wooding, D. S. (1996). The relationship between the locations of spatial features and those of fixation made during visual examination of briefly presented images. *Spatial Vision, 10,* 165-188.

McConkie, G.W. (1991). *Perceiving a stable visual world.* In Proceedings of the Sixth European Conference on Eye Movements, pages 5-7. Leuven, Belgium: Laboratory of Experimental Psychology.

McConkie, G. W., & Rayner, K. (1975). The span of the effective stimulus during a fixation in reading. *Perception & Psychophysics, 17,* 578-586.

McConkie, G. W., & Zola, D. (1979). Is visual information integrated across successive fixations in reading? *Perception & Psychophysics, 25,* 221-224.

McPeek, R. M., Skavenski, A. A., & Nakayama, K. (2000). Concurrent processing of saccades in visual search. *Vision Research, 40,* 2499-2516.

Morris, R. K. (1994). Lexical and message-level sentence context effects on fixation times in reading. *Journal of Experimental Psychology:*

Learning, Memory, and Cognition, 20, 92-103.

Morrison, R. E., & Rayner, K. (1981). Saccade size in reading depends upon character spaces and not visual angle. *Perception & Psychophysics, 30,* 395-396.

Najemnik, J., & Geisler, W. S. (2005). Optimal eye movement strategies in visual search. *Nature, 434,* 387-391.

Neider, M. B., & Zelinsky, G. J. (2006). Scene context guides eye movements during search. *Vision Research, 46*(5), 614-621.

Nelson, W. W., & Loftus, G. R. (1980). The functional visual field during picture viewing. *Journal of Experimental Psychology: Human Learning and Memory, 6,* 391-399.

Nodine, C. E, Carmody, D. P., & Herman, E. (1979). Eye movements during visual search for artistically embedded targets. *Bulletin of the Psychonomic Society, 13,* 371-374.

Oliva, A. (2005). Gist of the scene. In L. Itti, G. Rees, & J. K. Tsotsos (Eds.), *The encyclopedia of neurobiology of attention* (pp. 251-256). San Diego: Elsevier.

O'Regan, J. K., Rensink, R. A., & Clark, J. J. (1999). Change blindness as a result of 'mudsplashes'. *Nature, 398,* 34.

Parker, R. E. (1978). Picture processing during recognition. *Journal of Experimental Psychology: Human Perception and Performance, 4,* 284-293.

Parkhurst, D. J., & Niebur, E. (2003). Scene content selected by active vision. *Spatial Vision, 16,* 125-154.

Parkhurst, D., Law, K., & Niebur, E. (2002). Modeling the role of salience in the allocation of overt visual attention. *Vision Research, 42,* 107-123.

Peterson, M. S., Kramer, A. F., Wang, R. F., Irwin, D. E., & McCarley, J. S. (2001). Visual search has memory. *Psychological Science, 12,* 287-292.

Pollatsek, A., Rayner, K.,& Collins,W. E. (1984). Integrating pictorial information across eye movements. *Journal of Experimental Psychology: General, 113,* 426-442.

Pollatsek, A., Rayner, K., & Henderson, J. M. (1990). Role of spatial location in integration of pictorial information across saccades. *Journal of Experimental Psychology: Human Perception and Performance, 16,* 199-210.

Pollatsek, A., Reichle, E. D., & Rayner, K. (2006). Tests of the E-Z Reader model: Exploring the interface between cognition and eye-movement control. *Cognitive Psychology, 52,* 1-52.

Posner, M. I. (1980). Orienting of attention. *Quarterly Journal of Experi-*

mental Psychology, 32, 3-25.
Potter, M. (1999). Understanding sentences and scenes: The role of conceptual short-term memory. In V. Coltheart (Ed.), *Fleeting memories* (pp. 13-46). Boston: MIT Press.
Rayner, K. (1975). The perceptual span and peripheral cues in reading. *Cognitive Psychology, 7*, 65-81.
Rayner, K. (1978). Eye movements in reading and information processing. *Psychological Bulletin, 85*, 618-660.
Rayner, K. (1995). Eye movements and cognitive processes in reading, visual search, and scene perception. In J. M. Findlay, R. Walker, & R.W. Kentridge (Eds.), *Eye movement research: Mechanisms, processes and applications* (pp. 3-22). Amsterdam: North Holland.
Rayner, K. (1998). Eye movements in reading and information processing: 20 years of research. *Psychological Bulletin, 85*, 618-660.
Rayner, K., Ashby, J., Pollatsek, A., & Reichle, E. D. (2004). The effects of frequency and predictability on eye fixations in reading: Implications for the E-Z Reader model. *Journal of Experimental Psychology: Human Perception and Performance, 30*, 720-732.
Rayner, K., & Bertera, J. H. (1979). Reading without a fovea. *Science, 206*, 468-469.
Rayner, K., & Duffy, S. A. (1986). Lexical complexity and fixation times in reading: Effects of word frequency, verb complexity, and lexical ambiguity. *Memory & Cognition, 14*, 191-201.
Rayner, K., & Fisher, D. L. (1987a). Eye movements and the perceptual span during visual search. In J. K. O'Regan, & A. Levy-Schoen (Eds.), *Eye movements: From physiology to cognition* (pp. 293-302). Amsterdam: North Holland.
Rayner, K., & Fisher, D. L. (1987b). Letter processing during eye fixations in visual search. *Perception & Psychophysics, 42*, 87-100.
Rayner, K., Inhoff, A. W., Morrison, R. E., Slowiaczek, M. L., & Bertera, J. H. (1981). Masking of foveal and parafoveal vision during eye fixations in reading. *Journal of Experimental Psychology: Human Perception and Performance, 7*, 167-179.
Rayner, K., Liversedge, S. P., & White, S. J. (2006). Eye movements when reading disappearing text: The importance of the word to the right of fixation. *Vision Research, 46*, 310-323.
Rayner, K., Liversedge, S. P., White, S. J., & Vergilino-Perez, D. (2003). Reading disappearing text: Cognitive control of eye movements. *Psychological Science, 14*, 385-389.
Rayner, K., McConkie, G. W., & Ehrlich, S. F. (1978). Eye movements

and integrating information across saccades. *Journal of Experimental Psychology: Human Perception and Performance, 4,* 529-544.

Rayner, K., McConkie, G. W., & Zola, D. (1980). Integrating information across eye movements. *Cognitive Psychology, 12,* 206-226.

Rayner, K., & Pollatsek, A. (1989). *The Psychology of Reading.* Englewood Cliffs, NJ: Prentice Hall.

Rayner, K., & Pollatsek, A. (1992). Eye movements and scene perception. *Canadian Journal of Psychology, 46,* 342-376.

Rayner, K., Reichle, E. D., & Pollatsek, A. (1998). Eye movement control in reading: An overview and model. In G. Underwood (Ed.), *Eye guidance in reading and scene perception* (pp. 243-268). Oxford, England: Elsevier.

Rayner, K., Slowiaczek, M. L., Clifton, C., & Bertera, J. H. (1983). Latency of sequential eye movements: Implications for reading. *Journal of Experimental Psychology: Human Perception and Performance, 9,* 912-922.

Rayner, K., Warren, T., Juhasz, B. J., & Liversedge, S. P. (2004). The effect of plausibility on eye movements in reading. *Journal of Experimental Psychology: Learning, Memory, and Cognition, 30,* 1290-1301.

Rayner, K., & Well, A. D. (1996). Effects of contextual constraint on eye movements in reading: A further examination. *Psychonomic Bulletin & Review, 3,* 504-509.

Reichle, E. D., Pollatsek, A., Fisher, D. L., & Rayner, K. (1998). Toward a model of eye movement control in reading. *Psychological Review, 105,* 125-157.

Reichle, E. D., Pollatsek, A., & Rayner, K. (2006). E-Z Reader: A cognitive-control, serial-attention model of eye-movement behavior during reading. *Cognitive Systems Research, 7,* 4-22.

Reichle, E. D., Rayner, K., & Pollatsek, A. (2003). The E-Z Reader model of eye movement control in reading: Comparison to other models. *Behavioral and Brain Sciences. 26,* 507-526.

Rensink, R. A., O'Regan, J. K., & Clark, J. J. (1997). To see or not to see: The need for attention to perceive changes in scenes. *Psychological Science, 8,* 368-373.

Saida, S., & Ikeda, M. (1979). Useful field size for pattern perception. *Perception & Psychophysics, 25,* 119-125.

Sereno, S. C., O'Donnell, P. J., & Rayner, K. (2006). Eye movements and lexical ambiguity resolution: Investigating the subordinate bias effect. *Journal of Experimental Psychology: Human Perception and Performance, 32,* 335-350.

Tanenhaus, M. K., Chambers, C. G., & Hanna, J. E. (2004). Referential domains in spoken language comprehension: Using eye movements to bridge the product and action traditions. In J. M. Henderson, & F. Ferreira (Eds.), *The interface of language, vision, and action: Eye movements and the visual world* (pp. 279-318). New York: Psychology Press.

Torralba, A., Oliva, A., Castelhano, M. S., & Henderson, J. M. (2006). Contextual guidance of attention in natural scenes. *Psychological Review, 113*, 766-786.

Van Diepen, E. M. J., & d'Ydewalle, G. (2003). Early peripheral and foveal processing in fixations during scene perception. *Visual Cognition, 10*, 79-100.

Van Diepen, E. M. J., Wampers, M., & d'Ydewalle, G. (1998). Functional division of the visual field: Moving masks and moving windows. In G. Underwood (Ed.), *Eye guidance in reading and scene perception* (pp. 337-356). Oxford, England: Elsevier.

Van Zoest, L. J. F. M., Donk, M., & Theeuwes, J. (2004). The role of bottom-up control in saccadic eye movements. *Journal of Experimental Psychology: Human Perception and Performance, 30*, 746-759.

Vaughan, J. (1982). Control of fixation duration in visual search and memory search: Another look. *Journal of Experimental Psychology: Human Perception and Performance, 8*, 709-723.

Vlaskamp, B. N. S., & Hooge, I. T. C. (2006). Crowding degrades saccadic search performance. *Vision Research, 46*, 417-425.

Williams, C. C., Henderson, J. M., & Zacks, R. T. (2005). Incidental visual memory for targets and distractors in visual search. *Perception & Psychophysics, 67*, 816-827.

Williams, R. S., & Morris, R. K. (2004). Eye movements, word familiarity, and vocabulary acquisition. *European Journal of Cognitive Psychology, 16*, 312-339.

Yarbus, A. (1967). *Eye movements and vision*. New York: Plenum Press.

Zelinsky, G. (2005). Specifying the components of attention in a visual search task. In L. Itti, G. Rees, & J. Tsotsos (Eds.), *Neurobiology of attention* (pp. 395-400). Elsevier, Inc.

Zelinsky, G. J., Rao, R. P. N., Hayhoe, M. M., & Ballard, D. H. (1997). Eye movements reveal the spatiotemporal dynamics of visual search. *Psychological Science, 8*(6), 448-453.

Section 2

Models of eye movements in reading

Chapter 2

The E-Z Reader model of eye movement control in reading

Alexander Pollatsek, Keith Rayner, and Erik D. Reichle

About 100 years ago, Huey (1908) wrote a wonderful book about the psychology of reading. In it, he said:

> *To completely analyze what we do when we read would almost be the acme of a psychologist's achievements, for it would be to describe very many of the most intricate workings of the human mind, as well as to unravel the tangled story of the most remarkable specific performance that civilization has learned in all its history. (p. 9).*

We think this statement is not only true, but it also indicates that, in spite of the large amount of good research about the process of reading in the last 30-40 years, we are still a long way from anything like a complete understanding of the reading process. Thus, in attempting to construct a quantitative model of reading, it would seem foolhardy to attempt to model everything that occurs when people read. However, researchers have made more progress in some areas of processing of language than in others, largely because the issues are better defined and easier to study. In particular, the area of word identification, and in particular the identification of visually presented words, seems much better understood than how grammatical or discourse structures are understood. Thus, it seemed to us that this was a good place to start modeling the reading process.

Of course, just because one has a pretty good understanding of the word identification process, this doesn't necessarily mean that one can build even a tentative model of reading based on it alone. However, it seemed that there was a conception of reading in which it made sense to assume that word identification is the basic "engine" that drives the eyes forward in text. This conception relies on a few basic facts about reading and eye movements. The first is that a typical fixation in reading is on the order of about 200-250 ms (Rayner, 1978). The second is that eye movement programming and execution is not instantaneous; that is, even the most rapid saccades driven by physical input (such as moving to a sudden onset of a bright stimulus) take on the order of 180 ms (Becker & Jürgens, 1979; Rayner, Slowiaczek, Clifton, & Bertera, 1983). Thus, if "moving on" in reading (i.e., moving to the right in most Western alphabetic orthographies) depends, at least to some extent, on having processed the word that has just been fixated, then there isn't a lot of time for processing it before a decision to move the eyes has to be made. It thus seems unlikely that this decision of whether to move on to the next word or not is based on really deep processing of a word (e.g., revising the grammatical parse of the sentence or adding to the discourse structure). Instead, it would seem more probable that a "preliminary check" of whether the word has been processed adequately enough so that it is likely that subsequent processing will be successful would be the signal to move ahead in the text. Whether we arrive at an acceptable definition of what this state would be is, of course, an open question.

Before moving on to characterize what this state would be and how it could fit into a model of reading, however, we need to discuss two issues. The first is whether one even needs such a mechanism to explain reading. That is, one solution to the problem of how to model eye movements in reading (Reilly & O'Regan, 1998; Yang & McConkie, 2001, 2004) is to deem that they are in fact too rapid for serious cognitive operations to drive them, and instead, to posit that eye movements are programmed "automatically" and targeted to the next word. We think this solution is woefully inadequate, as it ignores the large literature (see Rayner, 1998) that indicates that the fixation time on a word varies depending on the word's frequency in the language (and other variables that would influence the time to identify the word). Thus, we will not consider this alternative view any further.

The second issue is how closely tied fixating a word is to processing it. That is, the way we posed the problem above was to suggest that eye movements (on average) take about 180 ms to execute after a simple signal such as the sudden onset of a stimulus on a blank background, so that if one assumed something like 90 ms for such a signal to reach primary visual cortex and initiate a saccadic program, then the programming time for the eye movement would be approximately 90 ms. Thus, whatever the identification processes of the word are that are influencing the eye movement have to be completed within something like 250 ms (a reasonable estimate of how long it takes to access a word's meaning; Rayner & Pollatsek, 1989) minus the 90 ms it takes to program a saccade, or about 160 ms. (In fact, the latest versions of our model assume that the motor programming time is 125 ms.) However, this extremely short estimate of how quickly the processing of words can take place during a fixation (160 ms) tacitly assumes that word identification begins when the word is fixated. Thus, some of the time pressure would be reduced if part of the work of word identification is done parafoveally before the word is fixated.

One can ensure that word processing begins when the word is fixated using the *moving window* paradigm (McConkie & Rayner, 1975). In this paradigm, there is normal text in only a specified region around the fixation point, and all other letters are changed to "garbage" (e.g., random letters or Xs). In one experiment using this technique (Rayner, Well, Pollatsek, & Bertera, 1982), there was a one-word window; that is, only the fixated word was normal text and all other words were replaced by nonsense, although the spaces between the words were preserved. Thus, in this situation, readers were forced to start processing a word when they fixated it. The finding was that fixation times in this condition were appreciably longer (roughly 50 ms) than in normal reading. This indicates that part of the work of word identification is indeed done parafoveally and that slowing the process of word identification is delaying the signal to move to the next word. This finding, together with a large amount of evidence from the *boundary* paradigm (in which a nonsense preview is typically replaced by a real word when the reader's eyes fixate the word; Rayner, 1975) makes clear that encoding of a word in normal reading does not begin when a word is fixated, and that readers often get preview information from the parafovea about a word before it is fixated.

A key issue that models of reading differ on is how to explain this fact. Most other models of reading (e.g., Glenmore: Reilly & Radach, 2003, 2006; SERIF: McDonald, Carpenter, & Shillcock, 2005; SWIFT: Engbert, Nuthmann, Richter, & Kliegl, 2005) assume that words are processed in parallel. That is, they assume that at any given point in time, the attention of the reader is distributed over a region larger than a single word. For example, in SWIFT (see the chapter by Risse, Engbert,

& Kliegl, this volume), this region is approximately four words (although it is defined by a given number of character spaces) whereas in Glenmore, the effective window is the fixated word and the word to the right. In contrast, the E-Z Reader model assumes that processing of words is serial: that processing of letter information at any given point in time is only on a single word. We think that this assumption is reasonable and is the most parsimonious explanation of the data. Moreover, we think that if one abandons this assumption, quantitative modeling of reading is likely to turn into an empty exercise because a model assuming parallel processing will essentially be a deus ex machina (i.e., it will be flexible enough to explain any possible data—including phenomena that don't occur in reading). Given that serial processing is a crucial assumption in the E-Z Reader model, we clearly need to document the assertions just made.

Is serial processing of words a reasonable assumption?

The first claim made above is that serial processing of words is consistent with all the data on reading to date. How can this be reconciled with the fact that more than one word is processed on a fixation? Our assumption is that attention at any given time is devoted to encoding a single word, but that when the encoding of that word is completed, covert attention moves to the next word before the saccade to the next word is executed. (We'll specify the details of how this is implemented in our model below.) This attentional shift allows time for processing of the next word before it is fixated, and thus is a simple explanation for parafoveal preview of a word. As a result, the typical pattern posited in our model is that the reader extracts information from a word before it is fixated, finishes processing of that word while it is being fixated, and then begins processing of the next word. However, our model also allows for the possibility that parafoveal processing of the next word (word n+1) can be completed before a saccade away from the fixated word (word n) is executed, so that occasionally there will be parafoveal processing of the word two words ahead of the fixated word (word n+2). (This latter mechanism is related to explaining how words are skipped, and we will specify the details of how this is accomplished below.)

Our model thus explains how preview benefit can naturally occur even though words are processed serially: All that is needed is the assumption that covert attention shifts occur before saccades are executed. Are there any other data that demand parallel processing? One of the major phenomena that people who posit parallel processing point to is so-called "parafoveal-on-foveal effects". That is, it is claimed that parafoveal information is not only extracted, but that it guides eye movements in a manner that is inconsistent with the assumptions of a serial processing model. We should quickly point out that our serial model does predict one version of a "parafoveal-on-foveal" effect that was just mentioned: word skipping. That is, skipping of word n+1 is determined—at least in part—by its linguistic properties, such as its frequency in the language and its predictability from the prior text. (We will make clearer how the E-Z Reader model explains word skipping below; however, the essential idea is that a command to fixate word n+1 can be cancelled by a later command to fixate word n+2.) On the other hand, what is inconsistent with a serial model, such as E-Z Reader, is if linguistic properties of word n+1 can influence the fixation time on word n when word n+1 is subsequently fixated and thus was presumably not fully processed when word n was fixated.

There is now a large literature trying to document such parafoveal-on-foveal effects. Our view is that there are few, if any, effects that are consistently replicable. In particular, it is our view that it has not been documented that aspects of word n+1 that might be termed "linguistic" indeed influence fixation patterns on word n. A finding that seems to be more replicable is that if word n+1 is either (a) orthographically strange or (b) a nonword, then it has some influence on fixation times on word n. In the former case, that may have little to do with normal reading as detecting a strange-looking stimulus (because of some gross dissimilarity with what words look like) could result from some process other than the process of trying to identify a word. One thing we wish to make clear is that our model does not assume that all visual processing progresses from word to word in a serial manner. Among other things, such an assumption seems nonsensical, as it's clear that if the stimulus to the right of the word they were fixating was a word, a picture, or a blank space, people could easily determine which it was. In addition, in order for programming of eye movements to progress speedily, a target for the next saccade must be selected and, in alphabetic languages with spaces between words, it seems clear that these spaces are crucial in guiding the saccade (McConkie, Kerr, Reddix, & Zola, 1988). Thus, in our model, we posit that there is an early stage of visual processing in which all information is processed in parallel (although more inefficiently the farther the information is from the fovea), followed by the later word-identification stage (or stages) which are assumed to go one word at a time. Such a distinction between early, parallel stages, and later, serial processing has been a standard aspect of cognitive psychology theories since Broadbent (1958).

The finding that fixation time on word n is lengthened if word n+1 is a nonword does seem fairly consistent and is less likely to be ascribed to detecting low-level features of word n+1. However, this finding (and to some extent the above finding that presenting a "strange" looking stimulus as word n+1 influences fixation time on word n) has generally been observed only when fixations on word n are on the last letter or two of it. (In fact, in a recent attempt to replicate this finding, Drieghe, Rayner, and Pollatsek (2008) found inflated fixation durations on word n only occurred when the fixation was on the last letter.) However, fixations on a word that are near the end of the word are likely to include many fixations that were programmed to land on the next word, but fell short. (We will provide a mechanism for this below.) Hence, these lengthened fixations are likely to be examples of "parafoveal-on-foveal processing" only because of errors of eye-movement programming, and are thus not clear evidence that, in the normal course of reading, one is simultaneously processing word n and word n+1 in parallel.

In sum, we think that the assumption that words are lexically processed one word at a time is a reasonable one given the data at hand; we don't think that there are any compelling data that argue against it. Furthermore, as we will argue later, it is by far the most parsimonious assumption one can make in explaining how word identification is tied to the movements of the eyes during reading. In addition, if one abandons the serial-processing assumption, it makes understanding higher-order processes, such as syntactic parsing, almost impossible, as one then has little idea of when lexical processing of a word has been completed.

The E-Z Reader model

As indicated above, when we decided to try to model eye movements in reading, we started from two basic premises. The first is that, as it has already been established, the fixation time on a word is influenced by variables such as word frequency and the predictability of the word from prior context, so that it is clear that encoding of a word is a major influence on the decision of when to move to the next word in the text.

Second, as has been argued above, as there is no compelling evidence for simultaneous lexical processing of more than one word, it appeared that the natural starting point in modeling was to make the simplest assumptions: (a) that only one word is attended to at any given instant, and (b) that in the normal (forward) progress of the reader through the text, attention moves through the text in a strictly sequential manner (e.g., from left-to-right across a line of text in English). When we started modeling, we were not at all confident that we would be able to successfully model reading with these central assumptions using reasonable parameters for the time for lexical access and for the programming of saccades. Needless to say, we were quite pleased when we were successful at doing this. We now will detail how these key assumptions are implemented in the model together with the other assumptions of the model. Although we will present the latest version of the model, E-Z Reader 9 (Pollatsek, Reichle, & Rayner, 2006), the core assumptions of the model are the same as in the original model (Reichle, Pollatsek, Fisher, & Rayner, 1998).

Word encoding assumptions

Our formal modeling divides the time necessary to encode a word into three sequential stages. The first stage, *V*, is a (low-level) visual processing of the features of the word. In this stage, all information on the page is processed in parallel, and, among other things, the processing in this stage allows the outlines of words to be processed so that this information can be used in saccadic programming. The time that this stage is assumed to take (50 ms) can be thought of as the time for visual information to go from the retina to form coherent representations in primary visual cortex. We do not necessarily think of the next two stages, L_1 and L_2, as being qualitatively different from each other; instead, it is more reasonable to think of them as two different stages of encoding of the word, and that L_1 is a stage that (when completed) signals the saccadic system that lexical access is immanent and that it is "safe" to program a saccade to the next word (word n+1). (We should make clear that in outlining the model, word n refers to the word that is attended to at the beginning of the fixation; this will usually be the word actually fixated except for cases involving saccadic programming errors.) The completion of the third stage, L_2, is the completion of the identification of the word and is the signal to shift attention to word n+1.

Thus, an important feature of the E-Z Reader model is that the signal to program a saccade and the signal to shift attention are not the same.

This was introduced primarily to explain "spillover" effects (i.e., that variables like the frequency of word n not only influence fixation times on word n, but also have smaller effects on fixation times on word n+1). If saccade programming and attention shifting were yoked, this would not happen: all effects of the frequency of word n would be predicted to be on word n. However, if the duration of L_2 is also a function of the frequency of the word, then the model predicts that lower frequency words will be processed for a longer amount of time after the saccade program has been initiated and thus there will be less parafoveal processing of word n+1. By the same logic, the model also predicts that there will be less benefit of a preview of word n+1 when word n is low frequency (Henderson & Ferreira, 1990).

Our model does not contain a theory of word identification. Instead, one can view it as a framework for testing models of word identification in reading. Thus, we merely introduced assumptions about how linguistic variables would affect the durations of L_1 and L_2. To account for the two variables that have been most reliably shown to affect fixation times in reading, the written frequency of the word in the language and the predictability of a word from the prior text, we posited the following function for the duration of L_1, where α_1, α_2, and α_3 are parameters that are allowed to vary in the simulation.

(1) $t(L_1) = \alpha_1 - \alpha_2 \ln(\text{frequency}) - \alpha_3 (\text{predictability})$

Equation 1 ignores instances where word n is "guessed" from its sentence context [i.e., the duration of $t(L_1)$ is set equal to 0 ms], which for the sake of simplicity is assumed to occur with a probability equal to the word's normative cloze-task probability (i.e., the mean probability of guessing word n from all of the words preceding it). Although this assumption is largely limited to highly predictable function words (most often the word "the"), it is necessary to explain data from experiments involving 1-word moving "windows", where readers occasionally skip (and do not regress to) highly predictable words (Rayner et al., 1982). Another important fact about Equation 1 is that it is the "base form" of this equation in that it ignores where the fixation point is in relation to the word and it also ignores the length of a word (which has been shown to have an effect on the amount of time a word is fixated independent of the frequency of the word; Brysbaert & Vitu, 1998; Kliegl, Nuthmann, & Engbert, 2006; Rayner & McConkie, 1976). To deal with both of these problems in a parsimonious way, we assumed that this base rate of lexical processing is adjusted by multiplying it by the *rate coefficient* in Equation 2. The term in the exponent is the average distance of the letters in the word being processed from fixation, and in the case that a 1-letter word is fixated, the exponent would be zero and this coefficient would be equal to 1. Otherwise, the exponent is greater than one, and the farther (on average) the letters in the word are from fixation, the larger this exponent gets, and the slower lexical processing becomes. (Note that ε is a parameter we selected and was set to 1.15.) To see how word length (represented in Equation 2 by N) would affect the rate, consider a 3-letter word that is fixated on its middle letter versus a 7- letter word fixated on its middle letter. The average distance of letters from fixation for the 3-letter word is 2/3, whereas the average distance for the 7-letter word would be 12/7, and the rate coefficients would be 1.1 and 1.27. These rates are optimal for words of this length, however, as they were computed assuming that the word was fixated optimally (i.e., at its center). To see how the eccentricity would affect the rate, if a 3-letter word were seen parafoveally when fixating the prior word (assuming the center of the word was five characters from fixation), then the exponent would be 5 and the rate coefficient would be 2.01, which would represent an appreciable slowing of processing.

(2) $\text{rate} = \varepsilon^{\Sigma\,|\,\text{letter position} - \text{fixation position}\,|\,/\,N}$

Finally, we assumed that L_2 was a constant proportion of L_1, as in Equation 3 (where Δ is a free parameter whose value is set in the simulation). This is consistent with a fairly simple model of word identification, where processing proceeds at a relatively uniform rate. Thus, we realize that this simple assumption may have to be modified in the future. More to the point, however, is that these assumptions about lexical processing are oversimplified because there are other variables besides the frequency, predictability, and length of a word that influence processing time (e.g., the age of acquisition of the word, its "neighborhood" properties, and whether the word has more than one meaning, to name just a few). We will return later to discuss some of these issues.

(3) $t(L_2) = \Delta\, L_1$

Saccadic programming assumptions

Another key assumption of the E-Z Reader model is that there are two stages to the eye-movement program (actually three stages in the latest implementation of the model). The key idea is that saccadic programs can be cancelled in their early stages; this assumption is based on the work of Becker and Jürgens (1979; see also Leff, Scott, Rothwell, & Wise, 2001; McPeek, Skavenski, & Nakayama, 2000; Molker & Fischer, 1999; Vergilino & Beauvillain, 2000). This property is captured in the model by assuming two stages for saccadic programming: a *labile stage*, M_1, in which a subsequent saccadic program can cancel the program, followed by a *non-labile stage*, M_2, in which the program can no longer be interrupted and will invariably lead to a saccade. M_1 is assumed to have a duration of 100 ms and M_2 is assumed to have a duration of 25 ms. Furthermore, M_1 is broken down into two stages in our recent modeling (each taking 50 ms): the first stage is activating the saccadic system and the second stage is selecting a target. Thus, when a second saccadic program cancels the first one, the second program will not generally take the entire 125 ms to program, as the first stage will typically have already been partially completed by the first saccadic program.

As mentioned above, a key reason for introducing this cancellation assumption is to explain the fact that words are skipped, and skipped more often if they are easy to process (e.g., short, very frequent, or very predictable). (As we will see later, words are also skipped because of saccadic programming errors.) The way our cancellation assumption explains skipping of "easy" words is as follows. First, assume that the reader is fixating word n. It is typically the case that, in this situation, the reader started processing that word before it was fixated (via parafoveal preview), so that processing of word n will often be completed (i.e., L_2) within 100 ms of when it is originally fixated. Thus, when L_1 is completed, a saccade is programmed to word n+1 and relatively soon after that, attention shifts to word n+1 and lexical processing of it begins. (Note that the V stage of processing for word n+1 occurred in parallel with that for word n, at the beginning of the fixation on word n, making the V stage all but "invisible" except in cases involving display changes or very long saccades.) In most cases, L_1 processing of word n+1 is not complete before the end of the fixation, and hence there will be a saccade to word n+1 so that the processing of that word can continue after it has been fixated. However, if word n+1 is easy to process (i.e., the time for L_1 to complete is short), then this can occur while the saccadic program to word n+1 is still in the labile stage. In this case, a saccadic program is triggered to fixate word n+2, and this will cancel the saccadic program to fixate word n+1, causing word n+1 to be skipped.

The remaining key assumption of the model deals with refixations on words. That is, if the model only had the assumptions above, it would predict that all words that are fixated would receive exactly one fixation, which is clearly not the case in real reading data. To explain this, we assumed that there is a "clock" mechanism that will automatically program a refixation on a word when the word is initially fixated.

(Our latest version of the model has a slightly more complex assumption, but this difference is fairly minor.) Thus, through the same cancellation mechanism that explains skipping, the model handles refixations as well. That is, this automatic program to (re)fixate word n is made at the beginning of the fixation, but then if the subsequent program to fixate word n+1 is rapid enough to occur during the labile stage of the refixation program, the refixation is cancelled and the saccade will go to word n+1 (and word n will be fixated only once). This is clearly more likely to happen when word n can be processed more rapidly; thus the model predicts that a word is less likely to be refixated if it is short, frequent, or predictable (which is consistent with the data; Rayner, Sereno, & Raney, 1996).

Assumptions about "errors" in where saccades actually land

The final set of assumptions deals with where the saccades actually land. As we said above, the model assumes that the target for a saccade is the center of the word, which is a reasonable assumption in an alphabetic language like English where words are clear physical targets delimited by spaces. (We will comment briefly on saccade targeting in Chinese later in the chapter.) However, it is clear that all fixations do not land exactly in the middle of words. Thus, there must be some "random error" in saccadic programming, and the model indeed posits this.

In addition to random error in saccadic programming, and perhaps of greater importance, there is fairly clear evidence from McConkie et al. (1988) and others that there is also systematic "range error" in saccadic programming. That is, in some sense, there appears to be an "ideal" saccade length (Ψ in Equation 4) such that programmed saccades of this length do not have systematic error. As can be seen in Equation 4, if the programmed saccade length is equal to Ψ, the saccade will have no systematic error. (In our modeling, Ψ is set equal to 7, which is probably close to the average saccade length in reading.) However, all saccades that are programmed to be shorter than this value will have a systematic error that is positive (i.e., the saccades will tend to go further than intended, and will be overshoots) and all saccades that are programmed to be longer than this value will have a systematic error that is negative (i.e., the saccades will tend to fall short of their intended targets, and will be undershoots). One consequence of the systematic range error that we should quickly mention is that short words will not only tend to be skipped because they are easy to process but because they will tend to be overshot. However, this systematic range error is also modulated by the final term in Equation 4, so that saccades following longer fixations will tend to be less affected by the systematic error than saccades following shorter fixations. Finally, there is also random error in saccade programming, and as indicated in Equation 5, the standard deviation of the random error, σ, increases with the length of the programmed saccade. (Ω_1, Ω_2, η_1, η_2 are free parameters that are set in the simulations.)

(4) systematic error = (Ψ – intended length) $\{[\Omega_1 - \ln(\text{duration}_{n-1})] / \Omega_2\}$

(5) $\sigma = \eta_1 + \eta_2$ (intended saccade length)

Summary of assumptions

The above contains all the important assumptions of the E-Z Reader model. Although the model may sound complicated, it is in fact generally quite simple. It views reading as a process in which the reader identifies words one at a time, and when a word has been identified, the reader shifts attention to the next word. It is slightly complicated in that it assumes that the reader "cheats" and programs a saccade to the next word before fully identifying a word. It also assumes that refixations are (relatively) automatically programmed when the reader lands, presumably so that the reader doesn't get stuck viewing the word from a poor viewing location. (This is highly beneficial on those occasions where the initial fixation is far from the center of the word.) Then, the model assumes that saccade programs can be cancelled by later saccade programs (and this assumption allows us to explain word skipping and details about refixations). Lastly, there are natural assumptions about variability in saccadic programming. That's basically all there is to the model. However, before going on we wish to make one brief technical point and then a general comment about how we view what we have modeled so far. The technical point is that, when we were describing times in the equations above, these are mean durations (in milliseconds), but the actual times that are used during any given Monte-Carlo run of the model are assumed to be variable (i.e., random deviates sampled from gamma distributions).

The more general point, alluded to above, is that this is not intended to be a complete model of reading. Obviously, we have not said anything about how sentences or paragraphs are analyzed and understood or how this would impact on the reading process. An obvious symptom of this is that we have not said anything about *regressions*: eye movements going backward through the text. In its current instantiation, the model is limited to predicting some regressions due to saccadic error. For example, if a word is initially fixated near its end (due to an overshoot), then the refixation saccade will naturally tend to be backward as the target is the middle of the word. However, these are just intraword regressions. The model will also predict a few interword regressions. One example would be an extreme version of the last example, where a word is fixated near its end, but then the "refixation" (targeted towards the center of the word) overshoots and lands on the previous word. Another example would be where a word is skipped due to saccadic error, so that word n+1 is fixated but word n was the word that should have been fixated and is also the word that is attended to. In this case, the model would predict a "refixation" on word n, which would be a regression from word n+1 to word n. However, there is clearly much more to the phenomena of interword regressions than this, and they often indicate problems of misunderstanding of the syntax, such as in "garden path" sentences (Frazier & Rayner, 1982). Our model currently says nothing about such phenomena, although we will discuss later how we hope to expand the model to explain at least some of these phenomena.

As a result, in our modeling to date, we view our model as a highly schematic description of the "default" reading process that deals with the usual forward movement of the eyes through the text. We think it is not unreasonable to assume that these mechanisms are what operate until a signal of "non-understanding" comes from higher-up in the system telling the eyes to stop this forward movement and either remain fixated in a region or go backward to try to repair the damage. A consequence of this is that, in our modeling, we do not try to model interword regressions (even though, as indicated above, we could model a few). Thus, the data we model are sentences that have no interword regressions. In the next section, we will give some examples of our application of the model that should indicate how we see its role in helping to understand the reading process.

Applications of the model

Our first goal, when we developed the model, was to determine whether such a simple model could give a reasonable account of the pattern of eye movements in reading. To that end, we analyzed a large corpus of single sentences (Schilling, Rayner, & Chumbley, 1998) for which the eye-movement data had already been collected for other purposes. These were fairly simple sentences, and all of them were presented as one line of text on the computer screen. Another feature of these data was that the sentences had target words that were matched on length but varied on word frequency so that the effects of frequency on the fixations on the target words could be modeled as well as the overall pattern of eye movements. As the model incorporated the predictability of the word from the prior text as one relevant variable, we first collected predictability norms for this corpus of data (which is a fairly time-consuming process). In this norming study, we gave the participants a sentence up to word n-1, and had them guess word n for successive words in the sentence. Although the probability that people can guess the word without real time pressure is clearly not the same thing as how predictable a word is in the process of reading, it is clearly related to it closely enough to serve as a reasonable measure of the constraint on the word from the prior text.

Accordingly our initial step was to attempt to fit the eye movement data to the above corpus of text. Our modeling was word-based, so the indices from the data were eye-movement measures related to fixating on words. The duration measures of interest were: *first-fixation duration* (the duration of the initial fixation on a word during the first pass through the sentence), *single-fixation duration* (the fixation duration on a word conditional on it being fixated only once on the first pass), and *gaze duration* (the sum of the fixation durations on a word on the first pass before the eyes move on). (All of these measures are conditional on the word being fixated.) In addition, there were measures related to how many times a word was fixated: the probability of skipping the word, the probability of making exactly one fixation, and the probability of making two fixations on the first pass. (Words were virtually never fixated more than twice on the first pass.) As indicated above, we excluded all sentences in which the participant had regressed to a prior word. In addition, we did not attempt to model eye movements on the first or last word of the sentence; in the former case, there is "noise" in moving to the first word from the initial fixation location, and in the latter case, the eye movements are contaminated by the participant pushing the button indicating that the sentence has been read.

An example of one of our initial modeling efforts (Reichle et el., 1998) is shown in Table 2.1. In our primary analysis, we divided the words into five frequency classes and examined the measures averaged over these sets of words. The fits we obtained were very good; not only did they predict the mean fixation-duration measures well, but the model also simultaneously predicted both the probability of skipping and refixating the same set of words. Thus, the model was doing a good job in predicting both where the eyes went and how long they remained

Table 2.1 Observed and predicted values of gaze durations, and individual fixations, probability of skipping, making a single fixation, and making two fixations for E-Z reader 5 for five frequency classes of words.

Freq. class	Mean freq.	Gaze duration		First fixation duration		Single fixation duration	
		Observed	Predicted	Observed	Predicted	Observed	Predicted
1	3	293	291	248	251	265	274
2	45	272	271	234	253	249	263
3	347	256	257	228	246	243	252
4	4889	234	226	223	223	235	224
5	40700	214	211	208	210	216	210

Freq. class	Probability of skipping		Probability of making a single fixation		Probability of making two fixations	
	Observed	Predicted	Observed	Predicted	Observed	Predicted
1	0.10	0.09	0.68	0.73	0.20	0.17
2	0.13	0.16	0.70	0.76	0.16	0.07
3	0.22	0.27	0.68	0.68	0.10	0.04
4	0.55	0.49	0.44	0.50	0.02	0.01
5	0.67	0.68	0.32	0.32	0.01	0.00

on a fixation once they landed. (Subsequent modeling also examined the landing positions on words more carefully and gave a good account of that as well.) A secondary analysis on the target words mentioned above also indicated that the model predicted the fixation-duration data on them quite well. This success indicated to us that a serial model like this was a tenable model for how the eyes normally move forward in text and has led us to continue modeling efforts using this model as a framework.

We have continued to refine the assumptions of the model and test these refinements (e.g., Pollatsek et al., 2006), but this chapter does not seem like the best place to go into detail discussing these refinements (for an overview of this work, see Reichle, Pollatsek, & Rayner, 2006). However, it is perhaps worth mentioning three of them. The first is that it seemed to be against the logic of the model to posit that an automatic refixation could be programmed instantaneously before there was adequate visual information to program such a refixation. Thus, the refixation assumption was modified such that refixations are no longer programmed the instant that the fixation begins; in addition, the probability of programming a refixation is influenced by how far the fixation is from the center of the attended word. The second refinement is that we wanted to test assumptions about what processing went on during a saccade and how continuous the lexical processing was from one fixation to the next (Pollatsek et al., 2006). Basically, the issue explored was whether the processing of a word on a fixation had to wait for the visual information on that fixation to arrive at the cortex or whether the first 50 ms or so of a fixation (and of the saccade prior to it) was spent continuing to process the word attended to on the prior fixation. Our modeling (Pollatsek et al., 2006) suggests that the latter is the case, and that assuming a "dead time" to wait for the new visual information at the beginning of a fixation is probably not tenable. The third is, as indicated above, the M_1 (labile) stage of the eye movement program was divided into two sub-stages. The results of a simulation using this more recent version of the model are shown in Table 2.2 (Pollatsek et al., 2006). Although the quality of the overall fit to this data set is only slightly better (using a root-mean-squared error measure) with the later model than the earlier model, it is a distinctly superior model. In particular, the later version of the model (E-Z Reader 9) makes far superior predictions in display-change situations such as the moving window paradigm, the boundary paradigm, and the disappearing text paradigm (see below). We thus view the added complexity of E-Z Reader 9 (i.e., the fact that it includes more a priori theoretical assumptions than earlier versions of our model) as both increasing the theoretical scope of the model (by allowing it to explain more phenomena) and increasing its overall plausibility (by incorporating more realistic assumptions and parameter values). Finally, it is also worth noting that our modeling strategy has generally been to develop "nested" or "cumulative" models (Grainger & Jacobs, 1998), so that each new version of our model accounts for some new phenomena, as well as all of the phenomena that could be explained by prior versions. (We hedge and use "generally" because we have also occasionally used our model as a framework to test hypotheses in the manner described by Seidenberg & Plaut, 2006; one recent example of this is our attempt to simulate readers' eye movements during the resolution of lexical ambiguity; Reichle et al., 2007.)

We should also mention that the E-Z Reader model was not only intended as a model of eye movements in reading English, but more generally of reading any printed alphabetic language. One article reported reasonably good fits of data in French (Miellet, Sparrow, & Sereno, 2007; Sparrow, Miellet, & Coello, 2003). However, these were obtained without any serious fitting of parameters, so the fits were likely to have im-

Table 2.2 Observed and predicted values of gaze durations, and individual fixations, probability of skipping, making a single fixation, and making two fixations for E-Z reader 9 for five frequency classes of words.

Freq. class	Mean freq.	Gaze duration		First fixation duration		Single fixation duration	
		Observed	Predicted	Observed	Predicted	Observed	Predicted
1	3	293	295	248	251	265	259
2	45	272	275	234	239	249	244
3	347	256	241	228	225	243	226
4	4889	234	220	223	217	235	217
5	40700	214	216	208	214	216	215

Freq. class	Probability of skipping		Probability of making a single fixation		Probability of making two fixations	
	Observed	Predicted	Observed	Predicted	Observed	Predicted
1	0.10	0.09	0.68	0.75	0.20	0.15
2	0.13	0.12	0.70	0.74	0.16	0.13
3	0.22	0.19	0.68	0.65	0.10	0.06
4	0.55	0.47	0.44	0.52	0.02	0.01
5	0.67	0.58	0.32	0.42	0.01	0.00

proved beyond what is reported there if there had been. (There is no reason to expect either that the parameters of the model would be the same for English and French or the same for any group of readers even within the same language.) We have also extended the E-Z Reader to Chinese (Rayner, Li, & Pollatsek, 2007; see also this volume), and have done so with reasonable success assuming the same basic processes as in English. However, this is just a first step, and further efforts are needed to explore certain mechanisms—most notably, exactly how the eyes are targeted in an orthography where there are no spaces between words.

Another use of the E-Z Reader model has been to provide testable predictions. Two of these that directly follow from the basic assumptions of the model and do not rely on specific parameter assumptions are: (a) that skipping word n increases fixation times on word n-1, and (b) that skipping word n also increases fixation times on word n+1. The rationale for the latter prediction is fairly obvious. If one skips word n, word n+1 has been seen from a worse vantage point (word n-1) than if one had not skipped word n; thus, there will be less information extracted from the parafovea, resulting in longer fixations on word n when it is fixated. The rationale for the former prediction is less obvious and stems from the assumption about a later saccade program canceling an earlier one. That is, in the model, a skip of word n occurs because a program to fixate word n+1 has cancelled a program to fixate word n. Thus, on average, fixations before skips will be longer than fixations before non-skips. Both of the predictions have been shown to be generally true (Pollatsek, Rayner, & Balota, 1986; Pynte, Kennedy, & Ducrot, 2004; Rayner, Ashby, Pollatsek, & Reichle, 2004; Reichle et al., 1998; but see Kliegl & Engbert, 2005). (These arguments are slightly oversimplified and ignore skips made due to saccadic programming error and individual differences among readers.)

The above example was one in which a specific prediction of the model was tested in existing data. Another, perhaps more exciting aspect of the model has been that it has inspired experiments to test some of its basic assumptions. One (Reingold & Rayner, 2006) was a test of the assumption that the duration of L_1 (the processing stage that triggers the eye movement) only affects the fixation time on word n, and does not affect later processing. This assumption was tested by manipulating the font of a target word. The logic was that if the font of the word was changed in such a way that it would only plausibly affect early stages of lexical processing, then only the duration of the fixations on word n would be affected. In fact, when the font of word n was made quite faint, it produced a sizeable effect on the gaze duration on word n, but had no effect on the fixation durations on word n+1 or later on in the text. More generally, this experiment also supports the serial processing assumption of E-Z Reader.

The second test of the E-Z Reader model (Liversedge, Rayner, White, Vergilino-Perez, Findlay, & Kentridge, 2004; Rayner, Liversedge, White, & Vergilino-Perez, 2003) was essentially a test of whether lexical processing of the fixated word is the major contributor to how long a word is fixated. In this experiment, whenever a word was fixated, it disappeared after 60 ms (this time has been shown in masking studies to be sufficient to allow words to be identified; Ishida & Ikeda, 1989). The key question, obviously, is how this disappearance affects fixation time on the word. The answer is that the disappearance, assuming it was late enough so that the visual information was fully registered, had virtually no effect on fixation times. Moreover, the word frequency effect on selected target words was also unaffected by the disappearance of the word. Thus, it appears that two key assumptions of the E-Z Reader model are valid: (a) that lexical processing—rather than responding to incidental visual aspects of the text—is the primary determinant of how long a fixation is, and (b) that this processing continues independent of whether the visual information is still present. A third interesting finding from these studies is that when the word to the right of fixation (word n+1) is masked after 60 ms, there is a substantial interference effect (in contrast to there being no interference when word n is masked). This naturally follows from the serial processing assumptions of the E-Z Reader model. That is, because attention shifts to word n+1 only after word n is processed (which would often be after more than 60 ms), the visual information from word n+1 will have often disappeared before attention has shifted to it. In contrast, we suspect that most parallel processing models would predict a greater cost when word n disappears than when word n+1 disappears.

Recent work and future directions

As previously indicated several times, we are definitely not claiming that the E-Z Reader model is a complete model of reading. Most notably, at present, it does not explain anything about language processing in reading beyond processing of individual words—with the possible exception of being able to model effects due to how predictable a word is. This obviously makes the model quite incomplete, as there is now an accumulating literature on how difficulties in syntactic parsing and in understanding the meaning of the discourse affect comprehension and eye movement behavior (Rayner, 1998). However, expanding our model (or any model of reading) to explain even some of these effects will be a huge enterprise, as it will necessitate including a theory of sentence processing into the model. In addition, at the motor level, it will require a serious model of what events trigger regressions and what the targets of these regressions are. Therefore, it is likely that anything resembling a complete model of how even single sentences are processed (not to mention how discourse is processed) is not likely in the immediate future. Thus, we think that the process of expanding the model is best done in small incremental steps.

One way we have tried to "deepen" the model is to try to explain some relatively "local" effects that relate to processing the meanings of words. One phenomenon that seemed appropriate to tackle was lexical ambiguity effects (Reichle, Rayner, & Pollatsek, 2007). *Lexical ambiguity* refers to a printed word having two quite distinct meanings. For example, in English, *port* can either mean a city with a harbor or a type of wine. In general, historically, the fact that the two words are spelled the same way is completely accidental (e.g., the wine is called 'port' as a shortening of either Portugal or the city of Oporto). As a result, this differs markedly from subtle differences in meaning of a word or from metaphoric uses of words where there is some semantic tie between the different meanings.

The role of lexical ambiguity in reading has been studied extensively by Rayner, Duffy, and others (1986; Duffy, Kambe, & Rayner, 2001; Duffy, Morris, & Rayner, 1988). (We will assume in what follows that there are only two distinct meanings of these words, although in some cases, there could be more.) Rayner and Duffy distinguished between (a) *balanced* ambiguous words (e.g., *case*) in which the two meanings occurred with almost equal frequency in the written language, and (b) biased ambiguous words (e.g., *port*) in which one of the meanings is much more frequent than the other (e.g., the harbor meaning of 'port' is much more frequent than the wine meaning). In both cases, the ambiguous word was paired with an unambiguous word (having the same orthographic frequency) that would naturally fit into the same sentence frame as the lexically ambiguous word. They also manipulated the type of sentence frame. In some of the sentence frames, there was *prior biasing context* (i.e., the text prior to the ambiguous word made clear which of the two meanings of the ambiguous word was intended). In the others, where there was no prior biasing context, so that the text prior to the ambiguous word was neutral with respect to which meaning was intended, only the later context made clear which meaning was intended. In all cases, the *less* frequent meaning of the word was the one consistent with the sentence context.

The basic results of these experiments can be stated fairly simply. First, when there was no prior biasing context, fixation times on the biased ambiguous words were about the same as for the unambiguous control words, but fixation times on the balanced ambiguous words were longer than on their unambiguous control words. Second, when there was prior biasing context, the pattern reversed: fixation times on the biased ambiguous words were longer than the controls, but the ones on the balanced ambiguous words were about the same as the controls. We should also quickly add that, in the case of no prior context, there was evidence of fairly serious disruption later on for the biased ambiguous words, indicating that these words had often been initially encoded as the more frequent meaning and that correcting this initial encoding took significant processing time. (There was a similar but much smaller effect in later processing for the balanced ambiguous words.)

The first important feature of these data is that these ambiguity effects surface early—even on first-fixation duration. In our earlier modeling papers, we had been fairly neutral about the interpretation of L_1 and L_2 and had suggested various possible interpretations including that L_1 might reflect the encoding of the orthographic and phonological form of the word. However, these data make clear that if the E-Z Reader model is a viable model of reading, then L_1 cannot be merely a stage in which the orthographic or phonological form of the word is processed, but that encoding of the word's meaning has to be part of the process. What is the best way to conceptualize how the processing of the meaning enters into the encoding process to explain these fixation-time data? One hypothesis that has been offered is that one considers the two meanings as independent entries, and thus that the fixation time on the word is dependent on the frequency of the meaning extracted. This hypothesis can explain some of the data qualitatively. For example, because the frequency of either of the meanings of a balanced ambiguous word would be approximately half that of the control, the hypothesis would predict longer fixation times on the balanced ambiguous words than the control words. However, this hypothesis is not satisfactory as, for example, it doesn't explain why prior context then causes fixation times on the balanced words to be equal to those on the control words.

Instead, a model in which there is an initial common stage for both meanings (influenced by the orthographic frequency of the word) followed by a second stage in which there is competition between the two meanings provided a much more satisfactory account and fit the data well. Briefly, this competition was assumed to be influenced by (a) the difference in the frequencies of the two meanings and (b) by the prior context. That is, we assumed that there was little competition when the two meaning frequencies were quite different, but that prior context could either lower the strength of the meaning inconsistent with prior context or raise the strength of the meaning of the word consistent with prior context. (The assumption of lowering the strength of the meaning inconsistent with prior context seems more reasonable given that the prior sentence contexts rarely primed the correct meaning.) Although we did not seriously attempt to model the processing in the later sentence, the model predicted that biased ambiguous words with no prior context would be usually encoded as the more frequent meaning—consistent with the later processing difficulty for these sentences.

The lexical ambiguity data make it clear that the processing of meaning is rapid enough to affect first-fixation durations on words. On some level, this is quite amazing. To quantify "rapid", consider that eye-movement programming time probably takes at least 100 ms, and that most fixation durations in reading are well under 300 ms. This means that within 200 ms of the beginning of the fixation (and probably well within 150 ms of it), the effects of lexical ambiguity have progressed far enough to affect eye movements. Even if one posits that something like 30-50 ms of the processing has been done parafoveally, it is quite remarkable that enough processing is going on so that the meaning of the word is processed fully enough such that it matters whether this meaning is consistent with the prior context in the sentence. We think we have modeled this phenomenon fairly well, but there are likely a set of phenomena involving how well a word fits into the immediate discourse context that should be the goal of our next modeling efforts. We will conclude by discussing one such phenomenon to illustrate that expanding the model to explain it will not be straightforward and will involve considerable thought.

The phenomenon is that, if a word doesn't make sense given the prior context, then there is often quite an immediate effect on eye movements. One classic example is syntactic "garden path" sentences, in which there are two possible parses of a sentence up to a target word, but one of the parses is highly preferred and is likely the "default" parse. When the target word is consistent with the other parse and inconsistent with the preferred parse, there is usually an immediate effect on the target word, including long fixation times and immediate regressions back in the text (Frazier & Rayner, 1987). Another example that we will focus on that is perhaps easier to model (because it won't require putting a serious theory of parsing in the model) is where a word is semantically strange (Rayner, Warren, Juhasz, & Liversedge, 2004). Consider the following three sentences.

(1) John used the pump to inflate the large carrots for dinner last night. (*Anomalous*)

(2) John used an axe to chop the large carrots for dinner last night. (*Implausible*)

(3) John used a knife to chop the large carrots for dinner last night. (*Normal*)

The finding is that having a context that makes *carrots* strange causes disruption in reading. Although this is not surprising, what is of primary interest is that the effects could be quite immediate: gaze durations on *carrots* in the anomalous sentences were significantly longer than in the "knife" sentence. In contrast, significant decrements in performance in the implausible sentences only appeared on fixation measures on the next region (e.g., *for dinner*). This suggests that the type of difficulty influences how soon the difficulty signals a regression; however, because the total interference effect was so much bigger in the anomalous sentences than in the implausible sentences, the apparent difference in timing may be largely due to the difficulty in observing an immediate small effect for the implausible sentences. This phenomenon seems like a good next step for modeling, as the effect of the context is clear (i.e., making it more difficult to fit in the meaning of the word in with the prior context) and the effects are relatively localized. However, there are some fairly deep issues that need to be dealt with in order to model this phenomenon. The first is how to model interword regressions. As mentioned above, the current model has no mechanism for this except those relating to errors in eye movement programming. The second issue is that generally introducing such anomalies in the sentence has varied effects; sometimes they cause quite long fixations but then the reader moves forward, whereas other times they cause regressions. The third, possibly related, issue is the timing of the effects. That is, if the type of difficulty produces a difference in the timing of the effect, it suggests that there may be more than one cognitive event that signals "I'm having trouble" and that is interrupting the normal reading process we have modeled so far.

We think that this kind of phenomenon is the appropriate arena in which to expand our modeling efforts. On the one hand, it will be a difficult endeavor, as we suspect that regressions will not be easy to model. On the other hand, as indicated above, the effects are all relatively "local" (e.g., most of the regressions just go a word or two back), so that one can keep one's focus on modeling what happens in a small region and not have to introduce detailed assumptions about sentence processing. We look forward to the challenge.

Summary

In this chapter, we have tried to explain the E-Z Reader model. In the first part, we discussed the rationale for the simplicity of the processing assumptions, focusing on the assumption of serial processing of words in text. We then gave an overview of the model and indicated the basic assumptions. We then discussed how it has been used. First, we gave an example of its success in fitting eye movement data, and followed that with some examples of how the model has been used as a heuristic device to generate testable predictions (which have been confirmed). In conclusion, we attempted to give some sense of where the modeling enterprise is going.

References

Becker, W., & Jürgens, R. (1979). An analysis of the saccadic system by means of double-step stimuli. *Vision Research, 19,* 967-983.

Broadbent, D. E. (1958). *Perception and communication*. London: Pergamon.

Brysbaert, M., & Vitu, F. (1998). Word skipping: Implications for theories of eye movement control in reading. In G. Underwood (Ed.), *Eye guidance in reading and scene perception* (pp.125-147). Amsterdam: Elsevier.

Drieghe, D., Rayner, K., & Pollatsek, A. (2008). Mislocated fixtions can account for parafoveal-on-foveal effects in eye movements during reading. *Quarterly Journal of Experimental Psychology, 61,* 1239-1249.

Duffy, S. A., Kambe, G., & Rayner, K. (2001). The effect of prior disambiguating context on the comprehension of ambiguous words: Evidence from eye movements. In D. S. Gorfein (Ed.), *On the consequences of meaning selection* (pp. 27-43). Washington, DC: APA Books.

Duffy, S. A., Morris, R. K., & Rayner, K. (1988). Lexical ambiguity and fixation times in reading. *Journal of Memory and Language, 27,* 429-446.

Engbert, R., Nuthmann, A., Richter, E., & Kliegl, R. (2005). SWIFT: A dynamical model of saccade generation during reading. *Psychological Review, 112,* 777-813.

Frazier, L., & Rayner, K. (1982). Making and correcting errors during sentence comprehension: Eye movements in the analysis of structurally ambiguous sentences. *Cognitive Psychology, 14,* 178-210.

Frazier, L., & Rayner, K. (1987). Resolution of syntactic category ambiguities: Eye movements in parsing lexically ambiguous sentences. *Journal of Memory and Language, 26,* 505-526.

Grainger, J., & Jacobs, A. M. (1998). On localist connectionism and psychological science. In J. Grainger, & A. M. Jacobs (Eds.), *Localist connectionist approaches to human cognition* (pp.1-38). Mahwah, NJ: Erlbaum.

Henderson, J. M., & Ferreira, F. (1990). Effects of foveal processing difficulty on the perceptual span in reading: Implications for attention and eye movement control. *Journal of Experimental Psychology: Learning, Memory, and Cognition, 16,* 417-429.

Huey, E. B. (1908). *The psychology and pedagogy of reading.* New York: Macmillan. (Republished: Cambridge, MA: MIT Press, 1968.)

Ishida, T., & Ikeda, M. (1989). Temporal properties of information extraction in reading studied by a text-mask replacement technique. *Journal of the Optical Society A: Optics and Image Science, 6,* 1624-1632.

Kliegl, R., & Engbert, R. (2005). Fixation durations before word skipping in reading. *Psychonomic Bulletin & Review, 12,* 132-138.

Kliegl, R., Nuthmann, A., & Engbert, R. (2006). Tracking the mind during reading: The influence of past, present, and future words on fixation durations. *Journal of Experimental Psychology: General, 135,* 12-35.

Leff, A.P., Scott, S.K., Rothwell, J.C., & Wise, R.J.S. (2001). The planning and guiding of reading saccades: A repetitive transcranial magnetic stimulation study. *Cerebral Cortex, 11,* 918-923.

Liversedge, S. P., Rayner, K., White, S. J., Vergilino-Perez, D., Findlay, J. M., & Kentridge, R. W. (2004). Eye movements when reading disappearing text: Is there a gap effect in reading? *Vision Research, 44,* 1013-1024.

McConkie, G. W., Kerr, P. W., Reddix, M. D., & Zola, D. (1988). Eye movement control during reading: I. The location of initial eye fixations in words. *Vision Research, 28,* 1107-1118.

McConkie, G. W., & Rayner, K. (1975). The span of the effective stimulus during a fixation in reading. *Perception & Psychophysics, 17,* 578-586.

McDonald, S. A., Carpenter, R. H. S., & Shillcock, R. C. (2005). An anatomically constrained, stochastic model of eye movement control in reading. *Psychological Review, 112,* 814-840.

McPeek, R. M., Skavenski, A. A., & Nakayama, K. (2000). Concurrent processing of saccades in visual search. *Vision Research, 40,* 2499-2516.

Mieller, S., Sparrow, L., & Sereno, S. C. (2007). Word frequency and predictability effects in reading French: An evaluation of the E-Z Reader model. *Psychonomic Bulletin & Review, 14,* 762-769.

Molker, A., & Fischer, B. (1999). The recognition and correction of involuntary prosaccades in an antisaccade task. *Experimental Brain Research, 125*, 511-516.

Pollatsek, A., Rayner, K., & Balota, D. A. (1986). Inferences about eye movement control from the perceptual span in reading. *Perception & Psychophysics, 40*, 123-130.

Pollatsek, A., Reichle, E. D., & Rayner, K. (2006). Tests of the E-Z Reader model: Exploring the interface between cognition and eye-movement control. *Cognitive Psychology, 52*, 1-52.

Pynte, J., Kennedy, A., & Ducrot, S. (2004). The influence of parafoveal typographical errors on eye movements in reading. *European Journal of Cognitive Psychology, 16*, 178-202.

Rayner, K. (1975). The perceptual span and peripheral cues in reading. *Cognitive Psychology, 7*, 65-81.

Rayner, K. (1978). Eye movements in reading and information processing. *Psychological Bulletin, 85*, 618-660.

Rayner, K. (1998). Eye movements in reading and information processing: 20 years of research. *Psychological Bulletin, 124*, 372-422.

Rayner, K., Ashby, J., Pollatsek, A., & Reichle, E. (2004). The effects of frequency and predictability on eye fixations in reading: Implications for the E-Z Reader model. *Journal of Experimental Psychology: Human Perception and Performance, 30*, 720-732.

Rayner, K., & Duffy, S. A. (1986). Lexical complexity and fixation times in reading: Effects of word frequency, verb complexity, and lexical ambiguity. *Memory & Cognition, 14*, 191-201.

Rayner, K., Li, X., & Pollatsek, A. (2007). Extending the E-Z Reader model of eye movement control to Chinese readers. *Cognitive Science, 31*, 1021-1034.

Rayner, K., Liversedge, S. P., White, S. J., & Vergilino-Perez, D. (2003). Reading disappearing text: Cognitive control of eye movements. *Psychological Science, 14*, 385-389.

Rayner, K., & McConkie, G. W. (1976). What guides a reader's eye movements? *Vision Research, 16*, 829-837.

Rayner, K., & Pollatsek, A. (1989). *The psychology of reading*. New Jersey: Prentice Hall.

Rayner, K., Sereno, S. C., & Raney, G. E. (1996). Eye movement control in reading: A comparison of two types of models. *Journal of Experimental Psychology: Human Perception and Performance, 22*, 1188-1200.

Rayner, K., Slowiaczek, M. L., Clifton, C., & Bertera, J. H. (1983). Latency of sequential eye movements: Implications for reading. *Jour-*

nal of Experimental Psychology: Human Perception and Performance, 9, 912-922.

Rayner, K., Warren, T., Juhasz, B. J., & Liversedge, S. P. (2004). The effect of plausibility on eye movements in reading. *Journal of Experimental Psychology: Learning, Memory, and Cognition, 30,* 1290-1301.

Rayner, K., Well, A. D., Pollatsek, A., & Bertera, J. H. (1982). The availability of useful information to the right of fixation in reading. *Perception & Psychophysics, 31,* 537-550.

Reichle, E. D., Pollatsek, A., Fisher, D. L., & Rayner, K. (1998). Toward a model of eye movement control in reading. *Psychological Review, 105,* 125-157.

Reichle, E. D., Pollatsek, A., & Rayner, K. (2006). E-Z Reader: A cognitive-control, serial-attention model of eye-movement behavior during reading. *Cognitive Systems Research, 7,* 4-22.

Reichle, E. D., Rayner, K., & Pollatsek, A. (2007). Modeling the effects of lexical ambiguity on eye movements during reading. In R. P. G. Van Gompel, M. F. Fischer, W. S. Murray, & R. L. Hill (Eds.), *Eye movements: A window on mind and brain* (pp. 271-292). Oxford, England: Elsevier.

Reilly, R., & O'Regan, J. K. (1998). Eye movement control in reading: A simulation of some word-targeting strategies. *Vision Research, 38,* 303-317.

Reilly, R., & Radach, R. (2003). Foundations of an interactive activation model of eye movement control in reading. In J. Hyona, R. Radach, & H. Deubel (Eds.), *The mind's eye: Cognitive and applied aspects of eye movement research* (pp. 429-455). Oxford, England: Elsevier.

Reilly, R., & Radach, R. (2006). Some empirical tests of an interactive activation model of eye movement control in reading. *Cognitive Systems Research, 7,* 34-55.

Reingold, E. M., & Rayner, K. (2006). Examining the word identification stages hypothesized by the E-Z Reader model. *Psychological Science, 17,* 742-746.

Schilling, H. E. H., Rayner, K., & Chumbley, J. I. (1998). Comparing naming, lexical decision, and eye fixation times: Word frequency effects and individual differences. *Memory & Cognition, 26,* 1270-1281.

Seidenberg, M. S., & Plaut, D. C. (2006). Progress in understanding word reading: Data fitting versus theory building. In S. Andrews (Ed.), *From inkmarks to ideas: Current issues in lexical processing* (pp. 25-49). New York: Psychology Press.

Sparrow, L., Miellet, S., & Coello, Y. (2003). The effects of frequency and prediction on eye fixations in reading: An evaluation of the E-Z Reader model. *Behavioral and Brain Sciences, 26*, 503-505.

Vergilino, D., & Beauvillain, C. (2000). The planning of refixation saccades in reading. *Vision Research, 40*, 3527-3538.

Yang , S. N., & McConkie, G. W. (2001). Eye movements during reading: A theory of saccade initiation time. *Vision Research, 41*, 3567-3568.

Yang, S. N., & McConkie, G. W. (2004). Saccade generation during reading: Are words necessary? *European Journal of Cognitive Psychology, 16*, 226-261.

Chapter 3

Eye movement control in reading: Experimental and corpus-analysis challenges for a computational model

Sarah Risse, Ralf Engbert, and Reinhold Kliegl

In eye movement research on reading, two major classes of models of eye movement control are typically distinguished: Models proposing that saccade targeting is guided by attentional gradients (GAG), which implicitly requires the assumption of distributed word processing across several words at a time (e.g., Engbert, Longtin, & Kliegl, 2002; Inhoff, Radach, Starr, & Greenberg, 2000), and those which assume serial attention shifts (SAS) from one word to the next in sequence (Reichle, Pollatsek, Fisher, & Rayner, 1998). During recent years, much progress has been made in translating these different theoretical perspectives into computational models to check their basic assumptions with simulations of empirical results. Meanwhile, experimental research and corpus analysis are delivering important empirical constraints that present quite formidable challenges to current models.

Box's (1979) statement "all models are wrong, some are useful", therefore, is an adequate characterization of computational models of reading. Although the options for adjusting the models to new constraints are far from having been exhausted, computational models are nevertheless advancing the scientific debate and have already proven to be extremely useful in deriving empirically testable hypotheses. And indeed, the research community has been prompt in its attempts to falsify critical assumptions (e.g., Inhoff, Radach, & Eiter, 2006; Kennedy & Pynte, 2005; Kliegl & Engbert, 2005; McDonald, 2006; Pollatsek, Reichle,

& Rayner, 2006b). Thus, current versions of computational models (e.g., E-Z Reader: Pollatsek, Rayner, & Reichle, this volume, Reichle et al., 1998; SWIFT: Engbert, Nuthmann, Richter, & Kliegl, 2005; Glenmore: Reilly & Radach, 2006; SERIF: McDonald, Carpenter, & Shillcock, 2005; see Reichle, Rayner, & Pollatsek, 2003, for a complete list and qualitative comparisons) and related theoretical proposals (i.e., Inhoff et al., 2000; Pynte & Kennedy, 2006; Vitu, Lancelin, Jean, & Farioli, 2006) stimulate a productive debate on a variety of theoretical issues and encourage the execution of challenging experiments as well as the set up of advanced corpus analyses.

One theoretically contentious issue in the comparison of parallel and serial models concerns the nature of preprocessing words to the right of the current fixation. Models based on GAG like SWIFT (Engbert et al., 2005, 2002; Kliegl & Engbert, 2003) assume that all words within the perceptual span are processed in parallel and thus predict preprocessing effects of all parafoveal words that fall into the span. In contrast, models based on SAS like E-Z Reader (Pollatsek, Reichle, & Rayner, 2006a; Rayner, Ashby, Pollatsek, & Reichle, 2004; see also Engbert & Kliegl, 2001) basically assume that preprocessing depends on complete processing of the currently fixated word followed by an attention shift to the next word to the right of fixation. However, due to an additional preattentive visual stage, low level information of parafoveal words (e.g., word length or orthographic irregularity) might be extracted even before attention is shifted onto this word (Pollatsek, Rayner, & Reichle, this volume; Rayner, White, Kambe, Miller, & Liversedge, 2003; Pollatsek, Reichle, & Rayner, 2003).

In this chapter, we elaborate on the issue of preprocessing effects of words to the right of fixation, emphasizing the potential of combining experimental, computational, and corpus-analysis methods to arrive at a more consistent picture of preprocessing in reading. First, we describe the qualitative predictions of GAG and SAS approaches concerning two different types of preprocessing effects, that is, the preview benefit effect and the parafoveal-on-foveal effect. For this chapter, we focus on effects stemming from word n+2, the word two words to the right of fixation. In our view, such effects represent a strong and challenging test case for both theoretical and computational modeling. Second, we introduce the dynamic of the current SWIFT version as one representative computational model based on the parallel processing approach and show the complexity of such a dynamical model for predicting preprocessing effects of word n+2. Third, we present both the existence and limitations of such effects in a corpus analysis of word patterns similar to those used in experimental studies and, finally, discuss the results with an outlook on further adjustments of SWIFT's mechanisms.

Sketch of preprocessing effects in GAG and SAS models

With respect to preprocessing words to the right of fixation, two types of effects have to be distinguished: preview benefit and parafoveal-on-foveal effects. In general, these preprocessing effects are in agreement with both parallel and serial processing accounts.

Preview benefit effects

By assuming an attentional gradient, models based on GAG necessarily assume distributed (parallel) processing of all words falling within the perceptual span[1]. Moreover, since processing efficiency decreases with increasing eccentricity from the current fixation position, preprocessing a word two words to the right of the current fixation (i.e., word n+2) is expected to be less efficient than for the direct fixation neighbor (i.e., word n+1). As a consequence, the dynamical behavior of SWIFT can be approximated by the activation of only three words (word n, word n+1, and word n+2; Engbert et al., 2005, Appendix C, pp. 811-813). Therefore, distributed processing is limited to only a few words at a time despite the general assumption of parallel processing.

SAS models like E-Z Reader account for the same effects with serial word-by-word processing. After the currently fixated word (i.e., word n) is completely processed and attention is shifted to the next word to the right of fixation, preprocessing of word n+1 can occur for the time it takes to finish programming the saccade from word n to word n+1. Moreover, if word n+1 is completely processed before the saccade from word n to word n+1 is executed, attention is shifted towards word n+2 while the saccade is reprogrammed to now land on word n+2. During reprogramming, word n+2 can be preprocessed. From this perspective, preprocessing effects will manifest themselves in word processing times for the thus previewed word (i.e., the preview benefit effect).

1 Recently, however, Engbert et al. (2005, p.803) proposed a possible variant of SWIFT with a serial lexical completion stage of word processing. In this approach, the dichotomy between serial and parallel processing was replaced by a continuous scale from strictly serial to fully parallel.

Parafoveal-on-foveal effects

Several words in the perceptual span are processed in parallel in the GAG framework, although at a decreasing rate with increasing distance. Given this premise, it seems also plausible that difficult (i.e., low frequency) parafoveal words attract relatively more attention than easy (i.e., high frequency) words. Thus, lexical properties of words to the right of fixation like their frequency may have an additional immediate impact on foveal word processing. Moreover, such effects may decrease with increasing distance from the current fixation position.

In SAS-models like E-Z Reader a preattentive visual stage allows for the perception of visual properties of parafoveal words (e.g., Pollatsek et al., this volume). Thus, orthographic irregularity or word length information of words to the right of fixation may pose an effect on processing the word in foveal vision (e.g., Inhoff, Starr, & Shindler, 2000; Inhoff, Radach, Eiter, & Juhasz, 2003). However, an attention shift to the next word is needed for higher level word processing. Since attention is not shifted until the currently fixated word is completely processed, the neighboring word's lexical properties (i.e., its frequency) cannot influence the processing of the fixated word anymore. Consequently, from a serial processing perspective, lexical parafoveal-on-foveal effects have to be explained by additional assumptions, for example mislocated fixations (Engbert, Nuthmann, & Kliegl, 2007; Nuthmann, Engbert, & Kliegl, 2005; Rayner, Warren, Juhasz, & Liversedge, 2004), that might have to be stretched even further to account for effects stemming from word n+2.

In summary, preview benefit and parafoveal-on-foveal effects can both be accounted for in the frameworks of GAG and SAS models. To explain the immediate influence of lexical properties of parafoveal words on the current fixation, SAS models must assume additional processes, whereas GAG models produce both preprocessing effects with a single mechanism.

Preprocessing effects from different methodological points of view

Traditionally, preprocessing effects are demonstrated with the gaze-contingent display-change technique where a critical target word is not revealed until the eyes cross an invisible boundary (Rayner, 1975). Most studies have been conducted to investigate effects of masking word n+1, the word directly to the right of the boundary. The target word (i.e., word n+1) typically shows a preview benefit effect with shorter fixation durations if preview of word n+1 was available, rather than denied, during fixations on the previous word n. Although less consistent, there is also evidence for parafoveal-on-foveal effects reflecting the influence of properties of the parafoveal word n+1 on fixation durations on the currently fixated word n (for a review on parafoveal preprocessing see Rayner et al., 2003).

Effects of gaze-contingent display changes of word n+2, the word two words to the right of fixation, have only recently been examined. Three studies (Rayner, Juhasz, & Brown, 2007; Kliegl, Risse, & Laubrock, 2007; Yang, Wang, & Rayner, 2006) agree in finding no preview benefit on the target word n+2. However, Kliegl et al. (2007) reported a small effect of preview of word n+2 in fixation durations on the previous word n+1. In addition, they found a comparably small parafoveal-on-foveal effect of word n+2 on word n (see also Yang et al., 2006). Thus, although more research is needed to solve this controversy, there is intriguing evidence that some preview information can be gained even from word n+2.

From a methodological point of view, there is broad agreement on the potential of the boundary technique in demonstrating preview benefit effects in reading (e.g., Drieghe, Rayner, & Pollatsek, 2005; McDonald, 2006; Inhoff et al., 2003). Manipulating only the target preview while keeping the rest of the sentence constant provides a straightforward experimental approach to examine the effect of preprocessing the target on its later, final processing time. However, preview benefits reflect a rather indirect measure of preprocessing. The effect of preprocessing word n+1 (or word n+2) during fixations on the prior word n is shown by shorter subsequent fixations only when the eyes finally reach this word. Although there is agreement on interpreting the shorter fixation durations as reflecting benefits from providing preview of the target word during prior fixations, longer fixation durations in case of preview denial can likewise be viewed as costs depending on whether the non-word (i.e., former case) or the identical preview condition (i.e., latter case) is used as the baseline condition.

An alternative and more direct test of preprocessing upcoming words lies in analyzing their immediate influence on the currently fixated word n. In this case, the preprocessing effects are measured in fixation durations directly on the word where preprocessing of the neighboring words takes place. Such parafoveal-on-foveal effects have also been examined in boundary experiments, but corpus analysis of eye-movement fixations provide a complementary and statistically more powerful alternative. There is ample evidence for parafoveal-on-foveal effects of word n+1 frequency and predictability in corpus analyses (e.g., Kennedy & Pynte, 2005; Kliegl, 2007; Kliegl, Nuthmann, & Engbert, 2006). These effects are apparently stronger than those observed in experimental studies (see Henderson & Ferreira, 1993; Rayner, Fischer, & Pollatsek, 1998). The differences may be related to the larger range of frequency and predictability present in corpus analyses, frequently low stastistical power of experimental manipulations, selection of different words for the analysis, or a combination of them (see Rayner, Pollatsek, Drieghe, Slattery, & Reichle, 2007; Kliegl, 2007, for a discussion). In light of the controversial n+2 effects from boundary experiments, corpus analyses are important for understanding parafoveal-on-foveal effects.

Parafoveal-on-foveal n+2 effects in a computational model like SWIFT

With respect to the importance of parafoveal-on-foveal effects in the theoretical framework of distributed parallel processing models, it is a promising challenge to investigate the behavior of computational models. In this section, we introduce the current version of SWIFT as one representative of computational models of parallel word processing implementing the concept of an attentional gradient. Moreover, we focus on how SWIFT might account for the empirical findings of parafoveal-on-foveal effects of word n+2.

Outline of the SWIFT model

SWIFT's mechanisms are formulated mathematically to map onto psychologically and physiologically plausible assumptions. Here we introduce the theoretical assumptions in SWIFT and illustrate the dynamics between the different mechanisms, skipping the mathematical formalism (for details see Engbert et al., 2005; Richter, Engbert, & Kliegl, 2006).

Modeling fixation positions: The spatial pathway

In agreement with neurophysiological findings, SWIFT distinguishes between spatial and temporal pathways of saccade generation (Findlay & Walker, 1999; see Figure 3.1). The (spatial) mechanism of saccade-target selection derives from a dynamic field of activations (see Erlhagen & Schöner, 2002, for a general discussion) establishing a dynamic saliency map. As a first approximation in SWIFT, the activation value assigned to each word represents the current progress on word processing.

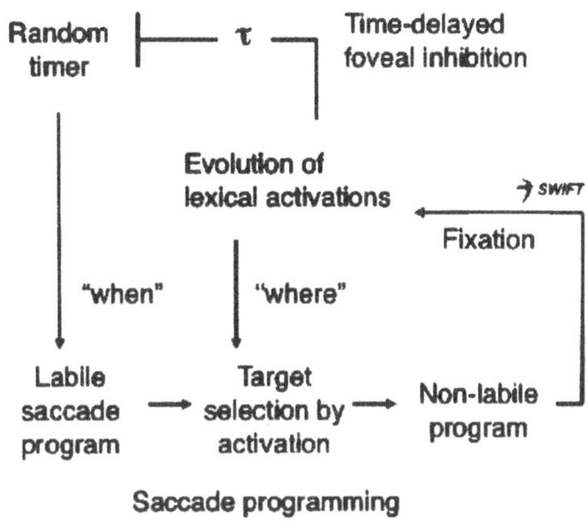

Figure 3.1 Outline of the SWIFT model. Saccade programming is guided by separate temporal ("when") and spatial ("where") pathways. An autonomous random timer triggers new saccade programs and is itself influenced by foveal inhibition. The set of lexical activations of all words in a sentence evolves dynamically and can be conceived of as a saliency map.

More technically, word processing evolves as a dynamic field of activations via three cognitive factors: a preprocessing factor, a lexical processing rate, and an additional global decay process. First, lexical access is represented in two stages (see Figure 3.2). A preprocessing stage ensures a fast increase in lexical activations up to a maximum value determined by each word's difficulty, followed by a lexical completion stage with a slow decrease in lexical activations. Thus, for word recognition, lexical activations have to evolve from zero to a maximum value back to zero. Additionally, the preprocessing factor is modulated by word predictability. Such two-stage conceptions are quite common in theories of word recognition and there is one also implemented in E-Z Reader (see Reichle et al., 1998, for a discussion). Indeed, the design of SWIFT was inspired by and is quite similar to E-Z Reader in this respect.

Second, the lexical processing rate reflects a processing gradient with faster processing for foveal than parafoveal words due to visual acuity

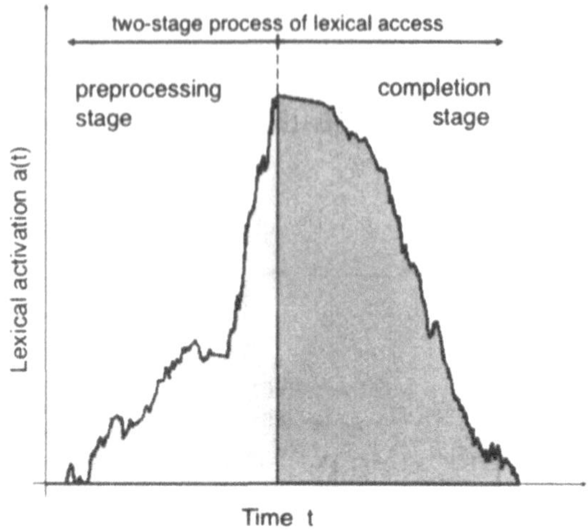

Figure 3.2 The preprocessing factor reflects a two-stage process. In the first preprocessing stage, lexical activation is increasing from zero to a processing maximum, whereas in the second completion stage lexical activation decreases back to zero.

decreasing with increasing eccentricity from the fixation position (see Legge, Hooven, Klitz, Mansfield, & Tjan, 2002). Moreover, the perceptual span is asymmetric around the fixation position with a greater spatial extent of letter-information extraction in the direction of reading (McConkie & Rayner, 1976; Rayner & Bertera, 1979). Thus, SWIFT determines the lexical processing rate for each word by the combination of its letter's eccentricities from fixation position with a rapid decrease for the word(s) to the left, a more shallow decrease for the word(s) to the right of fixation and a zero processing rate for all words outside this perceptual span (see Figure 3.3). It is important to note, however, that there is a nonlinear relation between processing rate at the word level and processing rate of its letters.

Third, an additional process simulates a constant memory decay of each word within the dynamic field of activations. This leads to a reduction of lexical activation of words even if the perceptual span has moved beyond them, that is, even if the word is assigned to a zero processing rate.

The dynamics between these mechanisms defines the evolution of the lexical activations of the words that determine saccade target selection. Basically, SWIFT assigns a selection probability to each word by its activation relative to the activations of all other words, which is a nonlinear mapping from activations to target-selection probabilities. Thus, the

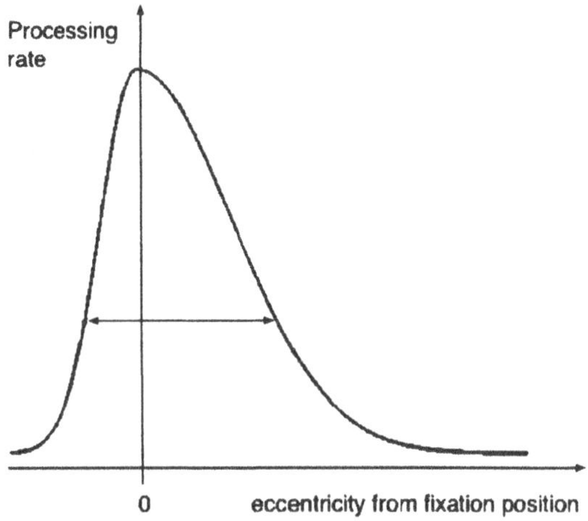

Figure 3.3 The lexical processing rate is assumed to follow an asymmetric Gaussian distribution with the highest processing rate at the current fixation position, a fast decrease to the left of fixation and a more shallow decrease to the right of fixation.

set of activations introduces a competitive process for saccade target selection (Engbert & Kliegl, 2003), i.e., the determination of the next fixation position.[2]

Modeling fixation durations: The temporal pathway

The temporal pathway is designed to model the pattern of fixation durations. An autonomous random timer produces time intervals that initiate the start of independent saccade programs (see Figure 3.4). Moreover, an inhibitory process can delay saccade initiation, that is, the start of a new saccade program. In the current SWIFT version, foveal inhibition itself is represented by the amount of foveal lexical activation not only at the current point in time but as the sum of its previous development. At the end of each random time interval foveal inhibition is calculated as the integral of the past evolution of the lexical activation in fovea. Simulations show that foveal inhibition is active during, on average, about 10% of fixation time (Engbert et al., 2002). The foveal inhibition process reflects the delayed impact of the slower word recognition processes on the fast brainstem saccade generator (e.g., Sparks, 2002) and is able to account for spillover effects of word difficulty.

2 In the current SWIFT version, oculomotor errors are introduced by computing the actual saccade length as a function of the intended saccade length and by adding a (systematic) saccade range error and a random error component (McConkie, Kerr, Reddix, & Zola, 1988).

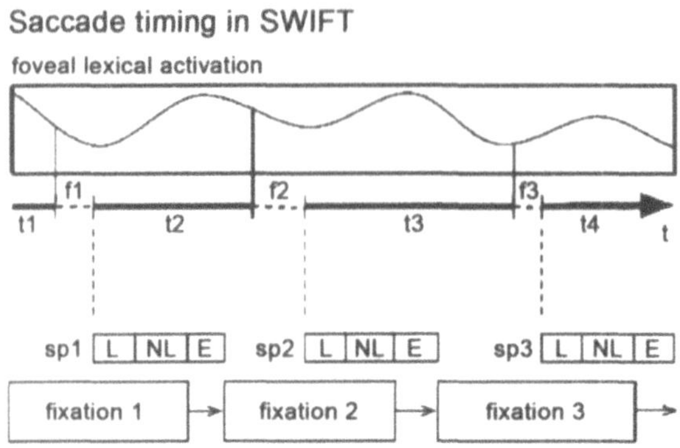

Figure 3.4 An example for saccade timing in SWIFT. Randomly selected time intervals (t) can be delayed by the current amount of foveal inhibition (f) and initiate the start of the next saccade program (sp). Saccade programming is a two-stage process with a labile (L) and non-labile (NL) stage. Execution (E) reflects the duration of the saccade moving the eye from one fixation position to the other.

The actual saccade programming mechanism initiated by the end of the random timer interval is designed as a two-stage process following findings on the double-step paradigm (Becker & Jürgens, 1979; in the context of reading see Reichle et al., 1998; Engbert & Kliegl, 2001). During the transition from the labile to the non-labile stage the saccade target is selected from the set of lexical activations according to the corresponding selection probabilities. Thus, the non-labile stage links the temporal and the spatial pathway (see Figure 3.1).

Fixation durations are generated in SWIFT as the time between two successive saccades. These durations depend on when the saccade landed on a word within the duration of the current random time interval, how long the next time interval is delayed due to foveal inhibition, and the time needed for the initiated saccade program. Since both the random time intervals and the saccade programming times are stochastic in nature, only the inhibitory process can account for systematic variation in first-fixation durations. This is an important aspect of the model for the discussion of parafoveal-on-foveal effects on fixation durations.

Although the above outline of SWIFT represents a highly descriptive level of the model's key principles without going into detail on the mathematical implementation, it shows the complexity of such a dynamic model of eye movement control.

Parafoveal-on-foveal predictions for word n

SWIFT's behavior is strongly determined by the evolution of the field of lexical activations incorporating all words within the perceptual span. If word n+1 is short—which increases the chance of word n+2 falling into the perceptual span and being preprocessed—word n+1 is likely to also be of high frequency and of low difficulty. Consequently, word n+1 will be easy to process with an average processing time shorter than those for its neighboring words n and n+2. Importantly, word difficulty has no direct effect on the slope of processing since the speed of lexical processing depends only on the word's distance from the current fixation position. Differences in lexical activations due to a word's difficulty can only result indirectly from the word's current stage of processing, that is, if the word is either far within its preprocessing stage leading to high lexical activation or already in its completion stage showing a continuous decrease in its activity. More specifically, easy words are assigned to a lower processing maximum thus needing less time to arrive in the completion stage with decreasing activation.

Spatial decision. During fixations on word n, this word is processed with a high processing rate which generates a fast increase in activation. At the same time, the rise of the activation of both parafoveal words n+1 and n+2 is slower. Moreover, as a result of its greater eccentricity from the current fixation position, lexical activation of word n+2 increases even slower than for word n+1. If fixation on word n is long enough for (almost) complete lexical access of the short and frequent$_{n+1}$ neighbor, lexical activation of word n+1 approaches zero and it drops out of the competition for being selected as the next saccade target. Thus, at the moment of saccade target selection, word n might still show higher lexical activation than word n+1 although it was processed with the highest processing speed. Moreover, whether word n is now selected as the next saccade target and thus will be refixated depends on its lexical activation still being higher than the slowly increasing activity of the parafoveal word n+2. If word n processing is in its completion stage and activation decreased enough to be lower than the rising degree of activity of word n+2 this will rather lead to immediate skipping word n+1. This makes it very difficult to predict which of the two words is the more competitive saccade target. However, if word n wins against its competitors and is refixated, the likelihood of subsequently skipping word n+1 increases even more.

Temporal decision. In its current version, SWIFT does not include a direct mechanism that can lengthen fixation durations due to the processing demands arising from words to the right of fixation; the only mechanism influencing fixation durations is foveal inhibition. As a consequence, SWIFT in its current version does not predict modulations in first-fixation durations on word n relative to word properties of the words to the right of fixation. Modulations are possible, however, as a consequence of target selection effects for cumulative measures of fixation durations (i.e., gaze duration, or total viewing time). Moreover, the SWIFT model accounts for preprocessing effects at least for word n+1 via accelerating the refixation probability of word n which necessarily leads to increasing gaze durations, the sum of all first-pass fixations.

In summary, the dynamical behavior of the SWIFT model seems highly compatible with preprocessing effects stemming from word n+1. In its current version, however, the model does not predict parafoveal-on-foveal effects on first or single fixations resulting from word n+2.

Parafoveal-on-foveal n+2 effects in the Potsdam Sentence Corpus

The purpose of the present analysis is to test parafoveal-on-foveal effects of word n+2 on word n, given a short word n+1 of 2 or 3 letters length. To preview the results, we indeed found a signficant effect of word n+2 on fixation durations of word n, that is an effect extending across word n+1. We also carried out a second analysis with 4-letter and 5-letter words n+1.

Method

Data base. Kliegl et al. (2006, also Kliegl, 2007) reported analyses of distributed processing during reading fixations using a corpus comprising 71,097 first-pass single fixations that were assigned to the same word in both eyes. These data were based on 222 readers (collapsed across nine experiments) who read 144 sentences each. Ignoring the first and last words of each sentences there are a total of 850 words; they actually represent 550 different words because some of them are repeated across sentences or even within a sentence (e.g., determiners and prepositions).

Data selection. For the following analyses we selected a subset of fixations on content words that were followed either by words of 2 or 3 letters length (main analysis) or by words of 4 or 5 letters length (control analysis). We also required that the saccade leaving word n had to be directed at word n+1 or word n+2 (see Figure 3.5 for illustration). For the obvious reason of word length, words n+1 were of much higher fre-

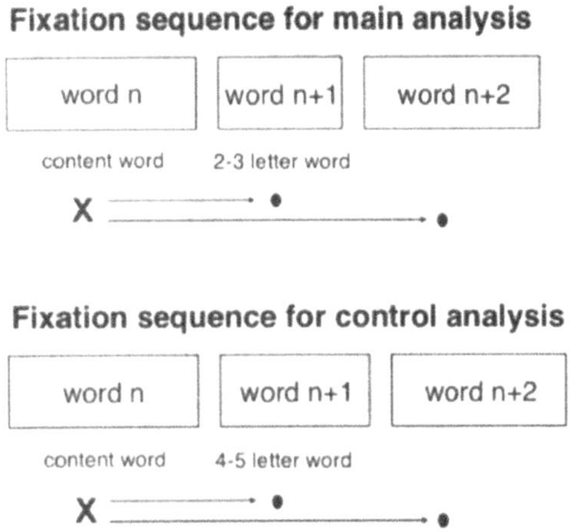

Figure 3.5 Illustration of data selection for the main and control analysis. Only fixation durations on content words n were considered followed either by a 2-3 letter (main analysis) or a 4-5 letter word n+1 (control analysis). Furthermore, fixations leaving word n either landed on word n+1 or the subsequent word n+2 skipping word n+1.

quency and predictability than the two neighboring words n and n+2. Mean and standard deviations are summarized in Table 3.1.

Dependent and independent variables. Fixation duration (log) on word n served as the dependent variable. Predictors were 1/length (of word) n [ln], logit predictability n [pn], log linear frequency n [fn] as well as log quadratic and cubic frequency n, skipping status n+1 [sn1], lexical status n+1 (i.e., content vs. function word) [fwn1], logit predictability n+1 [pn1], logit predictability n+2 [pn2], log frequency n+2 [fn2], and 1/length n+2 [ln2]. Parafoveal effects might be stronger for fixations close to the end of words. Therefore, we also specified closeness of fixation to the end of word n as a predictor (coded from the end of the word; i.e., fixations on the last letter of a word are coded as zero) [ep]. In addition, we included several strong predictors identified in previous analyses: (1) the relative position of letter position within words [rp] and its associated quadratic trend coding the inverted optimal viewing position effect, that is the fact that fixation durations are longer in the relative word center than at the edges of words (Vitu, McConkie, Kerr, & O'Regan, 2001; Nuthmann et al., 2005); (2) the log frequency of word n-1 (i.e., the lag-frequency effect) [fn-1], and (3) the amplitude of the incoming saccade [sac].

Statistical analysis. We used a series of linear mixed-effect models (lme) with partially crossed independent random effects associated with read-

Table 3.1 Descriptive information about fixations and word-triplets

Length of word n+1:	2 or 3		4 or 5	
Variable	M	SD	M	SD
Word n-1				
1 sacc-ampl.	-0.161	2.510	0.053	2.610
2 freq.	-0.073	1.251	-0.230	1.287
Word n				
3 length	5.990	2.080	6.170	1.950
4 freq.	-0.398	0.939	-0.481	1.010
5 predict.	-0.156	0.936	-0.337	0.861
Word n+1				
6 length	2.780	0.413	4.490	0.500
7 freq.	1.180	0.863	0.173	1.150
8 predict.	0.336	1.060	-0.232	1.120
9 skip	0.522	0.500	0.189	0.392
10 CW/FW	0.798	0.402	0.485	0.500
Word n+2				
11 length	6.240	3.350	4.840	2.430
12 freq.	-0.278	1.370	0.136	1.360
13 predict.	-0.121	1.170	-0.004	1.200
N of fixations	17592		13822	
N of readers	222		222	
N of sentences	119		93	
N of unique words	169		130	

Note: Frequency (freq.) and predictability (predict.) values are centered log and logit transformed values; "sacc-ampl." is centered amplitude of saccade from word n-1 to word n; "skip" is proportion of skipped words n+1; "CW/FW" is proportion of words n+1 that are function words. Length is number of letters.

ers [id], sentences [sn], and words [wid] to establish the significance of the predictors and their interactions.[3] Different from mixed-model F1-F2 ANOVA, correlations within subjects (here: reader) and within items (here:sentences) are considered simultaneously for the computation of the fixed-effect statistics in lme. In addition, we included words as a third random factor. Based on previous analyses (Kliegl, 2007), we spec-

3 Estimation was carried out with the *lmer* 4 package (Bates & Sarkar,2007) provided in the R environment for statistical computation (R-Core team, 2007) under the GNU 2 public license. Data preprocessing and graphical visualization relied or *reshape* and *ggplot* packages (Wickharn, 2005, 2006).

ified the effects of relative fixation position within words [o], log frequency n [fn], and logit predictability n [pn] as normally distributed across readers. In other words, we estimated the variances of these three effects and their associated covariances as additional random effects. The analyses occurred in three steps. First, we specified a baseline model with all predictors and including also all two-predictor interactions. Second, from this model, we eliminated all non-significant interaction terms. In a third set of analyses we checked the reliability of the random effects. In this context, the three variances, but only the covariance between frequency and predictability effects contributed significantly to the goodness of fit.

Results

The results for the final model are reported in Table 3.2. They are based on fixations on word n followed by 2 or 3 letter words n+1. The critical result of this analysis is the interaction between the length and the frequency of word n+2 (see Table 3.2); this interaction was also significant in the baseline model (not shown). There are a number of additional effects reported in Table 3.2 that mostly confirm previously reported lag-frequency, IOVP, and parafoveal-on-foveal frequency and predictability effects from word n+1. These effects have been described in Kliegl et al. (2006) and Kliegl (2007). The new result reported here is the interaction between length and frequency of word n+2 represented in the top left panel of Figure 3.6. Fixation durations on word n responded to the frequency of word n+2 when word n+1 was 2 or 3 letters long. Basically, there was a frequency effect for short words n+2.

In an additional set of analyses, we checked the dependency of this result on the length of word n+1. The interaction of frequency and length of word n+1 was no longer significant when word n+1 was 4 or 5 letters long (bottom left panel of Figure 3.6); also the frequency of word n+2 was not significant by itself. This n+2 parafoveal-on-foveal effect is important because it demonstrates that both word length and lexical information (or a sublexical correlate such as the frequency of initial letters) of word n+2 are extracted already during fixations on word n if word n+1 is a short word.

SWIFT simulation generates data at the word level. We can submit the simulation fixations to the same analyses as the human reading data. The right panels in Figure 3.6 are based on 300 simulations using the parameter specification published in Engbert et al. (2005); 32829 and 26509 fixations met the selection criteria applied in the analyses reported above for words n+1 with length 2-3 letters and 4-5 letters, re-

Table 3.2 Linear mixed-effects model results for 2&3-letter words n+1

AIC	BIC	logLik	MLdeviance	REMLdeviance
-135.4	90.09	96.7	-359.2	-193.4
Random effects:				
Groups	**Name**	**Variance**	**Std.Dev.**	**Corr**
id	(Intercept)	0.018	0.134	
id	o	0.020	0.142	
id	pn	0.001	0.030	
	fn	0.001	0.021	-0.614
wid	(Intercept)	0.005	0.071	
sn	(Intercept)	0.002	0.043	
Residual		0.053	0.229	
number of obs: 17592, groups: id, 222; wid, 169; sn, 119				

Fixed effects:

	Estimate	Std.Error	t value
(Intercept)	5.268	0.023	229.28
freq n-1 (fn-1)	-0.032	0.005	-6.62
sacc-ampl (sac)	0.025	0.001	28.04
lngth n (ln)	0.292	0.124	2.36
endpos(ep)	0.020	0.005	4.46
relpos(rp)	0.006	0.033	0.18
rp*rp	-0.239	0.038	-6.28
pred n (pn)	-0.028	0.007	-4.29
freq n (fn)	-0.005	0.010	-0.53
fn*fn	-0.003	0.005	-0.55
fn*fn*fn	-0.011	0.003	-4.19
pred n+1 (pn1)	0.011	0.006	1.84
skip n+1 (sn1)	-0.045	0.010	-4.66
FW n+1 (fwn1)	-0.012	0.017	-0.72
freq n+2 (fn2)	-0.013	0.007	-1.92
lngth n+2 (ln2)	0.133	0.095	1.41
pred n+2 (pn2)	0.035	0.016	2.17
ln*sn1	0.209	0.069	3.01
ep*sn1	0.009	0.003	3.38
fwn1*pn2	-0.046	0.018	-2.63
pn1*pn2	0.010	0.004	2.25
fn2*ln2	-0.159	0.053	-3.04

Note: Fit by Restricted maximum likelihood (REML); see text for explanation.

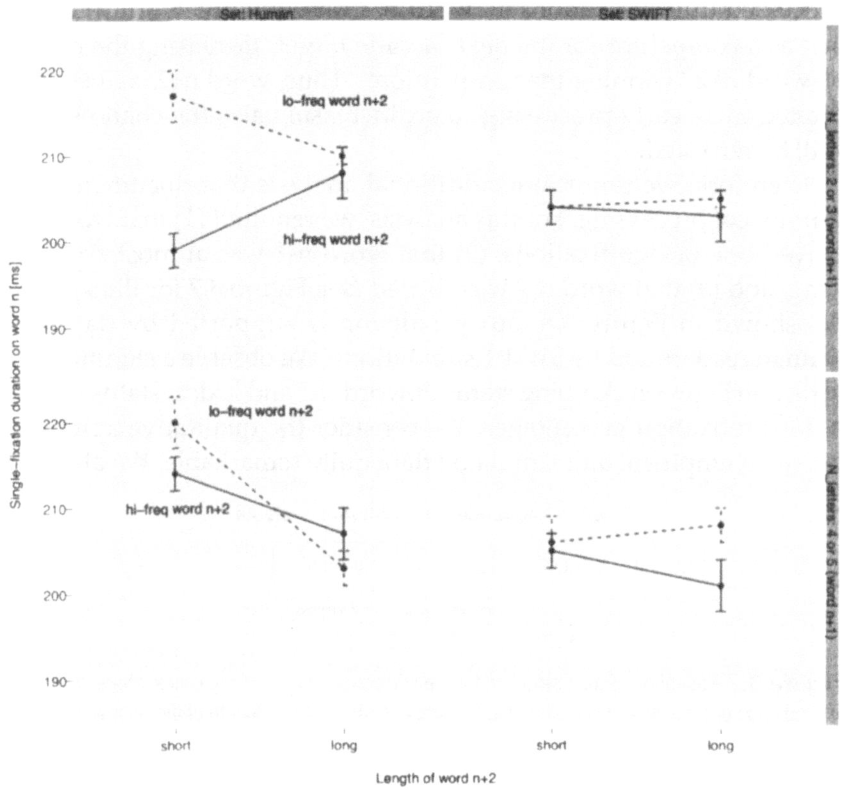

Figure 3.6 Interactions for length of word n+2 and frequency of word n+2 for fixations before words n+1 of length 2-3 or 4-5 letters (top and bottom panels, respectively). Empirical results are presented in the left and SWIFT simulation results in the right column. Error bars are 95% confidence intervals (two-tailed). Only the interaction in the top left panel was significant in a corresponding linear mixed-effects model with continuous predictors (see Table 3.2).

spectively. As expected from the earlier description of SWIFT dynamics, we did not obtain any n+2 effects on fixation durations on word n (see Figure 3.6). Thus, the parafoveal processing assumptions of SWIFT are in need of further development. We will outline a few options in the discussion.

Additional analysis

We have shown that SWIFT does not reproduce an empirical modulation of fixation durations to the frequency of short words n+2. All along, we have emphasized that SWIFT predicts quite a bit of parafoveal processing relating to the selection of saccade targets. In particular, we derived that, in SWIFT, function words in position n+1 are likely to be processed during fixations on word n. Consequently, word n+1 drops out as a competitor for the next saccade target, increasing the chances of word n+2 "winning the competition". Thus, word n+2 is likely to be fixated in an early processing stage, increasing also the chances that it will be refixated.

Therefore, we report one additional analysis that documents such parafoveal processing. For this analysis, we required (1) that word n received one or two fixations, (2) that word n-1 was at most six letters long, and (3) that word n-2 was fixated (see Figure 3.7 for illustration). As shown in Figure 3.8, our prediction is supported by data from human readers and by SWIFT simulations. We observe a significant interaction between skipping status of word n-1 and lexical status of word n-1 on refixation percentages. We consider the qualitative agreement between empirical and simulated data quite remarkable. We also note,

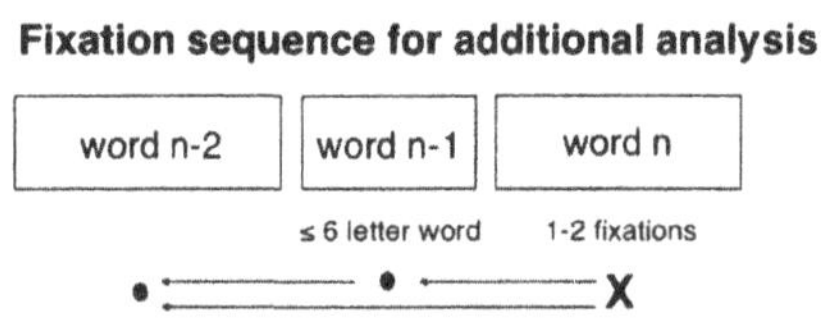

Figure 3.7 Illustration of data selection for the additional analysis. Only cases where word n was fixated once or twice where considered in the analysis. Additionally, length of the prior word n-1 was restricted to a maximum of six letters. The even preceding word n-2 had to be fixated whereas the intermediate word n-1 could have been either skipped or fixated.

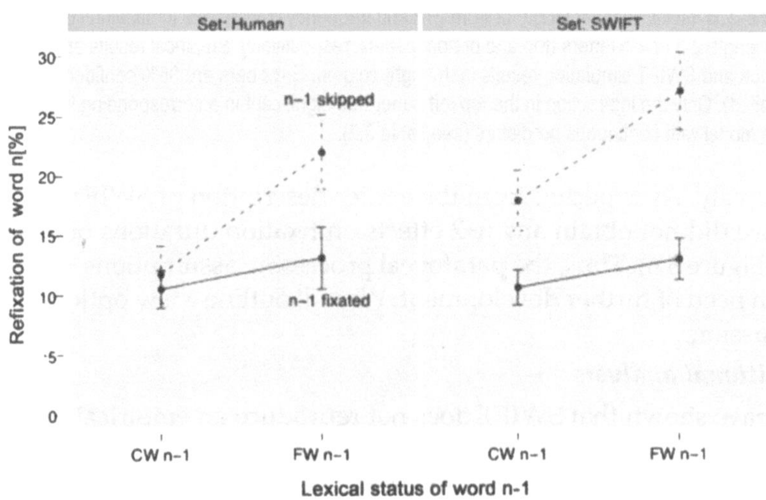

Figure 3.8 Preview benefit for refixation percentages. Readers and SWIFT show a larger percentage of refixations after skipped function words. SWIFT overestimates refixations after skipped words when compared to human eye-movements. Error bars are 95% confidence intervals (two-tailed).

however, that SWIFT overpredicts refixations after skipped words, irrespective of lexical status of word n-1.

In control analyses, we checked whether the interaction was due to an inverse pattern of means in terms of word n frequencies. This was not the case. There was only one reliable effect: Word n was of lower frequency if word n-1 was a function word. Thus, the difficulty of word n, in terms of its lexical frequency, cannot account for the interaction shown in Figure 3.8.

Discussion

The conjunction of computational, experimental, and corpus-analysis research deepens and improves insight into the complex dynamics underlying eye-movement control in reading. We presented the details of the distributed parallel processing assumptions of the SWIFT model in predicting immediate preprocessing effects on the current fixation, and contrasted them with empirical results and simulated data from a corpus analysis.

Corpus-analysis evidence

Selecting fixation patterns from an eye-movement corpus that is similar to those used in experimental studies, we demonstrated frequency effects of short words n+2 on fixation durations on word n if the intermediate word n+1 was restricted to a length of 2-3 letters. This result does not put to rest the controversy about preprocessing of parafoveal words, but it is another piece of evidence that—under special conditions of short n+1 neighbors—word n+2 is preprocessed; it is in agreement with Kliegl et al.'s (2007) report of preview effects of word n+2 in a boundary experiment where the length of word n+1 was fixed to three letters. Whereas the latter result could be interpreted as a parafoveal-on-foveal effect due to lower level visual properties of an orthographic irregular random string of letters in the condition of preview denial, the corpus-analysis results presented here support the notion that lexical information can also be extracted at least from short words n+2.

There is additional evidence from corpus studies analyzing fixation durations as a function of word frequency and predictability of the next word n+1 (Kliegl et al., 2006; Kennedy & Pynte, 2005). These successor effects—although in this case restricted to the neighboring word n+1—underline the notion of preprocessing as an immediate measurable event with an effect on current and not only subsequent word processing. Thus, parafoveal-on-foveal effects have been demonstrated both in experimental and corpus-analysis studies for both word n+1 and even word n+2. The source of contradictory results has to be ascertained from other research.

Parafoveal-on-foveal effects reflect only one type of preprocessing effects, namely the direct and immediate influence of preprocessing word n+1 or word n+2 on the current fixation of word n. These effects need to be distinguished from later indirect effects on the processing time of the previewed words (i.e., preview benefit). In parallel models, both the early parafoveal-on-foveal and the subsequently observed preview benefit effect require a single mechanism, namely the attentional gradient for distributed parallel processing of all words within the perceptual span. Since several words are lexically processed in parallel, although to different degrees relative to their eccentricity from the current fixation position, properties of parafoveal words should be visible in foveal fixations (i.e., the parafoveal-on-foveal effect). At the same time, preprocessing of parafoveal words should gradually reduce their later demand for processing, leading to benefits during subsequent fixations (i.e., the preview benefit effect).

Such later preprocessing benefits could be demonstrated in an additional analysis. Refixation probability of word n was higher when the previous function word was skipped. If the prior word n-1 (function or content word) is fixated there is an additional chance of gaining preview of the current word n. Skipping word n-1, however, implies that the last fixation prior to fixating word n reflects a situation in which word n is previewed as a parafoveal word n+2. Since preview from neighboring words n+1 is expected to be more efficient than from more distant words n+2, the effect in refixation probability on word n conditional on skipping word n-1 recovers a preview benefit effect in corpus analyses.

Parafoveal-on-foveal and preview-benefit effects represent test cases for parallel and serial processing models. Whereas parallel models can account for both effects by assuming one single mechanism (i.e., the attentional gradient), serial models require additional assumptions to allow for parafoveal-on-foveal effects. An additional preattentive stage scanning parafoveal words on a visual level before attention is shifted toward them captures parafoveal-on-foveal effects of visual word properties like orthographic irregularity (e.g., Pollatsek et al., this volume). However, lexical word properties like word frequency can only be perceived if attention is shifted toward them. Since an attention shift is triggered by complete lexical processing of the currently fixated word n, the frequency of the parafoveally preprocessed word cannot influence the fixation duration on word n. Effects of lexical properties of parafoveal words on fixations on word n are explained by mislocated fixations assuming that due to oculomotor error the fixation failed to land on the targeted word. Explaining the parafoveal-on-foveal frequency effect from short words n+2 on word n fixations with reference to mislocated fixations implies, however, a saccade error comprising the average length of word n+1.

Computational challenges

E-Z Reader's and SWIFT's success is primarily their account of a broad spectrum of eye-movement measures (e.g., various measures of fixation durations and fixation probabilities as a function of word frequency and length) collected during reading of isolated sentences (i.e., Schilling, Rayner, & Chumbley, 1998; Kliegl, Grabner, Rolfs, & Engbert, 2004). Every new empirical constraint identified with experimental or corpus-analysis methods is, however, an empirical challenge. Thus, analyzing SWIFT's behavior on capturing the results of immediate and later preprocessing effects of words to the right of fixation gives rise to the potential and limitations of its current development.

One may expect that SWIFT as a computational model based on the parallel processing assumption should necessarily lead to predictions of parafoveal-on-foveal effects from word n+1 or even word n+2 on fixations on word n. This, however, is not the case. Parafoveal preprocessing in SWIFT is likely to affect saccade targeting and, consequently, refixation and skipping probability but, in its present implementation, we did not expect a strong modulation of fixation durations on word n for parafoveal properties of word n+2 (more precisely, no effect on first-fixation durations, possibly weak effects for cumulative measures of fixation duration). With the simulated corpus data, we showed that, as expected, the current SWIFT model does not recover this new parafoveal-on-foveal effect in fixation durations.

However, SWIFT captures the empirically observed effect of an increased refixation probability on word n and shows that it is conditional on skipping a previous function word n-1. SWIFT's overestimation of refixations after skipped words points to its greater reliance on fixation positions than on lexical information (i.e., whether word n+1 is a content or a function word), consistent with the discussion in Engbert et al. (2005). Nevertheless, the model is still clearly useful because such new results offer some rather clear options for theory-guided model modifications. In the following we will discuss one such option. Obviously, this is speculation and without implementation we cannot be sure that it does not destroy some of the other effects the model is handling well so far.

Extending foveal inhibition to all words in the perceptual span

SWIFT's acronym derives from autonomous Saccade Generation With Inhibition by Foveal Targets. Ironically, in its present implementation foveal targets provide less inhibition than suggested by the acronym because inhibition is restricted to the fixated word, ignoring that the word to the right may actually be a foveal target as well (e.g., when the fixation is on the last letter of a word). If all words within the perceptual span are inhibiting the onset of the saccade program during a fixation on word n with a degree relative to their assigned processing rate, this would allow for direct prolonging the current fixation duration on word n conditional on the parafoveal word's properties. Thus, difficult words to the right of fixation would be able to exert some inhibition on initiating the saccade program on the currently fixated word n. Due to decreasing processing rates for words with increasing eccentricity from the current fixation position, the difficulty of word n+1 would place relatively stronger inhibition on the word n fixation durations than the processing demand of word n+2.

The implementation of this principle may still show only a very limited effect on fixation durations, because word difficulty is not directly influencing lexical activation, only indirectly via processing maxima. Thus, especially for word n+2 with a slow processing rate, differences in difficulty might not have an impact on the development of lexical activation of word n+2 in the early stages of preprocessing. SWIFT can just show an effect for extreme groups (very easy vs. difficult word n+2), if the very easy word n+2 already reaches its completion stage; its lower lexical activation could then really lead to less inhibition of the foveal word.

Other difficulties for SWIFT and parallel models in general arise from a corpus analysis conducted by McDonald (2005) who did not find cumulative preview benefit effects conditional on the duration and the eccentricity of fixations prior to a target word. These results appear to contradict SWIFT assumptions: Fixating closer and longer to a parafoveal target should increase its progress in parallel preprocessing. The critical inverse effect of eccentricity on the fixation duration on the target word, however, was found only for the first of two preceding fixations.

Thus, there was a second fixation before finally landing on the target word. Moreover, duration and eccentricity of this second fixation showed the expected effects on the target fixations. Since SWIFT's behavior on a word very strongly depends on its individual previous fixation sequences, it is not clear yet if the absence of such cumulative preview benefits might not also—under specific circumstances—be captured with SWIFT. Further research is necessary.

In summary, the undisputable usefulness of computational modeling is to translate complex theoretical assumptions into directly testable predictions. All models start out with mechanisms that are designed to account for a limited set of effects. In a best-case scenario, a model is able to predict—with these mechanisms—new empirical effects it was not designed to handle originally (e.g., see Figure 3.8). More often, however, models will have to be adjusted to cope with new empirical constraints. If these adjustments are theory-guided, the implementation of new mechanisms into a model will certainly extend its lifetime. The topic of preprocessing parafoveal words is a good example of how the combination of experimental research, corpus-analysis, and computational methods lead to an increasingly detailed picture and comprehensive understanding of eye-movement control in reading.

Acknowledgment

This research was supported by grant KL 955/6 from Deutsche Forschungsgemeinschaft.

References

Bates, D., & Sarkar, D. (2007). lme4: Linear mixed-effect models using S4 classes. R package version 0.9975-14.

Becker, W., & Jürgens, R. (1979). An analysis of the saccadic system by means of double step stimuli. *Vision Research, 19*, 1967-1983.

Box, G. E. P. (1979). *Robustness in the strategy of scientific model building.* In R.L. Launer, & G.N. Wilkinson (Eds.), *Robustness in Statistics*. Academic Press: New York.

Drieghe, D., Rayner, K., & Pollatsek, A. (2005). Eye movements and word skipping during reading revisited. *Journal of Experimental Psychology: Human Perception and Performance, 31*, 954-969.

Engbert, R., & Kliegl, R. (2001). Mathematical models of eye movements in reading: A possible role for autonomous saccades. *Biological Cybernetics, 85,* 77-87.

Engbert, R., & Kliegl, R. (2003). The game of word skipping: Who are the competitors? *Behavioral and Brain Sciences, 26,* 481-482.

Engbert, R., Longtin, A., & Kliegl, R. (2002). A dynamical model of saccade generation in reading based on spatially distributed lexical processing. *Vision Research, 42,* 621-636.

Engbert, R., Nuthmann, A., & Kliegl, R. (2007). An iterative algorithm for the estimation of the distribution of mislocated fixations during reading. In R. P. G. van Gompel, M. H. Fischer, W. S. Murray, & R. L. Hill (Eds.), *Eye movements: A window on mind and brain.* Oxford: Elsevier.

Engbert, R., Nuthmann, A., Richter, E., & Kliegl, R. (2005). SWIFT: A dynamical model of saccade generation during reading. *Psychological Review, 112,* 777-813.

Erlhagen, W., & Schöner, G. (2002). Dynamic field theory of movements preparation. *Psychological Review, 109,* 545-572.

Findlay, J. M., & Walker, R. (1999). A model of saccade generation based on parallel processing and competitive inhibition. *Behavioral and Brain Sciences, 22,* 661-721.

Henderson, J. M., & Ferreira, F. (1993). Eye movement control during reading: Fixation measures reflect foveal but not parafovela processing difficulty. *Canadian Journal of Experimental Psychology, 47,* 201-221.

Inhoff, A. W., Radach, R., & Eiter, B. (2006). Temporal overlap in the linguistic processing of successive words in reading: Reply to Pollatsek, Reichle, & Rayner (2006a). *Journal of Experimental Psychology: Human Perception and Performance, 32,* 1490-1495.

Inhoff, A., Radach, R., Eiter, B. M., & Juhasz, B. (2003). Distinct subsystems for the parafoveal processing of spatial and linguistic information during eye fixations in reading. *Quarterly Journal of Experimental Psychology, 56,* 803-827.

Inhoff, A. W., Radach, R., Starr, M., & Greenberg, S. (2000). Allocation of visuo-spatial attention and saccade programming during reading. In A. Kennedy, R. Radach, D. Heller, & J. Pynte (Eds.), *Reading as a Perceptual Process* (pp. 221-246). Amsterdam: Elsevier.

Inhoff, A. W., Starr, M., & Shindler, K. L. (2000). Is the processing of words during eye fixations in reading strictly serial? *Perception & Psychophysics, 62,* 1474-1484.

Kennedy, A., & Pynte, J. (2005). Parafoveal-on-foveal effects in normal reading. *Vision Research, 45,* 153-168.

Kliegl, R. (2007). Toward a perceptual-span theory of distributed processing in reading: A reply to Rayner, Pollatsek, Drieghe, Slattery,

& Reichle (2007). *Journal of Experimental Psychology: General, 136,* 530-537.

Kliegl, R., & Engbert, R. (2003). SWIFT explorations. In J. Hyönä, R. Radach, & H. Deubel (Eds.), *The mind's eye: Cognitive and applied aspects of eye movement research* (pp.103-117). Amsterdam: Elsevier.

Kliegl, R., & Engbert, R. (2005). Fixation durations in word skippings in reading eye movements. *Psychonomic Bulletin & Review, 12,* 132-138.

Kliegl, R., Grabner, E., Rolfs, M., & Engbert, R. (2004). Length, frequency, and predictability effects of words on eye movements in reading. *European Journal of Cognitive Psychology, 16,* 262-284.

Kliegl, R., Nuthmann, A., & Engbert, R. (2006). Tracking the mind during reading: The influence of past, present, and future words on fixation durations. *Journal of Experimental Psychology: General, 133,* 12-35.

Kliegl, R., Risse, S., & Laubrock, J. (2007). Preview benefit and parafoveal-on-foveal effects from word N+2. *Journal of Experimental Psychology: Human Perception and Performance, 33,* 1250-1255.

Legge, G. E., Hooven, T. A., Klitz, T. S., Mansfield, J. S., & Tjan, B. S. (2002). Mr. Chips 2002: New insights from an ideal-observer model of reading. *Vision Research, 42,* 2219-2234.

McConkie, G. W., Kerr, P. W., Reddix, M. D., & Zola, D. (1988). Eye movement control during reading: I. The location of initial fixations on words. *Vision Research, 28,* 1107-1118.

McConkie, G. W., & Rayner, K. (1976). Asymmetry of the perceptual span in reading. *Bulletin of the Psychonomic Society, 8,* 365-368.

McDonald, S. A. (2005). Parafoveal preview benefit in reading is initalic across multiple saccades. *Vision Research, 45,* 1829-1834.

McDonald, S. A. (2006). Parafoveal preview benefit in reading is only obtained from the saccade goal. *Vision Research, 46,* 4416-4424.

McDonald, S. A., Carpenter, R. H. S., & Shillcock, R. C. (2005). An anatomically constrained, stochastic model of eye movement control in reading. *Psychological Review, 112,* 814-840.

Nuthmann, A., Engbert, R., & Kliegl, R. (2005). Mislocated fixations during reading and the inverted optimal viewing position effect. *Vision Research, 45,* 2201-2217.

Pollatsek, A., Reichle, E. D., & Rayner, K. (2003). Modeling eye movments in reading: Extension of the E-Z Reader. In J. Hyönä, R. Radach, & H. Deubel (Eds.), *The mind's eye: Cognitive and applied aspects of eye movement research* (pp. 361-390). Amsterdam: Elsevier.

Pollatsek, A., Reichle, E. D., & Rayner, K. (2006a). Tests of the E-Z Reader model: Exploring the interface between cognition and eye-movement control. *Cognitive Psychology, 52,* 1-56.

Pollatsek, A., Reichle, E. D., & Rayner, K. (2006b). Attention to one word at a time in reading is still a viable hypothesis: Rejoinder to Inhoff, Radach, and Eiter (2006). *Journal of Experimental Psychology: Human Perception and Performance, 32,* 1496-1500.

Pynte, J., & Kennedy, A. (2006). Control over eye movements in reading can be exerted from beyond the level of the word: Evidence from reading English and French. *Vision Research, 46,* 3786-3801.

Rayner, K. (1975). Eye movements and the perceptual span in reading. *Cognitive Psychology, 7,* 65-81.

Rayner, K., Ashby, J., Pollatsek, A., & Reichle, E. D. (2004). The effects of frequency and predictability on eye fixations in reading: Implications for the E-Z Reader model. *Journal of Experimental Psychology: Human Perception and Performance, 30,* 720-732.

Rayner, K., & Bertera, J. H. (1979). Reading without a Fovea. *Science, 206,* 468-469.

Rayner, K., Fischer, M. H., & Pollatsek, A. (1998). Unspaced text interferes with both word identification and eye movement control. *Vision Research, 38,* 1129-1144.

Rayner, K., Juhasz, B. J., & Brown, S. J. (2007). Do readers obtain preview benefit from word n+2? A test of serial attention shift versus distributed lexical processing of eye movement control in reading. *Journal of Experimental Psychology: Human Perception and Performance, 33,* 230-245.

Rayner, K., Pollatsek, A., Drieghe, D., Slattery, T. J., & Reichle, E. D. (2007). Tracking the mind during reading via eye movements: Comments on Kliegl, Nuthmann, and Engbert (2006). *Journal of Experimental Psychology: General, 136,* 520-529.

Rayner, K., Warren, T., Juhasz, B. J., & Liversedge, S. P. (2004). The effect of plausibility on eye movements in reading. *Journal of Experimental Psychology: Learning, Memory, and Cognition, 30,* 1290-1301.

Rayner, K., White, S. J., Kambe, G., Miller, B., & Liversedge, S. P. (2003). On the processing of meaning from parafoveal vision during eye fixations in reading. In J. Hyönä , R. Radach, & H. Deubel (Eds.), *The mind's eye: Cognitive and applied aspects of eye movement research* (pp. 213-234). Amsterdam: North Holland.

R Development Core Team (2007). *R: A language and environment for statistical computing. (version 2.4.1).* R Foundation for Statistical Computing, Vienna, Austria. ISBN 3-900051-07-0.

Reichle, E., Pollatsek, A., Fisher, D. L., & Rayner, K. (1998). Toward a model of eye movement control in reading. *Psychological Review, 105,* 125-157.

Reichle, E. D., Rayner, K., & Pollatsek, A. (2003). The E-Z Reader model of eye movement control in reading: Comparisons to other models. *Behavioral and Brain Sciences, 26,* 446-526.

Reilly, R. G., & Radach, R. (2006). Some empirical tests of an interactive activation model of eye movement control in reading. *Cognitive Systems Research, 7,* 34-55.

Richter, E. M., Engbert, R., & Kliegl, R. (2006). Current advances in SWIFT. *Cognitive Systems Research, 7,* 23-33.

Schilling, H. E. H., Rayner, K., & Chumbley, J. I. (1998). Comparing naming, lexical decision, and eye fixation times: Word frequency effects and individual differences. *Memory & Cognition, 26,* 1270-1281.

Sparks, D. L. (2002). The brainstem control of saccadic eye movements. *Nature Reviews Neuroscience, 3,* 952-964.

Vitu, F., Lancelin, D., Jean, A., & Farioli, F. (2006). Influence of foveal distractors on saccadic eye movements: A dead zone for the global effect. *Vision Research, 46,* 4684-4708.

Vitu, F., McConkie, G. W., Kerr, P., & O'Regan, J. K. (2001). Fixation location effects on fixation durations during reading: An inverted optimal viewing position effect. *Vision Research, 41,* 3513-3533.

Wickham, H. (2005). Reshape: Flexibly reshape data. R package version 0.7.1. [Software].

Wickham, H. (2006). Ggplot: An implementation of the Grammar of Graphics in R. R package version 0.4.0. [Software].

Yang, J., Wang, S., & Rayner, K. (2006). *A test of serial attention shift versus distributed lexical processing models of eye movement control in reading: Evidence from Chinese.* Presentation at the Second China International Conference on Eye Movements, Tianjin, China, June 22, 2006.

Chapter 4

Modeling the eye movements of Chinese readers via E-Z Reader

Keith Rayner, Xingshan Li, and Alexander Pollatsek

A number of formal computational models of eye-movement control in reading have been proposed over the past few years. Among these models, E-Z Reader (Reichle, Pollatsek, Fisher, & Rayner, 1998; Reichle, Pollatsek, & Rayner, 2006; see Pollatsek, Reichle, & Rayner, this volume) and SWIFT (Richter, Engbert, & Kliegl, 2006; see Risse, Engbert, & Kliegl, this volume) are perhaps the most well-known. Other models include SHARE (Feng, 2006), Glenmore (Reilly & Radach, 2006), and the Competition/activation model (Yang, 2006). See Reichle, Rayner, and Pollatsek (2003) for an overview of the models and the differences between them.

These models differ on a number of dimensions including (a) the extent to which cognitive/lexical processing influences eye movements, (b) whether or not lexical processing drives eye movements or primarily serves to interrupt processing when something doesn't compute, and (c) the extent to which words are lexically processed serially or in parallel. Among the models listed here, E-Z Reader has the most lexical involvement and the Competition/activation model, which is generally described as an oculomotor model, has the least amount of lexical involvement. While E-Z Reader involves serial lexical processing of words, SWIFT and Glenmore allow for parallel processing of words. Despite differences between the models, most of them are able to account for certain benchmark data on eye movements during reading. Specifically, they generally account for the following effects (see Rayner, 1998 for a summary of studies supporting these effects): (a) readers spend less time fixating on high-frequency words than low-frequency words, (b) readers spend less time looking at predictable words than unpredictable words, (c) readers spend less time looking at a word when they have received a valid preview of the word than when they received an invalid preview, and (d) the initial fixation in a word tends to be halfway between the middle and the beginning of a word.

While these different models can account for much of the data, they all deal with the reading of alphabetic languages. One venue for testing the generalizibility of the models would be to determine how effectively they can account for the data on eye movements when reading a non-alphabetic language.[1] Given that Chinese is the most dramatically different from alphabetic writing systems like English, it seems like an ideal test case. In this article, we will discuss how the E-Z Reader model (Pollatsek, Reichle, & Rayner, 2006; Reichle et al., 1998; Reichle et al., 2003), which we developed for English, fared when we subjected it to Chinese (Rayner, Li, & Pollatsek, 2007). Such an endeavor is interesting in the context of models of eye-movement control in reading. But, it may also have broader significance in that there has recently been considerable interest in the extent to which cultural differences influence language processing and cognition in general (Chua, Boland, & Nisbett, 2005; Rayner, Li, Williams, Cave, & Well, 2007; see also the chapters in this volume by Boland et al. and by Li et al.).

The facts about Chinese are well-discussed throughout the present volume. However, we will briefly make some comments about Chinese writing and then provide a quick overview of what is known about the eye movements of Chinese readers (although other chapters in this volume do so as well). Chinese text is formed by strings of equally spaced box-like symbols called characters. It used to be printed from top-to-bottom (with the columns printed from right-to-left), but like English, it is now most typically printed horizontally from left-to-right. Unlike English (and other alphabetic writing systems), Chinese is written without spaces between successive characters and words. Also, individual characters vary in terms of complexity because they differ in (a) the number of strokes per character, (b) the number of radicals (or certain combinations of strokes that denote semantic or phonological informa-

1 Another way to test the generalizability of the models is to examine how well they account for the performance of readers who have different reading strategies; see Rayner, Reichle, Stroud, Williams, and Pollatsek (2006) and Laubrock, Kliegl, and Engbert (2006) for examples of how the E-Z Reader model and the SWIFT model (Engbert, Nuthmann, Richter, & Kliegl, 2005) account for the eye-movement data of older readers.

tion), and (c) the manner of construction (that is, radicals can be combined in different ways to form compound words). Basically, there are many visual details packed into a constant, box-shaped area for each character.

While the concept of a word is not as clearly defined in Chinese as it is in English (so that Chinese readers will disagree somewhat concerning where word boundaries are located), Chinese words obviously differ in the frequency with which they are encountered. Chinese characters are more like morphemes and most words are made up of two characters, though some words consist of only one character and some consist of three or more characters. Finally, Chinese words, like English words, vary in terms of how predictable they are from the preceding context.

A number of facts are known about the eye movements of Chinese readers. First, the perceptual span[2] for Chinese readers extends 1 character to the left of fixation to 2-3 characters to the right when reading from left-to-right (Chen & Tang, 1998; Inhoff & Liu, 1997, 1998);[3] in contrast, in English the span extends 3-4 letters to the left of fixation to about 14-15 letters to the right of fixation (Rayner, 1998). Second, and not surprisingly, average saccades are much shorter in Chinese (about 2.6 characters) than in English (about 7-9 letters) since the information is more densely packed in Chinese (Chen, Song, Lau, Wong, & Tang, 2003). Third, average fixation durations are similar (about 225-250 ms) for readers of Chinese and English (Chen et al. 2003; Sun & Feng, 1999; Rayner, 1998). Fourth, regression rate appears to be slightly higher in Chinese (about 15%) than English (about 10%) for skilled readers (Chen et al., 2003; Rayner, 1998). Fifth, the probability of skipping a word tends to be fairly similar in Chinese and English (Rayner, Li, Juhasz, & Yan, 2005).[4] Sixth, Chinese readers, like English readers, fixate longer on low-frequency words than on high-frequency words (Yan, Tian, Bai, & Rayner, 2006) and on low-predictable words than on high-predictable words (Rayner et al., 2005); like English readers, they also skip high-

2 The perceptual span refers to the region of effective vision during an eye fixation. It is usually determined via the use of the moving window technique (McConkie & Rayner, 1975; Rayner & Bertera, 1979) in which the number of letters/characters available on each fixation is manipulated.

3 If the perceptual span is measured in terms of words or "idea units" rather than characters, the spans are fairly equivalent.

4 Chen et al. (2003) reported that Chinese readers skipped 42% of the characters. However, other studies in which word skipping, as opposed to character skipping, is examined have yielded estimates around 10-25% depending on the predictability of the word (Rayner et al., 2005; Tsai, Lee, Tzeng, Hung, & Yen, 2004; Yan et al., 2006).

predictable words more than low-predictable words (Rayner et al., 2005) and high-frequency words more than low-frequency words (Yan et al., 2006). Finally, character frequency affects fixation time on a word, but only when word frequency is low (Yan et al., 2006).

The E-Z Reader model

We will first briefly describe the basic architecture of the E-Z Reader model (see also Pollatsek et al., this volume), and then turn to simulations to see how well it could account for the eye movements of Chinese readers (see Rayner, Li, & Pollatsek, 2007 for further details). A main motivation for E-Z Reader was to account for eye movements during reading in English (or a typical alphabetic orthography) making the fewest and simplest assumptions possible. In such orthographies, a salient visual entity is the word, which is delimited by spaces.[5] Thus, in E-Z Reader, the primary engine driving the eyes forward in the text is the encoding of a word, and the target for a saccade is the middle of a word. Given that words are not visually marked in Chinese, it is an open question whether a model that makes such assumptions will give a satisfactory account of reading in Chinese. On the other hand, there is good reason to believe that words are also quite salient for Chinese readers (even though the word boundaries are not clearly marked). The key encoding assumption of E-Z Reader with respect to encoding mechanisms is that words are lexically processed serially, one word at a time, although it is tacitly assumed that the component letters within a word are processed in parallel. Thus, covert attention is posited to be directed to a word (word n) and does not shift to the next word (word n+1) until encoding of word n is completed. A second key assumption is that the signal that triggers a saccade to a word is not the same signal that triggers an attention shift to that word. That is, lexical encoding is divided into two stages, L_1 and L_2, although they may not be distinct stages in the lexical processing system, but instead may reflect the crossing of two different thresholds of lexical activation. Completion of the earlier L_1 stage provides a signal to the eye movement system to make a saccade to the next word and completion of the later L_2 stage results in signal to the attention system to shift attention to word n+1. Both of these stages, in which words are processed serially, are assumed to be pre-

5 A possible counter-example is spaced compound words such as tennis ball, which are single words in some analyses.

ceded by a visual stage, V, in which visual information impinging on the retina (with acuity constraints) is assumed to be processed in parallel. Thus, low-level information, such as the spaces between words, is available early in a fixation to aid the planning of eye movements.

A third key assumption of the model is that both L_1 and L_2 are assumed to be functions of the frequency of the word in the language and its predictability from the prior text and thus that the speed of processing a word can influence the fixation time on it (see Equations 1 and 2 in Table 4.1). A fourth key assumption with respect to processing speed is that it decreases as words are farther from the fixation point. The form of Equation 3 (see Table 4.1), in which speed is modulated by the average absolute distance of the letters in a word from the fixation point implies: (a) words in the parafovea will be processed more slowly than those in foveal vision, (b) fixated words will be processed more slowly the farther the fixation point is from the center of the word,[6] and (c) that, all else being equal, longer words will take longer to process than

Table 4.1 Key assumptions of the E-Z Reader model

Equation 1:	$t(L_1) = \alpha_1 - \alpha_2 \ln(\text{word frequency}) - \alpha_3 (\text{word predictability})$
Equation 2:	$t(L_2) = \Delta\, t(L_1)$
Equation 3:	$\text{rate} = \varepsilon^{(\Sigma\, \mid \text{letter} - \text{fixation} \mid)\, /\, N}$
Equation 4:	$\text{systematic error} = (\Psi - \text{intended length})\, [\Omega_1 - \ln(\text{duration}_{n-1}) / \Omega_2]$

Notes:

In Equation 1, α_1, α_2, and α_3, are free parameters; the word frequency was obtained from corpus searches, and word predictability was obtained from a judgment experiment in which participants were given the sentence prior to word n, asked to guess word n, then were given word n, and asked to guess word n+1, etc.

In Equation 2, Δ is a free parameter relating the durations of L_1 and L_2. Note that this equation implies that L_2 has the same function form as L_1.

In Equation 3, the rate modifies the time computed from equation 1.

In Equation 4, Ψ is the medium saccade length at which there is no systematic error, and the other two parameters define the size of the error (which is reduced for longer fixation durations).

The values defined by the equations are means, and they are all posited to vary with gamma distributions.

---

6 Actually, single fixations on a word tend to be shorter on the ends of words than in the middle of words. This counterintuitive finding is accounted for within the E-Z Reader model via mislocalized fixations (see Pollatsek et al., 2006).

shorter words because, on average, the letters will be farther from fixation.

In addition to the encoding assumptions mentioned above, a second set of assumptions of the model deals with how signals are sent to, and executed by, the eye-movement system. The key assumption, which explains why words that are easier to process are skipped, is a saccade cancellation mechanism. This is realized in the model by positing two stages in the eye-movement planning time. That is, when a signal goes to the eye-movement system, there is a program immediately laid down, but it is in a labile state and can be cancelled by a subsequent eye-movement program; after a period of time has elapsed it goes into a non-labile state and can't be cancelled by a subsequent program.

In the normal course of affairs, when the reader is fixated on word n, a signal goes out to fixate word n+1 when L_1 is completed, and after both the labile and non-labile stages of the eye-movement program are complete, a saccade is executed whose target is word n+1. However, when word n+1 is easy to process (and thus its L_1 stage is short), a second eye-movement program can be initiated to fixate word n+2 (while the reader is still fixating word n) while the eye-movement program to word n+1 is still in the labile stage. In these cases, the eye movement program to fixate word n+1 will be cancelled, the program to fixate word n+2 will be executed (later), and thus word n+1 will be skipped. To handle refixations on words, it is assumed that an eye-movement program to refixate a word is initiated almost automatically at the beginning of a fixation. However, this refixation program can be cancelled (and will often be cancelled) by the initiation of the program to fixate word n+1. This cancellation will occur more often when L_1 is long, and thus the model predicts that words that are more difficult to process will be refixated more often.

The last set of assumptions deals with eye-movement targeting. As indicated above, eye movements are assumed to be directed to the middle of the targeted word (both refixation programs and programs targeting other words). However, because no motor programming is perfect there are errors in the execution of the eye-movement programs. First, random error is assumed, which is a gamma distribution whose standard deviation is proportional to the length of the programmed eye movement. Second, and perhaps more importantly, there is assumed to be bias: There is a preferred eye movement distance, and saccades that are programmed to be longer than this distance tend to be shorter than they were intended and saccades that are programmed to be shorter than this distance tend to be longer than intended (see Equation 4 in Table 4.1). Thus, short words can also be skipped just because they are short. However, if they are also reasonably easy to process (and thus the L_2 stage on word n+1 is complete before word n+2 is fixated), this will create no problems for the reader.

E-Z Reader and Chinese

An obvious question is whether the control of eye movements during reading in a language like Chinese is fundamentally different than in English. One way to test this is to try to apply E-Z Reader to Chinese. In the modeling, there are three obvious differences in the orthography that one has to consider. First, the concept of "word" in Chinese is perhaps less clear than in English as different readers of Chinese may disagree on where the word boundaries are. We believe, however, that there is still a reasonable amount of agreement on what words are, and thus the word boundaries we used (see Table 4.2 for examples) were based on the judgments of three native speakers of Chinese).[7] Second, there are no word boundaries signaled by the orthography similar to the spaces between words in English. Thus, it is far from clear how a Chinese reader would target the middle of a word. However, we de-

Table 4.2 Example Chinese sentences with vertical lines inserted between words to illustrate how the words were segmented. (The vertical lines were not present during reading). English translations of the sentences are provided.

昨天|晚上|，这|场|戏|的|首场|演出|在|剧院|里|举行。 The opening performance was played at the theater last night.
由于|这项|困难|的|任务|超出|了|他|的|体力|极限|，他|都|快|急|疯|了。 The difficult task was beyond his physical strength and he became frustrated.
这个|迷路|的|旅行者|仔细|检查|风向|以|确定|向|哪|条|路|走。 The lost hiker carefully checked the direction of the wind to figure out where to go.

7 There was initial disagreement on approximately 10% of the word boundaries in the sentences. Virtually all of the disagreements had to do with function words, and subsequent discussion among the three raters led to full agreement on the word boundaries used in the simulations.

cided to leave that part of the model unchanged. Third, a character is quite different from a letter, both visually and linguistically. However, again, to keep the change from English as little as possible, we treated it as an orthographic unit, just as in English.

The corpus of text simulated consisted of 36 Chinese sentences (see Rayner et al., 2005). Each sentence was on a single line. The 16 participants read each sentence and pressed a key when they had read the sentence, and were periodically asked questions that tested for their understanding of the sentence they had just read.[8] As with the simulations involving reading of English, we did not attempt to model fixations on the first or last words of the sentence. Moreover, as E-Z Reader does not attempt to explain higher order effects on eye movements (such as syntactic parsing), we also did not analyze sentences in which there were interword regressions (as per earlier simulations).

Some of the parameters in our model fitting were fixed and others were free to vary within certain constrained reasonable limits (see Table 4.4 for details on the parameters), and as there is no algebraic solution for a best fit, we simply repeated the simulation a number of times and found the best fit (i.e., that minimized the RMSD: the root mean squared deviation between observed and predicted values) within these constraints. As with our simulations in English, we divided the words in the text into five frequency classes, using a Chinese dictionary (National Languages Committee, 1997), and examined how well the model fit various indices of eye movements, such as first-fixation duration, gaze duration, and probability of skipping, for the five classes.

As seen in Table 4.3, E-Z Reader does a reasonable job of predicting the durations of fixations and the probabilities of fixating Chinese words as a function of their frequency. As with our simulations of English reading, the fit is not perfect, but there don't seem to be any serious anomalies. With the fixation durations, the major deviation between what was observed and what was predicted is for frequency class 4, and there it appears that the observed values are a bit anomalous as the mean individual fixation durations on class 4 words are actually less than on class 5 words. Moreover, the means are based on relatively little data, as skipping rates were high for these words. The model also appeared to be under-predicting the effect of frequency on the skipping rates a bit.

In evaluating the performance of the model, one would want the pa-

8 For reasons related to the counterbalancing of materials in the Rayner et al. (2005) study, only half of the data were used for the simulations.

Table 4.3 E-Z Reader fits of Chinese data

Freq. class	Gaze duration		First fixation duration		Single fixation duration		Probability of a single fixation		Probability of two fixations		Probability of skipping	
	Pred.	Obs.	Pred.	Obs.	Pred.	Obs.	Pred.	Obs.	Pred.	Obs.	Pred.	Obs.
1	302	299	257	259	254	257	0.53	0.57	0.10	0.14	0.35	0.29
2	282	281	235	249	236	249	0.50	0.55	0.08	0.10	0.42	0.35
3	275	263	237	244	237	245	0.48	0.51	0.08	0.07	0.43	0.43
4	255	235	240	231	240	225	0.41	0.33	0.03	0.01	0.56	0.66
5	234	229	225	225	224	227	0.33	0.30	0.02	0.00	0.65	0.70

RMSD = 0.1731. The RMSD for E-Z Reader 9 in English was 0.153 (Pollatsek et al., 2006).
Note: The skipping rate presented here is much higher than that reported by Rayner et al. (2005). All of the target words in Rayner et al. were 2-characters. In the present analysis of the data, words that were 1-character were also included leading to the higher overall skipping rates. Adapted from Rayner, Li, and Pollatsek (2007).

rameter values estimated to be defensible in terms of what is known about reading. As a result, we present in Table 4.4 the best fitting parameter values of the fit for Chinese compared with those in our latest full simulation of data in English. As can be seen, the parameters involved in the speed of lexical access are all fairly similar to the English values. The parameters that are notably different, Ψ, Ω_1, Ω_2, η_1, η_2, deal with systematic and random errors in programming; however, these parameters were scaled in terms of characters and letters for Chinese and English, respectively, so that it makes sense that most of the values should be larger for English. The parameter η_2, indexing the random error component of targeting saccades, indicates that saccade targeting is more variable for larger planned saccades in Chinese (which we think is quite reasonable). Only the eccentricity parameter, ε, appears to be at all anomalous: It is about the same size in the two simulations even though the unit is the character in Chinese and the letter in English. Our attempts to force this value to be bigger in the Chinese simulations, so that the eccentricity parameters would be approximately equal when scaled in terms of degrees of visual angle, were unsuccessful. Apparently, Chinese readers are more successful at extracting relevant information about characters farther from fixation (in terms of visual angle) than were readers of English. This could be because there is lower spatial frequency information in Chinese orthography that plays a significant role in character and word identification, whereas analogous

Table 4.4 Best fitting parameters for the Chinese version of E-Z Reader

Parameter	Best fitting value in current simulation	Best fitting value in simulation of English (Pollatsek et. al, 2006)
α_1	138	122
α_2	3.4	4
α_3	18	10
Δ	0.5	0.5
ε	1.17	1.15
Ψ	2.2	7
Ω_1	3.9	7.3
Ω_2	1.1	3
η_1	0.10	0.5
η_2	0.67	0.15
M_1	100	100
M_2	25	25
λ	0.12	0.09
V	50	50
R	138	117
S	25	25
$\sigma\gamma$	0.22	0.22

Notes:

$\alpha_1, \alpha_2, \alpha_3, \varepsilon, \Omega_1, \Omega_2, \Psi, \eta_1, \eta_2$ were free to vary when fitting, all of the other parameters were fixed.

V = duration of visual stage; M_1 and M_2 are durations of labile and non-labile stages of eye-movement programming; R is the mean refixation decision time; S is the assumed time for a saccadic movement; η_1 and η_2 are the slope and intercept of the random error component of saccadic programming; $\sigma\gamma$ sets the SDs of the processing distributions to 0.22 times the mean; controls refixation probabilities as a function of distance from the center of the word. Adapted from Rayner, Li, and Pollatsek (2007).

information (e.g., word shape) appears to play little or no role in English.

Another issue that our initial simulation did not consider was whether character frequency plays an important role in determining eye-movement behavior apart from word frequency. There are several ways to test this. The one we chose was to include character frequency as a predictor as well as word frequency and word predictability in the equation for the duration of L_1. (All other aspects of the model were unchanged, although the parameter values were free to vary as in the above fit.) When we applied this version of the model (see Rayner, Li, & Pollatsek, 2007 for details) to the data, the fit was actually slightly worse than with the model that used only word frequency and word predictability in spite of having two more free parameters. This suggests that character frequency may not play an important role in Chinese reading apart from word frequency. However, it is possible that some alternative equation combining the effects of word frequency and character may do a better job.

General discussion

In this chapter, we have reported the results of simulations using the E-Z Reader model to account for both when (i.e., how long readers look at words) and where (i.e., which words are skipped) Chinese readers move their eyes. Basically, the simulations were fairly successful. We thus think that our simulations indicate that the hypothesis that the control of eye movements in reading Chinese is similar to that in reading an alphabetic language such as English is a reasonable one. Obviously, however, more sophisticated tests need to be done. A major question that needs to be explored, of course, is the mechanism by which saccades in Chinese are targeted given that there are no obvious cues for word boundaries. In simulations mentioned here, we assumed that they were appropriately targeted as if these cues were present. The one indication that something different was going on was that the η_2 parameter was substantially larger in Chinese indicating more variability in programming, especially for larger saccades. Given this, it is reasonable to consider alternatives to targeting words. However, they are far from obvious. Given that the probability of skipping a word in Chinese is influenced by the predictability of a word with word length held constant (Rayner et al., 2005), one can not reasonably posit that Chinese readers simply target saccades a fixed distance forward. Thus, they appear to have some sort of target based on what they have read. One possibility is that they do in fact have a fairly good idea where the end of a word is that has been encoded and program the next saccade to be something like 1-2 characters ahead of that (or possibly something like 1 degree of visual angle past the last word encoded). The answers to these questions require better knowledge of what kinds of visual information Chinese readers have on-line when they are reading.

Finally, by simulating the eye movements of Chinese readers in the context of the E-Z Reader model, we do not mean to imply that other models of eye-movement control in reading could not do likewise. Our goal with the present simulations was not to suggest that E-Z Reader can do it, and the other models can't. We do suspect that any type of purely oculomotor control model, in which the eyes move forward a set number of characters and pause for variable amounts of time to input the information, would have a difficult time accounting for the data. However, it seems at least plausible that other models which allow for cognitive/lexical influences on eye movements during reading could provide simulations that would capture the data pattern.

Acknowledgments

This work was supported by Grant HD26765 from the National Institute of Health and a Grant from Microsoft.

References

Chen, H. C., Song, H., Lau, W. Y., Wong, K. F. E., & Tang, S. L. (2003). Developmental characteristics of eye movements in reading Chinese. In C. McBride-Chang, & H. C. Chen (Eds.), *Reading development in Chinese children* (pp. 157-169). Westport, CT: Praeger.

Chen, H. C., & Tang, C. K. (1998). The effective visual field in Chinese. *Reading and Writing, 10,* 245-254.

Chua, H. F., Boland, J. E., & Nisbett, R. E. (2005). Cultural variation in eye movements during scene perception. *Proceedings of the National Academy of Sciences, 102,* 12629-12633.

Engbert, R., Nuthmann, A., Richter, E., & Kliegl, R. (2005). SWIFT: A dynamical model of saccade generation during reading. *Psychological Review, 112,* 777-813.

Feng, G. (2006). Eye movements as time-series random variables: A stochastic model of eye movement control in reading. *Cognitive Systems Research, 7,* 70-95.

Inhoff, A. W., & Liu, W. (1997). The perceptual span during the reading of Chinese text. In H. C. Chen (Ed.), *The cognitive processing of Chinese and related Asian languages.* Hong Kong: The Chinese University

Press.
Inhoff, A. W., & Liu, W. (1998). The perceptual span and oculomotor activity during the reading of Chinese sentences. *Journal of Experimental Psychology: Human Perception and Performance, 24,* 20-34.
Laubrock, J., Kliegl, R., & Engbert, R. (2006). SWIFT explorations of age differences in eye movements during reading. *Neuroscience and Biobehavioral Reviews, 30,* 872-884.
McConkie, G. W., & Rayner, K. (1975). The span of the effective stimulus during a fixation in reading. *Perception & Psychophysics, 17,* 578-586.
National Languages Committee. (1997). *Chinese dictionary: Character and word frequency statistics report.* (in Chinese). Taipei: Author.
Pollatsek, A., Reichle, E. D., & Rayner, K. (2006). Tests of the E-Z Reader model: Exploring the interface between cognition and eye-movement control. *Cognitive Psychology, 52,* 1-56.
Rayner, K. (1998). Eye movements in reading and information processing: 20 years of research. *Psychological Bulletin, 124,* 372-422.
Rayner, K., & Bertera, J. H. (1979). Reading without a fovea. *Science, 206,* 468-469.
Rayner, K., Li, X., Juhasz, B. J., & Yan, G. (2005). The effect of word predictability on the eye movements of Chinese readers. *Psychonomic Bulletin & Review, 12,* 1089-1093.
Rayner, K., Li, X., & Pollatsek, A. (2007). Extending the E-Z Reader model of eye movement control to Chinese readers. *Cognitive Science, 31,* 1021-1034.
Rayner, K., Li, X., Williams, C. C., Cave, K. R., & Well, A. D. (2007). Eye movements during information processing tasks: Individual differences and cultural effects. *Visual Research, 47,* 2714-2726.
Rayner, K., Reichle, E. D., Stroud, M. J., Williams, C. C., & Pollatsek, A. (2006). The effect of word frequency, word predictability, and font difficulty on the eye movements of young and older readers. *Psychology and Aging, 21,* 448-465.
Reichle, E. D., Pollatsek, A., Fisher, D. L., & Rayner, K. (1998). Toward a model of eye movement control in reading. *Psychological Review, 105,* 125-157.
Reichle, E. D., Pollatsek, A., & Rayner, K. (2006). E-Z Reader: A cognitive-control, serial-attention model of eye-movement behavior during reading. *Cognitive Systems Research, 7,* 4-22.
Reichle, E. D., Rayner, K., & Pollatsek, A. (2003). The E-Z Reader model of eye-movement control in reading: Comparisons to other mod-

els. *Behavioral and Brain Sciences, 26,* 445-476.

Reilly, R., & Radach, R. (2006). Some empirical tests of an interactive activation model of eye movement control in reading. *Cognitive Systems Research, 7,* 34-55.

Richter, E. M., Engbert, R., & Kliegl, R. (2006). Current advances in SWIFT. *Cognitive Systems Research, 7,* 23-33.

Sun, F., & Feng, D. (1999). Eye movements in reading Chinese and English Text. In J. Wang, A. W. Inhoff, & H. C. Chen (Eds.), *Reading Chinese script: A cognitive analysis* (pp. 189-206). Mahwah, NJ: Erlbaum.

Tsai, J., Lee, C., Tzeng, O. J. L., Hung, D. L., & Yen, N. (2004). Use of phonological codes for Chinese characters: Evidence from processing of parafoveal preview when reading sentences. *Brain and Language, 91,* 235-244.

Yan, G., Tian, H., Bai, X., & Rayner, K. (2006). The effect of word and character frequency on the eye movements of Chinese readers. *British Journal of Psychology, 97,* 259-268.

Yang, S. (2006). A oculomotor-based model of eye movements in reading: The competition/activation model. *Cognitive Systems Research, 7,* 56-69.

Section 3

Eye movements and visual processing

Chapter 5

Binocular eye movements during reading

Simon P. Liversedge

In this chapter I will describe data from a series of recent experiments that my colleagues and I have conducted to investigate how people coordinate their eyes binocularly when they read text (Liversedge, White, Findlay, & Rayner, 2006; Liversedge, Rayner, White, Findlay, & McSorley, 2006; Juhasz, Liversedge, White, & Rayner, 2006; Blythe, Liversedge, Joseph, White, Findlay, & Rayner, 2006). I will present the experiments in three separate sections, and in each section I will describe work that examined different aspects of binocular coordination during reading. In the first section I will discuss studies that have examined the characteristics of adults' binocular eye movements as they read, and in the second section I will describe similar comparative data taken from children as they read. The data from these experiments are largely descriptive offering insight into the characteristics of how the eyes are moved in relation to each other (as well as in relation to the words of a sentence) when we read. In the third section I will describe an experiment in which we gave participants sentences containing a target word that was presented dichoptically. Using this manipulation we investigated how readers attained a unified perceptual representation of the text given disparate patterns of retinal stimulation. Together these studies provide a comprehensive picture of how the eyes work mechanically together, and how the visual system processes binocular input to produce a unified visual representation of the text that can be employed by the language processing system to facilitate fast and efficient comprehension.

Binocular coordination during reading in adults

The most basic characteristics of eye movements that are most often measured in experiments investigating reading are saccade directions (whether saccades are progressive or regressive), saccade magnitudes (i.e., the size of saccades in relations to launch and landing sites) and fixation durations (i.e., how long the eyes remain stable as information about the text is extracted). Within the field of eye movements and reading, it is widely assumed that, regardless of whether the movements of the left or the right eye are measured, these basic characteristic remain the same. Both eyes are assumed to move at the same point in time and to fixate the same location within the text. When reading, humans are assumed not to function in a chameleon like manner, whereby, each eye moves independently in order to fixate a different spatial location at different points in time. In fact, just by closely watching a person's eyes as they read, it is relatively easy to observe that they appear to move together, in a very regular and synchronised way. Thus, it is perhaps not surprising that most researchers in this field assume that the two eyes move in this perfectly coordinated manner in order to permit alignment of the visual axes on the same point within the visual array.

In the work that I will describe below we attempted to examine whether this assumption was correct. In particular, we were interested to know whether there was any variability in the precise location of the point of fixation of the two eyes in relation to each other. To say that a reader is fixating the same point within a word, it is generally assumed that they are fixating the same letter of a word. We have adhered to this convention throughout the entire series of experiments that we have undertaken in this area, and at this point it is perhaps worth clearly defining the terminology that I will use throughout this chapter. I will refer to fixations as *aligned* when the horizontal displacement between the point of fixation of the left and the right eye is less than a single character. When the horizontal displacement between the two eyes' points of fixation is greater than this, I will refer to those fixations as *unaligned*. Furthermore, unaligned fixations may be broken down into two subcategories, namely *crossed* fixations in which the right point of fixation is more than one character to the left of the left point of fixation, and *uncrossed* fixations, for which the right point of fixation is more than one character to the right of the left point of fixation. To use this terminology, in our experiments we were interested to investigate the extent to which aligned, crossed and uncrossed fixations occurred during reading.

Before embarking on our experiments, we searched through the literature to see whether there were any existing experimental studies in this area that had already been published. We were particularly keen to establish whether there were any experimental findings that may be suggestive of disparity in the location of fixations made by the two eyes during reading. Furthermore, if this was a possibility, then we wished to consider how such a finding might inform our understanding of the nature of human visual function in relation to reading.

Perhaps the most relevant study to the work that we undertook was reported by Heller and Radach (1999). Although only limited methodological detail was included in Heller and Radach's paper, it is extremely valuable in that it reports data that are consistent with the suggestion that readers do not always fixate the same location with both eyes. In their study eye movements were recorded binocularly as sentences and short passages of text were read. They found that fixations of the two eyes were approximately 1.5 characters apart. Heller and Radach provided no indication of the proportion of fixations that were crossed or uncrossed, however, they did note that vergence movements did not serve to correct the disparity between the points of fixation. Vergence movements are movements of the eyes that are relatively slow in comparison to saccadic eye movements and these occur during fixations. Interestingly, while one might intuitively imagine that vergence movements serve to bring disparate points of fixation together onto a single character during a fixation, Heller and Radach showed that they persisted even when one of the two eyes was occluded and viewing was monocular. Thus, it appears that vergence movements are an intrinsic part of eye movement behaviour and are not necessarily a product of binocular input. A final result that they reported was that fixation disparity was reduced when sentences were presented in MiXeD CaSe text. Mixed case text is more difficult to read than is text presented normally, and the reduced disparity that Heller and Radach observed caused them to tentatively suggest an inverse relationship between disparity magnitudes and reading difficulty such that the visual system is able to tolerate less visual disparity for text that is more difficult to process.

Heller and Radach's findings were sufficiently intriguing and suggestive for us to decide that a series of experiments to investigate binocular coordination during reading would be valuable. We, therefore, conducted a series of very carefully controlled experiments using very accurate left and right Dual Purkinje Image eyetrackers to obtain data that would provide a comprehensive description of binocular eye movement behavior during reading. It is these experiments that I will briefly summarize in the following sections of this chapter. In the first of our experiments (see Liversedge, White et al., 2006) we tested 15 adult participants as they read 72 sentences (along with comprehension questions to ensure good reading performance). Participants' head movements were minimized through the use of a head restraint and bite bar, and the left eye tracker was calibrated monocularly for the left eye, and the right tracker monocularly for the right eye. Additionally, calibrations were checked for each eye monocularly after each trial. This methodological point is non-trivial as it is vital to undertake monocular calibrations and monocular calibration checks in order to be maximally confident that each eye tracker is providing a veridical indication of exactly where each of the participant's eyes is fixating. After testing our participants, we were also extremely cautious in the way that we analyzed the data. We were careful when coding the beginnings and endings of saccades to ensure that any disparity observed during a fixation could not have been caused by contamination from saccadic movements. In practice, this meant marking the beginning of a fixation "late," and the end of a fixation "early." Thus, fixations were slightly truncated in duration. We also excluded unusually long or short fixations, as well as any fixations for which there was an unusually large disparity. We adopted this careful approach to be sure that we did not favor the hypothesis that we would observe disparity in our participants' fixations.

We first examined our data to investigate whether we did observe disparity during fixations, and if so, to quantify the magnitude of that disparity. When we averaged across all the fixations in our data set we found that the mean disparity was 1.1 characters, and when we considered only unaligned fixations (i.e., those fixations with a disparity of 1 character or more), the average fixation disparity was 1.9 characters. Disparity magnitudes were the same for crossed and uncrossed fixations. We also considered the data for each of our participants in turn and the effects were of a similar magnitude for each of them (between 0.75 and 1.6 characters on average overall). Having established that fixation disparity was occurring as our participants read the sentences, we then investigated what proportion of fixations were aligned, uncrossed and crossed. We found that 53% of fixations were aligned, 39% were uncrossed and 8% were crossed. An important point to note is that the difference in the proportion of crossed and uncrossed fixations indicates that it is extremely unlikely that these data simply reflect noise associated with the eyetracking equipment (i.e., poorly calibrated eyetrackers). If this were the case, then we would anticipate the proportion of crossed and uncrossed fixations to be of a similar order, but that clearly was not the case. To very briefly summarize our findings from this experiment, consistent with Heller and Radach (1999), we found that fixations were unaligned on a substantial proportion of fixations; however, beyond this we found significantly more uncrossed than crossed fixations. Additionally, for the unaligned fixations the magnitude of the disparity was about 2 characters regardless of whether they were crossed or uncrossed.

In a follow up study by Juhasz et al. (2006) we replicated and extended these findings. In this study we included two additional manipulations. Sentences were presented in mixed case as well as normally, and included a target word that was either high or low frequency. These manipulations were included to examine Heller and Radach's claim that fixation disparity was reduced when text was more difficult to read. As noted above, the basic findings that Liversedge, White et al. reported were replicated in this study. Furthermore, robust effects of frequency and of mixed case text were observed on fixation durations. However, Juhasz et al. found that neither word frequency, nor mixed case text modulated disparity magnitudes, and thus, we could find no evidence to support Heller and Radach's claim that binocular disparity was reduced for text that was more difficult to read.

Overall, it is clear that, contrary to a very prevalent assumption in the field of eye movements and reading, on a substantial proportion of fixations the two eyes do not fixate the same letter of a word. Note also that normal participants do not ordinarily experience diplopia (double vision) when they read. Therefore, these results indicate that somehow the visual system is constructing a unified perceptual representation of the text based on the disparate patterns of retinal stimulation associated with each eye. There appear to be two possible mechanistic explanations as to how the visual system achieves this. One possibility is that the visual system operates according to a process of suppression, whereby one of the disparate inputs is blocked and the other is taken as the basis for the single representation of the text. The alternative explanation is that the visual system creates a unified perceptual representation of the text through the fusion of the two disparate patterns of retinal stimulation from each eye. To discriminate between these two theoretical possibilities, we conducted another experiment that is described later in this chapter. Next, however, I will consider data from an experiment in which we examined the binocular eye movements of children as they read.

Binocular coordination during reading in children and adults

The nature of children's eye movements during reading is a developing area within the field of eye movement research. A number of laboratories have published papers, or currently have papers under submission at journals that report investigations into different aspects of children's oculomotor behavior during reading. Two studies are particularly relevant to the work I will describe in this chapter, and these provide comparative binocular data from children and adults (Fioravanti, Inchingolo, Pensiero, & Spanios, 1995; Yang & Kapoula, 2003). Note, however, that both these studies examined binocular coordination in non-reading tasks. In their study, Fioravanti et al. tested adults as well as child participants aged between 5 and 10 years. They required participants to make saccades between small light sources (LED's) during which binocular recordings were taken. They found a different pattern of effects for children than adults. While adults' eyes became diverged (i.e., uncrossed) during saccades, children's eyes became converged (i.e. crossed). They also reported greater disparity magnitudes in children than in adults. Similarly, Yang and Kapoula (2003) measured eye movements as participants made saccades between LED's arranged in two concentric circles. They also found that the magnitude of fixation disparities observed in child participants was significantly greater than those observed in adults. Thus, based on these studies, not only might one anticipate disparity magnitudes in children that are greater than those observed in adults, but also since children's eyes become crossed rather than uncrossed during saccades, we might anticipate more crossed than uncrossed fixations during reading (i.e., the reverse pattern to that observed for adults).

We (Blythe et al. 2006) conducted a reading experiment in which we recorded adults' and children's (aged 7-11 years) binocular eye movements as they read sentences. The methodological details were very similar to those of Liversedge, White, et al. (2006), and for brevity's sake

I will not repeat them. One important difference, however, concerned the sentences that were used in the experiment. We created a new set of sentences for the children that were more appropriate for their reading age. These sentences were shorter in length than those for the adults (maximum length 60 compared with 80 characters for the adults), and were comprised of words that were certain to be within the vocabulary of children as young as 7 years.

In addition to examining the binocular characteristics of children's eye movements, we also considered some basic eye movement measures of reading behavior. In particular, we examined the number of fixations, the mean duration of fixations and the total sentence reading time for children compared with adults. We found that children made more fixations than adults (15.5 vs. 13.7 on average), children's mean fixation durations were longer than those for adults (263ms vs. 231ms on average), and the total sentence reading time was longer for children than adults (5692ms vs. 4058ms on average). Note that the increased fixations and reading times for children held even though the sentences that they read were substantially shorter than those read by the adults. These findings are consistent with other studies that have examined children's eye movements during reading (e.g., McConkie, Zola, Grimes, Kerr, Bryant, & Wolff, 1991).

Turning now to the measures of binocular disparity, in support of our hypothesis we found that disparity magnitudes in children were greater (m = 1.58 characters based on all fixations) than those observed in adults (m = 1.26 characters based on all fixations). Recall that we also predicted that for the proportion of crossed and uncrossed fixations we might observe the reverse pattern of effects for the children than that observed for the adults. In fact, this hypothesis was only partially supported. As can be seen from Figure 5.1, the pattern of effects obtained by Liversedge, White, et al. (2006) for adults replicated nicely. Approximately half the fixations were aligned, and there were substantially more uncrossed than crossed fixations.

For the children we did not find more crossed than uncrossed fixations as predicted. In fact, the proportion of uncrossed fixations was approximately the same as that observed for adults; however, the proportion of crossed fixations was significantly greater in children than in adults with a corresponding decrease in the proportion of aligned fixations for children than adults. Thus, while the effects did not completely reverse for the children, there was certainly a shift in the pattern of means in the predicted direction.

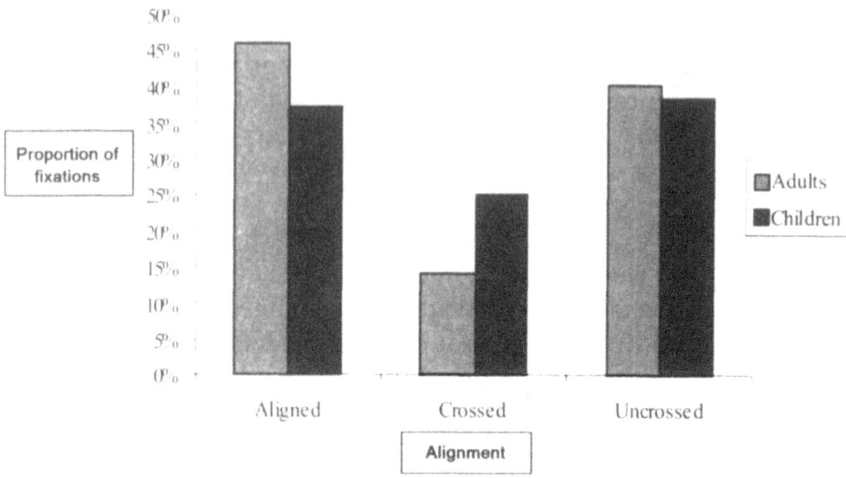

Figure 5.1 The proportion of aligned, crossed and uncrossed fixations for adults and children in the experiment reported by Blythe, Liversedge, Joseph, White, Findlay and Rayner, (2006). This Figure was originally published in *Vision Research*, *46*, 3898-3908.

Blythe et al.'s (2006) data are important in a number of respects. First, the data for the adults again replicated the findings of Liversedge, White, et al. (2006) and those of Juhasz et al. (2006), thereby firmly consolidating these findings. Secondly, the data for the children clearly demonstrated that the disparity effects obtained for adults also occurred for children. While perhaps not particularly surprising, these effects had not been demonstrated before in children's reading. Thirdly, the disparity effects obtained for children were greater than those obtained for adults. Finally, children exhibited crossed disparity to a greater degree than adults. These latter two points deserve further discussion in respect of why they occurred.

Given that the children and adults that we tested did not experience any difficulty reading, did not experience diplopia, produced standard patterns of eye movements and achieved high levels of comprehension (as indexed by correct answers to the comprehension questions), it seems reasonable to assume that they were reading normally and that any disparity effects were not disruptive to processing. What's more, the data indicate that the child participants are able to tolerate a greater degree of binocular disparity than adults (a finding that some may consider to be somewhat counter-intuitive). Quite why these effects occur is not entirely clear. What we do know is that Blythe et al. (2006) obtained very similar effects to those reported by Fioravanti et al. (1995), who employed a non-reading task. Given the similarity between the two data sets, it seems likely that the effects are not caused by higher order cognitive processes associated with the comprehension of language (otherwise why would they have also occurred for Fioravanti et al.?). Instead, it is likely that the effects reflect characteristic differences in the system responsible for low level oculomotor control regardless of the nature of the visual stimulus. Blythe et al. suggested that the effects possibly reflect the "ocular/visual immaturity" of the children's eye movement control mechanism relative to that of the adults. It is also not immediately clear why the children exhibited a greater proportion of crossed fixations than the adults. A possible explanation for this finding is that children do more of their "visual work" at a shorter viewing distance than adults. Under such circumstances children's eyes would be converged to a greater degree, and much more frequently, than would adults'. Given that children and adults read the sentences in our experiment at the same viewing distance, and that this viewing distance (1m) was perhaps further from the children than would ordinarily be the case if they were, say, reading a book, we would expect a higher proportion of crossed fixations for children than adults. This difference might, therefore, simply reflect vergence characteristics associated with different preferred viewing distances for reading in children and adults.

In the third section of this chapter I will now consider a final experiment in which binocular recordings were taken as adult participants read sentences containing a target word that was presented dichoptically.

Reading sentences containing dichoptically presented words

Liversedge, Rayner, et al. (2006) conducted an experiment to extend the basic descriptive account of binocular coordination in reading described in the first and second sections. Given the degree of disparity that exists on any particular fixation during reading, and the fact that readers do not ordinarily experience diplopia when reading, we were keen to investigate how the visual system constructed a single unified visual percept based on two disparate patterns of retinal stimulation. As mentioned earlier, there appear to be two possible mechanisms by which this might be achieved: suppression or fusion. To investigate this question, Liversedge, Rayner, et al. constructed sentences containing a target word that was a compound noun (e.g., cowboy) with 6, 8 or 10 letters. Binocular eye movements were recorded in the experiment using the Purkinje eyetrackers described earlier. However, in addition to this, the computer controlling the experimental procedure was interfaced with a pair of Cambridge Research Systems shutter goggles. These shutter goggles alternately open and close very rapidly (every 8 ms), such that when the left goggle is open, the right is closed, and vice-versa (see Figure 5.2).

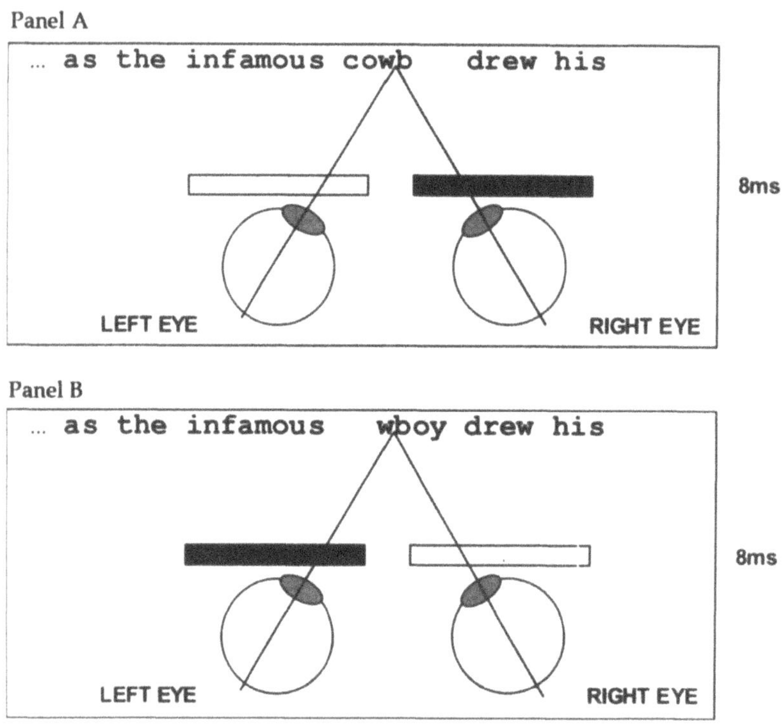

Figure 5.2 A schematic representation of the shutter goggle arrangement in the congruous dichoptic presentation condition. Panel A represents one 8ms time frame, and Panel B the next 8 ms time frame. The shutter goggles are represented by the horizontal bars in front of the eyeballs. A black bar represents a closed goggle and a white bar an open goggle. In Panel A the word portion *cowb* is presented to the left eye, and in Panel B, the word portion *wboy* is presented to the right eye. This Figure was originally published in *Current Biology, 16*, 1726-1729.

Such an arrangement allows the experimenter to block the visual input to each eye alternately. Additionally, if the visual image on the screen is also changed alternately in synchrony with the changes in the goggles, the experimenter is able to provide unique visual input to each eye. That is to say, the experimenter can present different text separately to each eye. In our experiment the only portion of the sentence that was presented dichoptically was the target word—the remainder of the sentence was shown in its entirety to both eyes. For the target word there were three presentation conditions: binocular, in which the whole word (*cowboy*) was presented to both eyes; congruous, in which the four initial letters (*cowb*) were presented to the left eye, and the four final letters (*wboy*) were presented to the right eye; and incongruous, in which the four initial letters (*cowb*) were presented to the right eye, and the four final letters (*wboy*) were presented to the left eye. Importantly, when part words were presented dichoptically, the letters were spatially extended such that they appropriately formed the full word cowboy (i.e., the "*w*" and "*b*" of *cowb* and of *wboy* were superimposed[1]).

These conditions allowed us to investigate how the dichoptic manipulation influenced saccadic targeting. When readers make a saccade to fixate a word, they do not land randomly on the string of letters that comprise that word. Instead, they target a point just left of the center of the word, the preferred viewing location (Rayner, 1979). Thus, we were able to formulate different experimental hypotheses regarding saccadic targeting based on the fusion, or the suppression account of the unified representation of text during reading. We reasoned that if the visual system attains a unified representation of the text through a process of suppression, then we might anticipate differential landing position distributions on the target word for the binocular, congruous and incongruous conditions. To be clear, if the input to one of the eyes was suppressed, then under the binocular condition, just left of the center of the whole word would be targeted, whereas under the congruous and incongruous conditions the center of the part word string that was not suppressed would be targeted. In other words, the landing position distribution on the target word would shift under the different viewing conditions. By contrast, if the visual system attains a unified representation of the text through a process of fusion, then regardless of the particular dichoptic presentation condition, the reader should always fuse the two complementary visual signals and therefore target exactly the same point in the word.

We conducted detailed analyses of both reading times and landing

---

1 The middle two letters of the target compound words always overlapped to ensure that the two halves of the word were anchored together and therefore the word's constituent letters were grouped appropriately.

positions on the target word. Early reading time measures such as first fixation duration, single fixation duration and gaze duration all showed significant effects of the dichoptic presentation conditions, with longer times in the congruous and incongruous conditions than the binocular condition. Clearly, the dichoptic manipulation was influential with respect to how long it took participants to read the word. The landing position data were quite different, however. There was a consistent difference of the same magnitude between the landing positions of the left eye and those of the right eye across the binocular, congruous and incongruous conditions. The right eye always landed almost a character further into the word than the left eye. This difference simply reflects the predominance of uncrossed fixations observed in the studies described in the first and second sections of this chapter. Critically, however, the distributions of landing positions on the target word were identical across the dichoptic presentation conditions. Regardless of whether the target word was presented binocularly, congruously or incongruously, the patterns of landing positions for the left eye were identical across conditions, as were the patterns of landing positions for the right eye. These data strongly suggest that saccade metrics associated with targeting the eye to an upcoming word in a sentence were computed on the basis of a unified perceptual representation of that word. Additionally, that unified perceptual representation appears to be attained through the fusion of disparate retinal signals, and is not attained through a process of suppression. Importantly, perceptual unification through fusion is critical to both processes associated with moment-to-moment saccadic control, as well as to successful language comprehension that occurs subsequent to the uptake of visual linguistic information.

Conclusion

To summarize, I have described a series of experiments undertaken in our laboratory to examine binocular coordination during reading. In these studies we have obtained a number of key findings. We have shown that fixation disparity of some magnitude does occur quite frequently during reading. Also, that disparity occurs mainly due to uncrossed fixations, though crossed fixations also occur on a minority of occasions. These effects are prevalent in children as well as adults, with disparity occurring more frequently, and with greater magnitude in children than in adults. Our data raised the question of how the visual system attains a single unified representation of the visual array, and we showed that dichoptically presented words embedded in sentences appear to be fused early during visual processing. Fused visual percepts, or whole word objects, are then used as the basis for computing the metrics required for saccadic targeting.

Acknowledgment

The research described in this chapter was supported by Grants F/00 128/AB and F/00 128/AG from the Leverhulme Trust and by Grant 519168 from the Biotechnology and Biological Sciences Research Council to Simon Liversedge, and by Grant HD26765 from the National Institute of Health to Keith Rayner. The work was entirely collaborative and the author gratefully acknowledges the contribution made by Hazel Blythe, John Findlay, Holly Joseph, Barbara Juhasz, Eugene McSorly, Keith Rayner and Sarah White. I am also thankful to Bob Metcalf for his programming assistance.

References

Blythe, H. I., Liversedge, S. P., Joseph, H. S. S. L., White, S. J., Findlay, J. M., & Rayner, K. (2006). The binocular coordination of eye movements during reading in children and adults. *Vision Research, 46,* 3898-3908.

Fioravanti, F., Inchingolo, P., Pensiero, S., & Spanios, M. (1995). Saccadic eye movement conjugation in children. *Vision Research, 35,* 3217-3228.

Heller, D., & Radach, R. (1999). Eye movements in reading: Are two eyes better than one? In W. Becker, H. Deubel, & T. Mergner (Eds.), *Current oculomotor research: Physiological and psychological aspects* (pp.341-348). New York: Plenum Press.

Juhasz, B. J., Liversedge, S. P., White, S. J., & Rayner, K. (2006). Binocular coordination of the eyes during reading: Word frequency and case alternation affect fixation duration but not fixation disparity. *Quarterly Journal of Experimental Psychology, 59,* 1614-1625.

Liversedge, S. P., Rayner, K., White, S. J., Findlay, J. M., & McSorley, E.

(2006). Binocular coordination of the eyes during reading. *Current Biology, 16,* 1726-1729.

Liversedge, S. P., White, S. J., Findlay, J. M., & Rayner, K. (2006). Binocular coordination of eye movements during reading. *Vision Research, 46,* 2363-2374.

McConkie, G. W., Zola, D., Grimes, J., Kerr, P. W., Bryant, N. R., & Wolff, P. M. (1991). Children's eye movements during reading. In Stein, J.F. (Ed.), *Vision and visual dyslexia* (pp.251-262). London: Macmillan Press.

Rayner, K. (1979). Eye guidance in reading: Fixation locations in words. *Perception, 8,* 21-30.

Yang, Q., & Kapoula, Z. (2003). Binocular coordination of saccades at far and near in children and in adults. *Journal of Vision, 3,* 554-561.

Chapter 6

Saccadic orienting in special populations

Valerie Benson

Much of psychology is about how we make sense of the world in order to interact with our environment. Information about the world arrives via the sense organs and is passed to the brain for processing. The sense organ for vision is the eye, which actively seeks out information in the visual environment to sample. In normal populations this is accomplished by saccadic orienting where the eye moves in a series of fast movements (saccades), interspersed with pauses (fixations), where the eye remains still. The brief pauses allow for detailed inspection of the point under fixation by the high acuity area of the retina known as the fovea. Thus, visual information is acquired during fixations. This stop-start-stop pattern of eye movements appears to be the default strategy to sample the visual environment and this chapter is concerned with how visual information is sampled in the absence of normal eye movement control.

Investigating eye movement control typically involves presenting stimuli on a computer screen with the request to fixate a target as quickly and as accurately as possible. Sometimes participants may be requested to move their eyes in the opposite direction to the target (Anti-Saccade task). Other paradigms require participants to search for a defined target set amidst an array of distractors (Visual Search), or more complex visual information is presented, such as real life scenes, which participants inspect under different instruction. For many low-level, and some higher level oculomotor paradigms, eye movement behavior can be predicted (for normal participants) in terms of saccade onset latencies, directional errors, eye landing positions, and eye scanpaths. Patterns of saccades and fixations can therefore reflect which features of a display drive the sequence of eye movements for a given task, and analysis of eye movements allows us to learn about the influence of different types of visual stimuli on visual and cognitive processing in normal and special populations.

If saccadic orienting is the default strategy for sampling the visual world then one might expect that problems with oculomotor control would result in problems with sampling the visual array, and consequently, problems with perceiving the world. In this chapter, data will be presented from two individual case studies to show, in the first instance, how the saccadic orienting system adapts to operate when there is damage to the muscles that normally allow the eyes to move, and in the second case, how it is affected when there is damage to the brain. Although one cannot extrapolate from individual case studies to the general population at large, findings from individual case studies can inform current theory in an area, and we can learn much about how damage to central or peripheral processing systems affects the ability to sample and perceive the world.

Case study 1

The first case study is of an individual (AI) who, as a result of congenital opthalmoplegia, has been unable to make eye movements from birth. Remarkably, this person is capable of doing most everyday tasks involving visual/cognitive processing without problems. It has recently been shown from a number of investigations that, for AI, the head moves in the same start-stop-start pattern as the eye, and the pattern of head movements for a range of visual/cognitive tasks is the same as that shown by normal participants' eye movement patterns (Gilchrist, Brown, & Findlay, 1997; Gilchrist, Brown, Findlay, & Clarke, 1998; Land, Furneaux, & Gilchrist, 2002). This achievement, it has been suggested, has come about as a result of adaptation of the neurophysiological mechanisms that normally control saccadic eye movements, to control this individual's head movements.

Congenital opthalmoplegia and saccadic orienting

At the time of testing AI was a 21-year-old female undergraduate, reading for a degree in English, who volunteered to take part in a project examining eye movements. AI was unable to participate in this project as she was actually incapable of making eye movements. Medical records reported that AI had a congenital opthalmoplegia. What this means is that although AI was equipped with the set of six extraocular muscles generally needed to move the eyes in the orbit (confirmed by ultrasonic imaging), when AI was born these muscles were thin and fibrotic and as a result she has not been able to make eye movements from birth. Apart from being unable to participate in sporting activities, and not being able to learn to drive, AI lives a normal life and has no problems with most everyday activities.

How can we be sure that AI makes no eye movements?

When normal participants are presented with a large field sinusoidal grating (a vertical stripe pattern moving from left to right) they find it impossible to keep the eyes fixated at the center of the screen, and instead the eyes move with the grating. This is known as an Optokinetic Nystagmus (OKN) response and can be used as a clinical diagnosis for residual eye movement function. AI was tested for an OKN response while her eye movements were recorded using a Dual Purkinjie eye-tracking machine. The records indicated that the standard OKN response was absent and only very small (less than half a degree) drift movements were present. AI's eyes remained fixed at the center of the display.

How does AI accomplish the task of reading?

AI was videoed while she was reading passages of text, and it was apparent that she moved her head across the text in what was thought to be a very similar way to the eye movements made by normal participants when reading. AI's reading speed was recorded for text passages with a range of difficulty levels and her mean reading speed was recorded as 257 words per minute (range 183 to 435). Although this is a relatively slow reading speed, it is within the range for 'normal' readers. In order to determine whether the pattern of head movements of AI were like the eye movements shown for normal populations when reading, her head movements were recorded during reading using a head-mounted search coil. It was found that AI's head movements, although slower, showed the same pattern of saccadic movements and fixation durations upon the text as that which would be expected from 'normal' readers (see Figure 6.1). Analysis of the distributions of 'saccade sizes' and 'fixation durations' showed that they were very similar to those of control participants, and those reported for normal participants (Gilchrist et al., 1997).

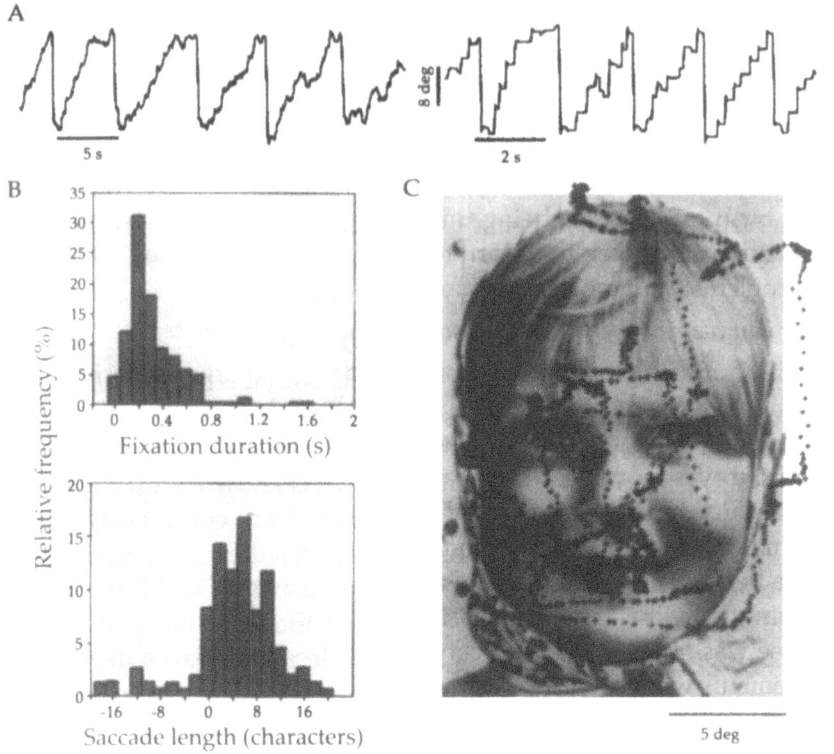

Figure 6.1 (A) head movement records for AI when she reads text and the eye movement records of a control participant reading text, (B) distributions of fixation durations and head movement size during reading the head fixate and (C) head saccade patterns for AI during picture scanning. (Figure reproduced from Gilchrist et al., 1997 with permission from Nature).

Do AI's head movements mimic eye movements in low-level visual paradigms?

AI's head movements were recorded for four robust low-level eye movement paradigms. From previously reported data for normal participants, it was anticipated that there would be automatic effects upon saccadic orienting in each paradigm, and that if AI showed a similar pattern of effects for her head movements, then this would indicate that AI's head movements could be controlled by the same neurophysiological mechanisms that control saccadic eye movements in normal populations.

The gap paradigm (Saslow, 1967) refers to a situation where participants have to saccade to a target presented at a peripheral location, and a central fixation stimulus is either removed prior to the onset of the target, or it remains on the display for some time after the target is presented. Saccade latencies to the target are significantly faster when there is a time gap between the removal of the fixation stimulus and the onset of the target, compared to when the fixation point remains on the display. The effects reflect activity in a region of the Superior Colliculus (SC), a well known mid-brain structure that is involved in the planning of eye movements, and is involved in maintaining fixation. AI's head movements showed a normal 'gap-effect' in this paradigm.

The RDE paradigm (Walker, Deubel, Schneider, and Findlay, 1997) requires participants to saccade to a target that is presented on its own, or accompanied by a distractor presented at a remote location from the target. Saccade latencies are significantly slower for distractor trials compared to single-target trials. This is known as the Remote Distractor Effect (RDE) and it is believed to result from activation in the fixation cells in the SC operating over a wide field. AI's head movements showed the characteristic RDE in this paradigm (Walker et al., 1997).

In the anti-saccade paradigm (Hallett, 1978), in one condition participants simply have to saccade to a peripherally presented target (pro-saccade condition), and in another condition they have to make an eye movement of an equal magnitude and in the opposite direction to the target on its appearance (anti-saccade condition). This is quite a difficult task, and impossible for some clinical populations (Guitton, Buchtel, & Douglas, 1985; Pierrot-Deseilligny, Rivaud, Gaymard, & Agid, 1991). For normal participants longer latencies and more variable landing positions would be expected for the condition where the request is to saccade in the opposite direction to the target. Additionally, it would be expected that saccades would be directed erroneously to the targets on a proportion of trials (about 20 percent). AI's head movements showed that she made the expected proportion of errors, and increased latencies in the anti-saccade, compared to the pro-saccade task.

In the saccadic suppression paradigm, stimuli are presented at the same time as an eye movement is initiated toward a target, and it would be expected that this would result in a reduction in the ability to detect such stimuli, compared to detection rates in trials where no eye movement is generated. When tested in this paradigm, AI showed saccadic suppression, in that her detection rates for a stimulus (a whole display flash) were reduced when she made a head movement, at the same time that the flash was presented, to simple targets located in the periphery.

From these standard visual experimental tasks, it was clearly demonstrated that for each paradigm AI showed a qualitatively similar pattern of head movements to that which has been shown for the eye movements of normal controls in the same paradigms. In the absence of eye movements, the neural mechanisms governing the preparation and initiation of saccades appear, in this case, to have adapted to control the head so that it moves in a stereotypical saccadic fashion.

How does AI perform an everyday task, such as making a cup of tea?

Tea drinking is an important part of the UK culture, and making a cup of tea involves activity in various areas of the brain. In hospitals in the UK a standard assessment for recovery from brain injury is to monitor the ability to 'make a cup of tea'. In order to complete the task successfully one has to locate, recognize, and manipulate the appropriate objects needed to do the job. A sequence of actions has to be performed in a particular order, and eye movement monitoring during a tea making task has shown that, in normal participants, saccadic orienting is used to accomplish the task, and that the eye leads each action by about 0.5 seconds (Land, Mennie, & Rusted, 1999).

AI's head movements were recorded while she made a cup of tea and the data were compared with that collected for three control participants. AI made a similar pattern of head saccades and fixations to the relevant objects in the scene (see Figure 6.2), and the time taken to complete the task was the same as that of the control participants. However, the number of fixations was a third less for AI, and the velocity of the saccades showed that AI was much slower at moving her head relative to those shown for the eye movements of the controls. AI also showed slow drift movements for up to 30degrees per second during fixation periods and this is an unusual finding that was not observed in the control data. It is suggested that this is a strategy adopted by AI to enable the uptake of visual information, albeit at a reduced resolution, to compensate for the slowness of executing head saccades (Land, Furneaux, & Gilchrist, 2002).

What can we conclude from the AI studies?

The original question of interest in this case study was how AI managed to 'see' if she was unable to sample the environment in the normal way, by moving her eyes in the preferred start-stop-start pattern of saccades and fixations. What has been shown in the investigation(s) of AI is that in the absence of eye movements, the head can be used successfully to orient in the same saccadic way as the eye does in normal populations. Moreover, the pattern of head 'saccades' for a range of high and low-level visual cognitive tasks is strikingly similar to eye saccades

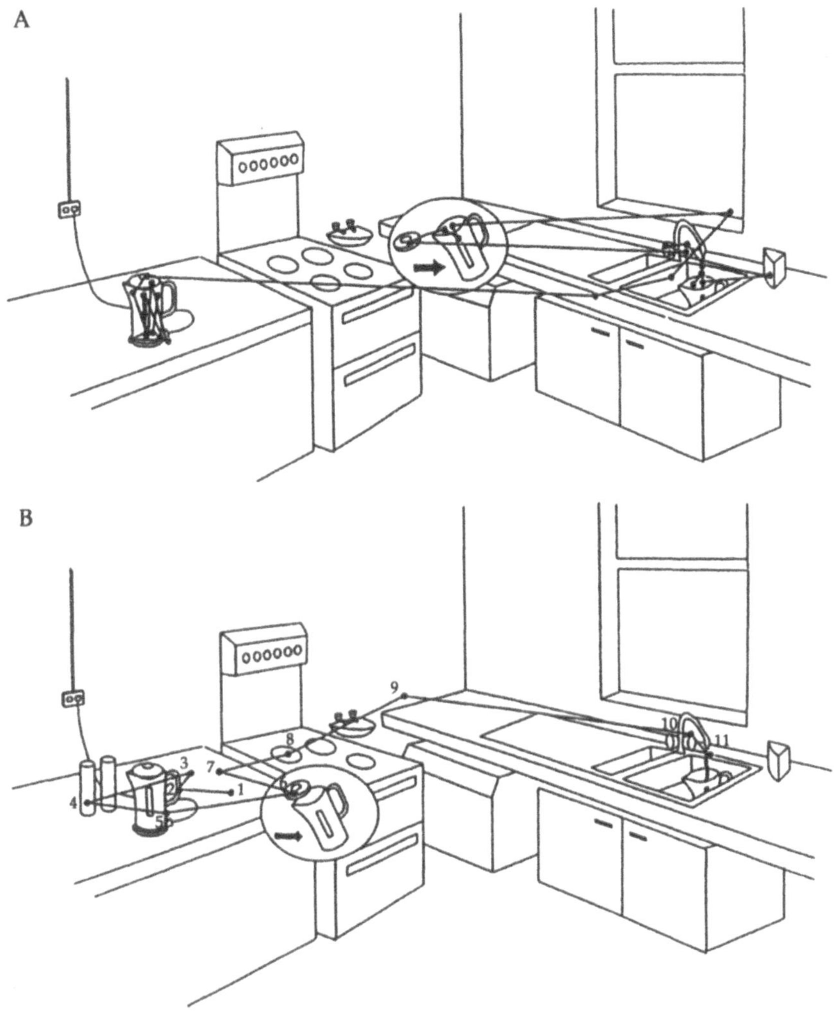

Figure 6.2 (A) eye fixations and gaze shifts in a control participant while making a cup of tea, and (B) eye fixations and gaze shifts for AI (who is only able to move her head for orienting). [Figure reproduced from Land et al., 2002 with permission from Taylor & Francis (UK) Journals].

in normal populations for the same tasks. Thus, this single case study has shown that the saccadic system can adapt to control the head, and although it is not known whether the neural mechanisms involved in the control of eye movements have adapted to control the head movements in AI, there is some neurophysiologial evidence examining combined movements of the eyes and head (gaze shifts) to support this idea, (see Freedman & Sparks, 1997).

It is not yet known whether similar adaptive mechanisms occur for cases of opthalmoplegia that have their onset later in life. Overall, the results from AI provide evidence to suggest that in the absence of the ability to make eye movements, the saccadic orienting system has adapted to control the head, and as such saccadic orienting is the optimal way to sample the visual environment.

Case study 2

The second case study is of an individual (MB), who as a result of damage to the right side of his brain following a stroke, is unable to always detect and perceive information presented to his left hemifield. This condition is known as unilateral neglect or hemi-neglect, and is observed most frequently and is of longer duration following a stroke to the right hemisphere of the brain (Halligan, Marshall, & Wade, 1989) resulting most commonly therefore, in the left side of space being 'neglected'. It is a condition in which a patient fails to respond to, orient towards, or report, stimuli located on the side of space contralesional to the brain damage in the absence of sensory motor deficits (Heilman, 1979). Although hemi-neglect does not result from a failure to scan the contralesional side of space, patients can show a range of deficits in making contralesional saccadic eye movements (e.g. Girotti, Casazza, Musicco, & Avanzini, 1983; Ishiai, Furukawa & Tsukagoshi, 1987; Walker & Findlay, 1996). This section of the chapter reports data from a detailed examination of eye-movement patterns in a single case study of neglect using both low and high-level visual cognitive tasks. These include the presentation of very simple single and double targets in either or both hemifields in order to elicit a Remote Distractor Effect (RDE), an examination of single sentence reading to investigate whether MB shows any systematic ordered scanning behavior during this high-level cognitive task, and the examination of patterns of saccades and fixations for scene inspection under different instruction. The data provide a detailed description of saccadic eye movement control in a participant with hemi-neglect, for a range of tasks that demand different levels of visual and cognitive processing.

There is some evidence to suggest that, although there may be a lack of awareness for visual information in the 'neglected' field, there is processing of this information at some level (Marshall & Halligan, 1988). The following case study reports experiments (Benson, Milner, Iestwaart, & MacIntosh, 2006) that examined oculomotor control in an individual with hemi-neglect to investigate whether there was any preserved processing of stimuli in an individual, in the absence of awareness of those stimuli, and whether distortions in perception for contralesional stimuli are reflected in impairments in the saccadic orienting system for low-level and higher level visual/cognitive tasks.

Visual neglect and saccadic orienting

At the time of testing MB was a 46-year-old left-handed male who had suffered a stroke in September 2005. A CT scan taken shortly after hospital admittance showed a large (4 cm) intracerebral haematoma with haemorrhagic stroke in the temperoparietal region of the right hemisphere. MB was screened six months post stroke, and showed visual neglect on a range of standard screening tests, including cancellation tasks, scene copying, and line bisection. Figure 6.3 (A) shows some of MB's screening data that show clear effects typical of those observed in hemi-neglect patients. For example, when asked to cross out all the lines on a piece of paper, MB fails to cross out those lines at the far left of the

A B C

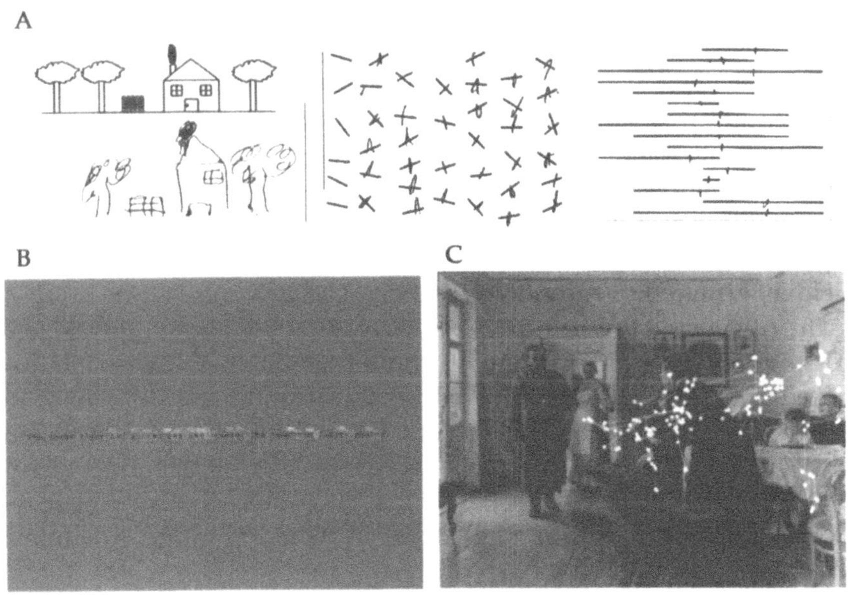

Figure 6.3 (A) screening data for MB for a cancellation task, a line bi-section task and a scene copying task, (B) the number, location and duration of fixations that were made by MB when reading a single sentence, and (C) the scanpath made by MB as he inspected the 'Repin' picture under free viewing conditions. (The Repin picture was downloaded from http://www.abcgallery.com/R/repin/repin46.JPG). (*See Plate 2.*)

paper, and when asked to copy a scene into the space below the scene, MB omits items from the scene that were on the left, and some left sides of objects in the scene, even when these were not presented to the left of MB's midline.

Does MB show any implicit processing for stimuli in his neglected field?

It is common for 'neglect' participants to be able to report a single stimulus presented for quite brief durations in their right or left visual field. However, when they are presented simultaneously with one stimulus in each hemifield, they report seeing only the one in the right visual field (e.g. Mattingley, Robertson, & Driver, 1998). This is known as extinction. To test whether MB showed extinction, single or bi-lateral targets were presented at five degrees to the left or the right from the center of the display for varying durations (50-5000 ms), and MB had to verbally report what he had 'seen'. This verbal detection task revealed that at presentation durations of 1 s MB detected 100 percent of single right targets, 77 percent of single left targets, and 44 percent of bi-lateral targets. At durations of 400 ms and below MB detected 100 percent of single right targets, no single left targets, and no bi-lateral targets. The verbal detection task confirmed that MB was unaware of single left targets when these were presented for less than 400 ms. At 800 ms his detection rate was still under 50 percent for single left targets and he reported only the right target when presented with bi-lateral targets at that presentation duration. MB does not show the classic extinction pattern in this task, but his self report measures have allowed us some insight into how long stimuli have to be presented in MB's 'neglected' field for him to show awareness of their existence.

In order to assess whether MB showed any evidence for implicit processing of stimuli presented in his contralesional field of view, he was tested using the RDE paradigm (as previously outlined). Since the RDE occurs when participants are instructed which target to saccade to, and also when they are free to move their eyes to either target under bi-lateral presentation, it has been assumed that the effect is an automatic reflexive property of the saccadic system (Walker, Kentridge, & Findlay, 1995).

Assessment of RDE magnitudes in MB would show whether low-level oculomotor behavior in the RDE paradigm was normal in the absence of conscious awareness of the contralesional stimuli. Although some work has been conducted in this area (e.g. Walker & Findlay, 1996; Brown, Walker, Gray, & Findlay, 1999), surprisingly the studies have not attempted to manipulate attentional orienting. Since hemi-neglect is thought to reflect an attentional bias toward the ipsilesional side of space, the RDE paradigm provides an opportunity to examine in detail the effects of the prior allocation of attention to either ipsilesional or contralesional space, on saccadic orienting in a case of hemi-neglect. Additionally, this task enabled an evaluation of whether there was any dissociation between the saccadic orienting system and conscious awareness for stimuli presented in the 'neglected' hemifield of MB. For example, if MB showed preserved processing of contralesional stimuli in the RDE paradigm this would provide evidence that in the absence of awareness of such stimuli, those stimuli still produced a behavioral effect.

MB was presented with small black square targets, positioned at 5° eccentricity from the center of the display, and instructed to look at the target as quickly and accurately as he could. On some trials a distractor (also a small black square) was presented at the same time as the target, and this was positioned in the hemifield opposite to the target at an equal eccentricity from the display midline. For each experimental condition there were three target types, single target on the right, single target on the left, and a bi-lateral target (one in each hemifield). Whenever a single target appeared MB had to look at it, but before each block of trials MB was given a different instruction for the bi-lateral target trials. MB was instructed to always go to the right bi-lateral target for one block of trials, always go to the left bi-lateral target for another block of trials, and for a third block of trials MB was free to saccade to either target when there were two possible targets to choose from.

MB did not show the characteristic RDE effect of an increase in saccade onset latencies for bi-lateral target presentation (compared to single target presentation) when distractors were presented in his contralesional hemifield and in his ipsilesional hemifield, although there were very few occasions in which MB moved his eyes to the left target in bilateral trials in this condition. This suggests that there was no implicit processing of the distractor in the contralesional hemifield.

What MB did show was a pattern of overall slower saccades to left targets, and these saccades were smaller in amplitude compared to saccades made to targets on the right. Additionally, MB was unable to ignore the distractor in his good hemifield when he was instructed to go left in the bi-lateral target presentation condition, and he moved his eyes to the distractor (positioned in his right hemifield) on 89 percent of the trials where a target and distractor were simultaneously presented. Similarly, in the condition where he was free to go to either possible target, he moved his eyes to the right target on 88 percent of trials. These data show that the attentional bias to the right shown by MB appears not to be under voluntary control.

However, what is of special interest here is to compare MB's responses in the verbal detection task with his saccade onset latencies in the RDE task. This comparison showed that although MB could not verbally report single left targets in his contralesional hemifield at durations of 400 ms; in the RDE task, eye movement recordings demonstrated that he was able to make saccades to single left targets, and that the average latency for those saccades was 313 ms. This means that MB is capable of moving his eyes to a target for which he shows no awareness in the verbal detection task, at the same presentation duration.

Taken together, the findings from the RDE task and the verbal detection task reveal an interesting dissociation between conscious awareness for visual information in MB's neglected field and saccadic orienting responses to that information. Although MB does not show the characteristic RDE effect of an increase in saccade latencies for trials where the target is accompanied by a distractor in the opposite hemifield, MB is still able to make saccades to single left stimuli, and furthermore the mean latency for such saccades is around 300 ms, at which duration he is unable to verbally detect such stimuli. This shows that the saccadic orienting system is responding to stimuli for which MB has no conscious visual perception.

How does MB accomplish the task of reading?

Neglect dyslexia is the term given to observed errors made in reading, where either whole words, or the left part of words are mispronounced or omitted (Ellis, Flude, & Young, 1987) and it is established that hemineglect can result in this condition. Anecdotally, MB has reported that he is an avid reader of novels. Given that MB neglects information on the left, how is he able to accomplish the task of reading novels? The points of interest in this study were whether MB exhibited a normal pattern of saccades for reading, and if not, could he comprehend what he read? To investigate these questions MB was presented with 20 single sentences, one at a time, positioned in the center of a computer screen, and he had to read each one silently while his eye movements were recorded. A comprehension question was asked at the end of each sentence. For ten of the sentences the information needed to answer the question correctly was positioned on the far left of the screen (at the beginning of the sentence), and for the other ten sentences the information was on the far right of the display (at the end of the sentence).

MB made no errors to the comprehension questions when the information required to answer these was on the right of the display, but answered only half of them correctly when the information was on the left of the display. MB's eye movement recordings showed an abnormal pattern of saccades during reading, revealing that he was unable to locate the beginning of a sentence with his first saccade, that he made fewer saccades to the left side of the display, but when he did fixate the left side of the display his fixation durations were longer compared to those made to the portion of the sentence on the right side of the display. Furthermore, MB's incorrect answers suggest that he made inferences related to those portions of the sentence he actually read. Also of interest is the observation that he makes many more regressive movements back along the sentence, compared to an age-matched control, presumably in an attempt to find what he considers to be a suitable word from which to start reading and making sense of the sentence. For some sentences the information on the left of the screen needed to answer the question was actually fixated, but MB still gave the wrong answer.

In normal populations there is a very stereotypical pattern of eye movements during reading (Rayner, 1998). The pattern of saccades and fixations is influenced by a variety of linguistic variables. MB's abnormal pattern of saccadic orienting in this task shows that he is not able to move his eyes using the optimal strategy for reading, but that in an attempt to comprehend what he is reading, MB makes repetitive regressive saccades. He is not able to read sequentially from left to right. Figure 6.3 (B) shows the pattern of fixations made by MB while reading one of the sentences where he answered the comprehension question incorrectly. MB did not fixate the critical information in this sentence. The question he was asked was "What ignored the tourists?" and MB responded, "The people lying in the sun."

MB was also asked to read sentences out loud, and his performance on this task was quite good, although he made some left word omissions, and mispronounced the left portions of some of the words presented on the far left of the display. Given that we know that MB was unable to locate the beginning of the sentence, and that he showed much more frequent regressive movements back and forth along the sentence, this seems to be a remarkable achievement.

Can MB orient to critical information presented in scenes?

In a classic study (Yarbus, 1967) participants were presented with the same scene (the 'unexpected visitor' painted by the Russian artist Repin) several times, with a different inspection instruction for each presentation. What Yarbus showed, using fairly primitive eye movement recording techniques, was that a different pattern of eye movements was exhibited for each inspection instruction. This study revealed what is known in much more detail today, namely, that patterns of saccades and fixations revealed by eye-movement recordings can provide an online measure of the cognitive processing associated with different tasks.

The question of interest was whether MB could make eye movements to fixate some critical information in his neglected field if he was made aware that the information was located there. The Repin picture was presented to MB several times for a period of 20 s, and the same inspection instructions as those used in the Yarbus study were given to MB. However, in addition, the picture was flipped in the horizontal plane for half the trials such that the 'unexpected visitor' appeared on the left half of the time, and on the right of the picture for the other half of the presentations. MB was informed of the manipulation prior to testing.

Plots of MB's scan paths during each inspection showed that he was able to scan and fixate both sides of the picture, although there were occasions where he failed to fixate relevant items/people in the scene. However, one of the most interesting aspects of the data was that although MB was able to scan and fixate the left half of the scene, this was never done in an immediate way. For example, for the first trial, which was a free viewing inspection of the scene MB scanned the right half of the picture for over 10 s before he made a fixation to the left to begin inspecting the 'unexpected visitor' who was positioned on the left of the scene in that trial. By contrast, a control participant with right brain damage but no hemi-neglect fixated the 'unexpected visitor' in the same position and under the same inspection instruction, in less than 2 s.

Even when MB was given the same instruction but presented with the picture in both orientations, he was unable to locate and fixate the relevant information quickly. For example, for one of the instructions the display was presented in its normal orientation, and at the end of the session, after a break, it was presented again in the opposite orientation to the first presentation. For both of these presentations MB and a control participant were asked to "estimate how long they thought the 'unexpected visitor' had been absent for". There was a qualitative difference between MB and the control participant in the pattern of saccades for each viewing. An analysis over the time of each trial showed that regardless of orientation, the control participant fixated the 'unexpected visitor' in less than 2 s. For MB, when the unexpected visitor appeared on the right of the display (first presentation) MB fixated him within 2 s, he also made no saccades to the far left of the display and he failed to fixate the two children sitting at a table in that location during that presentation. When the unexpected visitor appeared on the left of the display (second presentation) MB saccaded to and fixated every person in the picture. However, in this condition MB took over 8 s to fixate the 'unexpected visitor.' What this shows is that MB is unable to move to the critical information in the scene immediately, despite consciously knowing the location of the critical information based on previous alternating picture orientations.

What can we conclude from the MB studies?

The original question of interest in this case study was to investigate whether MB showed any preserved processing of stimuli, in the absence of awareness of such stimuli. The RDE paradigm was used to assess this and the findings supported previous work which shows that hemi-neglect does not produce the characteristic RDE. However, the saccade onset latencies for single left targets in this task provide evidence of a dissociation between MB's perceptual and saccadic orienting systems, since he was clearly able to move his eyes to targets in his contralesional hemifield faster than at presentation durations where he was unable to verbally report such targets.

A further question of interest was whether distortions in perception for contralesional stimuli would be reflected in impairments in the saccadic orienting system for some higher level visual/cognitive tasks. This was the case for both reading and scene perception where MB showed abnormal patterns of orienting in each task.

Conclusion

Two very different case studies have been presented to show how the saccadic orienting system operates when there is damage to either central or peripheral components of the system. In the absence of eye movements (Case study 1) the head can adapt to function in a saccadic fashion. The work with AI provides evidence to suggest that saccadic orienting is the optimal way to sample the visual environment. In the absence of awareness (Case study 2), the saccadic system is unable to sample the visual environment in the normal way and there is no evidence for preserved processing of contralesional stimuli. Data from MB show defective saccadic orienting for a range of tasks, and provide evidence to support the view that not only is an intact saccadic orienting system needed to sample the world, but that saccadic orienting may well be central to vision itself.

References

Benson, V., Milner, A. D., Iestwaart, M., & MacIntosh, R. (2006, June). *Eye movements in a case of visual neglect*. Paper presented at the 2nd International China Conference on Eye Movements, Tianjin Normal University, China.

Brown, V., Walker, R., Gray, C., & Findlay, J. M. (1999). Limb activation and the rehabilitation of unilateral neglect: Evidence of task specific effects. *Neurocase, 5,* 129-142.

Ellis, A. W., Flude, B. M., & Young, A. W. (1987). "Neglect dyslexia" and the early visual processing of letters in words and nonwords. *Cognitive Neuropsychology, 4,* 439-464.

Freedman, E. G., & Sparks, D. L. (1997). Activity of cells in the deeper layers of the superior colliculus of the rhesus monkey: Eevidence for a gaze displacement command. *Journal of Neurophysiology, 78,* 1669-1690.

Gilchrist, A. D., Brown, V., & Findlay, J. M. (1997). Saccades without eye movements. *Nature, 390,* 130-131.

Gilchrist, I. D., Brown,V., Findlay J. M., & Clarke, M. P. (1998). Using the eye movement system to control the head. *Proceedings of the Royal Society B: Biological Sciences, 265,* 1831-1836.

Girotti, F., Casazza, M., Musicco, M., & Avanzini, G. (1983). Oculomotor disorders in cortical lesions in man: The role of unilateral neglect. *Neuropsychologia, 5,* 543-553.

Guitton, D., Buchtel, H. A., & Douglas, R. M. (1985). Frontal lobe lesions in man cause difficulties in suppressing reflexive glances and in generating goal-directed saccades. *Experimental Brain Research, 58,* 455-472.

Hallett, P. E. (1978). Primary and secondary saccades to goals defined by instructions. *Vision Research, 18,* 1279-1296.

Halligan, P. W., Marshall, J. C., & Wade, D. T. (1989). Visuospatial neglect: Underlying factors and test sensitivity. *Lancet, 2,* 908-911.

Halligan, P. W., & Marshall, J. C. (1993). The history and clinical presentation of neglect. In I. H. Robertson, & J. C. Marshall, (Eds.), *Unilateral neglect: Clinical and experimental studies* (pp.1139-1167). Hillsdale, N J : Lawrence Erlbraum Associates.

Heilman, K. M. (1979). Neglect and related disorders. In K. M. Heilman, & E. Valenstein (Eds.), *Clinical neuropsychology*. New York: Oxford University Press.

Ishiai, S., Furukawa, T., & Tsukagoshi, H. (1987). Eye-fixation patterns in homonymous hemianopia and unilateral spatial neglect. *Neuropsychologia, 25*, 675-679.

Land, M. F., Mennie, N., & Rusted, J. (1999). The roles of vision and eye movements in the control of activities in daily living. *Perception, 28*, 1311-1328.

Land, M. F., Furneaux, S. M., & Gilchrist, I. D. (2002). The organisation of visually mediated actions in a subject without eye movements. *Neurocase, 8*, 80-87.

Marshall, J. C., & Halligan, P. W. (1988). Blindsight and insight in visuospatial neglect. *Nature, 336*, 766-767.

Mattingley, J. B., Robertson, I. H., & Driver, J. (1998). Modulation of covert visual attention by hand movement: Evidence from parietal extinction after right hemisphere damage. *Neurocase, 4*, 245-253.

Pierrot-Deseilligny, C., Rivaud, S., Gaymard, B., & Agid, Y. (1991). Cortical control of reflexive visually-guided saccades. *Brain, 114*, 1473-1485.

Rayner, K. (1998). Eye movements in reading and information processing: 20 years of research. *Psychological Bulletin, 124*, 372-422.

Saslow, M. G. (1967). Effects of components of displacement-step stimuli upon latency for saccadic eye movement. *Journal of the Optical Society of America, 57*, 1030-1033.

Walker, R., & Findlay, J. M. (1996). Saccadic eye movement programming in unilateral neglect. *Neuropsychologia, 34*, 493-508.

Walker, R., Kentridge, R. W., & Findlay, J. M. (1995). Independent contributions of the orienting of attention, fixation offset and bi-lateral stimulation on human saccadic latencies. *Experimental Brain Research. 103*, 294-310.

Walker, R., Deubel, H., Schneider,W. X., & Findlay, J. M. (1997). The effect of remote distractors on saccade programming: Evidence for an extended fixation zone. *Journal of Neurophysiology, 78*, 1108-1119.

Yarbus, A. (1967). *Eye movements and vision*. New York: Plenum.

Chapter 7

Using eye movements to understand complex visual comparisons

Kyle R. Cave, Andrew L. Cohen, Caren M. Rotello, Anthony McCaffrey, Michael G. Ross, Min Zeng, Matthew Zivot, Xingshan Li, and Kris Evans

Much of visual cognition relies on a core ability to encode information from complex visual patterns, store it, and compare it against other visual patterns encountered later. In the study reported in this chapter, we explored the encoding and comparison of visual patterns. The memory component was minimized because the patterns to be compared were presented simultaneously, side by side. Eye movements were tracked during the comparison to provide information about the comparisons as they proceeded. Eye movements were the focus of this study because of their potential to reveal whether the visual patterns were compared holistically, as complete units, or whether they were broken down into component parts and compared in a more piecemeal fashion. If the comparison is done piece by piece, then the eye movements should also provide evidence as to how the patterns are broken down for comparison.

The stimuli to be compared in this task were pairs of abstract patterns. Across different trials, the number of components in the patterns varied, as did the spatial relationships among them. In addition to these two factors, we also varied the orientation of one pattern relative to the other on some trials, which makes mental rotation relevant to the task. The ability to compare rotated shapes was first explored by Shepard and Metzler (1971), and since then a long series of studies has explored different aspects of mental rotation. Shepard and Metzler's main finding, replicated many times, is that the time to compare two objects increases with their degree of rotational offset.

Just and Carpenter (1976) used the mental rotation comparison task while tracking eye movements. They found that the eyes moved back and forth multiple times between the two shapes to be compared, and that the number of saccades from one shape to the other increased with the difference in orientation between the two shapes. Based on a subjective categorization of the eye movement patterns into different stages, they concluded that there were many eye movements back and forth between corresponding parts of the two objects, suggesting a systematic part-by-part comparison process (see Hakki et al., this volume, for further discussion).

Most of the comparison stimuli in mental rotation tasks have been objects (letters, 3-dimensional shapes). More recently, a handful of studies have considered mental rotation tasks with complex scenes, such as an array of objects (Diwadkar & McNamara, 1997) or a desktop scene (Nakatani, Pollatsek, & Johnson, 2002; Nakatani & Pollatsek, 2004).

Diwadkar and McNamara (1997) had subjects learn an array of objects as perceived from one orientation. They then presented subjects with a test display that had been rotated horizontally (as if the subjects' position at a table had changed). On some trials, some of the objects' relative positions had been changed, and subjects made same-different decisions. Reaction times were a linear function of angle of rotation of the test display. Although Diwadkar and McNamara did not record eye movements in their task, Nakatani and colleagues did. They presented subjects with complex study scenes (schematic desktops) and rotated comparison scenes. The comparison scene could be rotated along one of 4 axes (x, y, z, and an oblique axis). In addition, the changed scenes differed from the study scenes in one of two ways: either the locations of two objects were exchanged, or objects were themselves rotated. There was no simple relationship between angle of rotation and reaction time. Moreover, their eye-movement data indicated that subjects did not engage in any sort of analogue mental rotation until very late in the trial. Instead, Nakatani and Pollatsek (2004) argued that subjects mainly determined their same-different decisions by evaluating the positions of the objects from three perspectives: viewer-centered, desk-centered, and object-centered. The last of these was the least reliable, and the most likely to be followed up with a second, "checking" stage of mental comparison involving mental rotation.

The results of Nakatani's experiments were fairly complex, reflecting the complex comparison of the perception of the test stimulus and memory for the study stimulus. To make the problem more tractable, we minimized the memory requirement and focused on the actual comparison process itself that allows subjects to decide whether two displays are the same or not. We also eliminated rotations in depth and included only rotations in the picture plane.

Experiment

On each of the 540 trials of the experiment, subjects viewed one pair of stimuli, with one on the left and one on the right, separated by a line. Each of the two patterns fit within a square that was 13.79° of visual angle across, and there was a 3.47° space between these two squares. Subjects fixated at the center of the display before the stimuli appeared, but were free to move their eyes and look for as long as they liked once the stimuli appeared. They rated the similarity between the two stimuli on a scale of 1 (low) to 6 (identical); they were given no instructions about which aspects of the patterns they should consider when making their ratings.

Each of the two stimuli was a pattern created by randomly positioning a set of circles, or "nodes", and connecting some node pairs with straight lines. The stimuli appeared in black on a white background. Figure 7.1 shows an example of a stimulus pair.

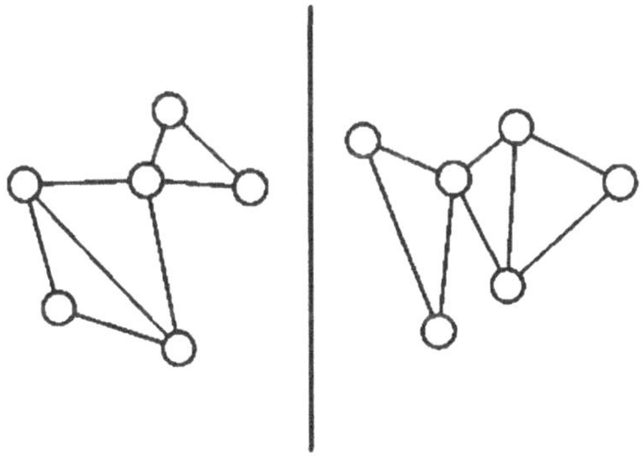

Figure 7.1 Example stimulus pair

Each stimulus pattern had four, six, or eight nodes; both stimuli in a pair had the same number of nodes but varied in the number and pattern of connections (lines) between nodes. The two stimuli presented on each trial could be identical, generated independently, or, to keep the comparison from being trivially easy, they could differ in one of three ways. First, one stimulus could be rotated relative to the other by 60°, 120°, 180°, 240°, or 300°. Second, some of the nodes' locations could be moved, or "perturbed," from one pattern to the other. None, half (randomly selected), or all nodes could be perturbed. Third, the stimuli could be subject to both perturbation and orientation changes. The three levels of perturbation (none, half, all) were equally represented across trials and were fully crossed with the six rotations and the three levels of node number. The number of nodes, the amount of rotation, and the amount of perturbation varied randomly from trial to trial. Finally, for some pairs of stimuli the two patterns were generated independently. They had the same number of nodes, but varied in the number and pattern of connections between nodes.

Subjects' eye movements were recorded using a 500 Hz EyeLink II head-mounted system, which was calibrated every 180 trials or as needed.

Ratings

The similarity ratings that the subjects assigned to each stimulus pair give clues to how they performed the comparison task. The ratings primarily depended on the amount of perturbation between one pattern and the other within the pair, as shown in Figure 7.2. Orientation had a much weaker effect on the ratings. The pairs with no orientation difference were rated as somewhat more similar than the others. Among the pairs with an orientation difference, the ratings were about the same whether the difference was 60° or 180°, as shown in Figure 7.3. Thus, to a large extent, subjects were generalizing across different orientations when assessing similarity.

Fixated locations

As the two patterns were being compared, there were numerous fixations on both stimuli, but the fixations were not evenly distributed across the entire pattern. On many trials, multiple fixations would be lo-

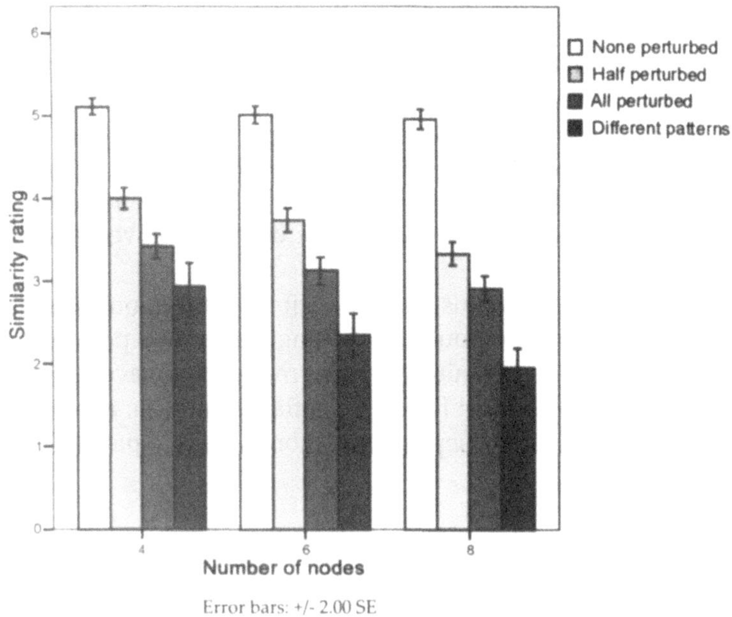

Figure 7.2 The effect of node position perturbation on similarity ratings

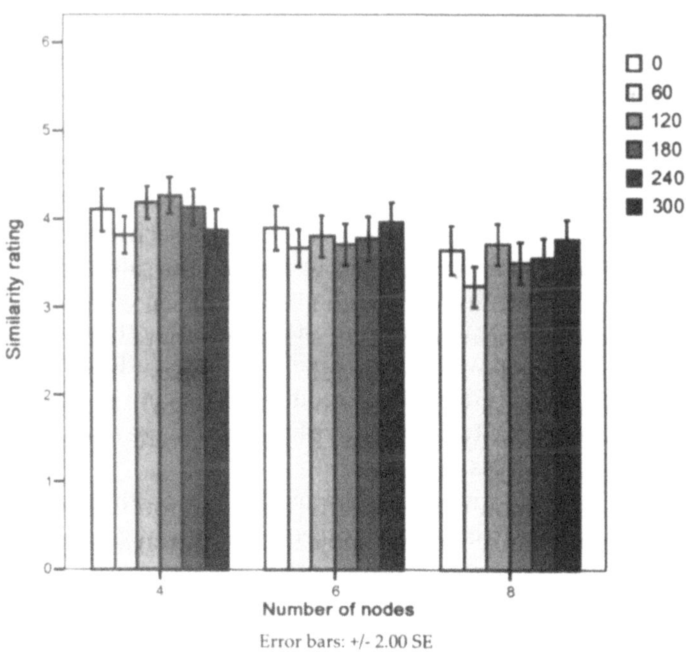

Figure 7.3 The effect of rotation on similarity ratings

cated in one region of a pattern, whereas other large regions of the pattern were never fixated. There tended to be more fixations in the upper regions of the display than in the lower region, and more fixations near the midline separating the two patterns. Together, these biases result in a concentration of fixations in the upper right corner of the left pattern, and in the upper left corner of the right pattern. This fixation pattern minimizes the lengths of the saccades between patterns, although it is not clear why the top part of the display is favored over the bottom.

The absence of fixations in large regions of the stimulus patterns suggests that, within the bounds of a single stimulus pattern, acuity did not pose a major constraint on performance. However, if the fixations are not driven by a need for high spatial resolution, then it is not clear why there are so many separate fixations within a pattern.

Saccade types

Recall that the goal of this experiment was to use eye movements to determine how complex patterns are compared. We hypothesized that subjects would use saccades within a pattern to gather spatial information about that pattern, and would then saccade to the other stimulus pattern to make mental comparisons. To test this idea, we categorized the saccades into "within" saccades, which started and ended within a single pattern on one side of the display, and "cross" saccades, which started in one pattern and crossed the midline to end in the other pattern. There was an average of about 4 to 6 cross saccades on each trial, so that the number of cross saccades was about the same as the number of nodes in each stimulus. This high number of saccades suggests that the comparison is done in a series of steps, and that the number of necessary steps increased with the complexity of the patterns. The average number of within saccades ranged from 6 to 12, again depending on the number of nodes in the two patterns. Thus, there were almost two within saccades for every cross saccade.

Given the large amount of eye traffic back and forth between the two patterns, we might surmise that subjects are splitting the patterns into separate parts or regions, and comparing the regions separately. This regional approach is a bit difficult to reconcile with the observation that many regions received no fixations, but nonetheless we tested this possibility by looking at the beginning and end points of the cross saccades.

We identified "corresponding" cross saccades, as those that start at one location on one pattern and end near the corresponding location in the other pattern. The idea was that saccades to the corresponding location in the other stimulus would be made during detailed stimulus comparisons.

One pattern could be rotated relative to the other, and the locations of individual nodes could be perturbed. Nonetheless, the two stimuli were topologically equivalent, so it was possible to identify the (X, Y) coordinates in one stimulus that were equivalent to the coordinates (X′, Y′) in the other. For each stimulus pair, we used a warping algorithm to determine the correspondence-mapping between the points in the two patterns (see Figure 7.4). A saccade was labeled as a "corresponding" cross saccade if its endpoint was within 80 pixels of the location that corresponded to its beginning point; the 80 pixels allowed for the possibility of imperfectly-targeted saccades. These corresponding saccades linked one part of one pattern with the matching part of the other pattern.

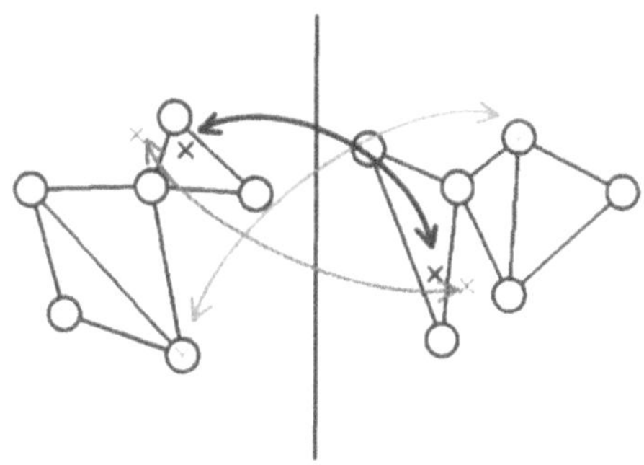

Figure 7.4 The warping algorithm is used to rotate, squeeze, and stretch the pattern on one side to match the pattern on the other side. Once this mapping between the two patterns is established, then for any point on one side, the algorithm can identify the corresponding point on the other side.

Figure 7.5 shows the mean number of corresponding, non-corresponding cross saccades, and within saccades, as a function of the number of nodes in each pattern of the pair. Of the four to six cross saccades in each trial, about two are corresponding saccades, and this number remains fairly constant across patterns of different sizes. Adding more nodes to the patterns increases the number of within saccades and non-corresponding cross saccades, but not the number of corresponding cross saccades.

The relatively constant number of corresponding saccades across trials, and the large regions of the stimuli that were never fixated at all,

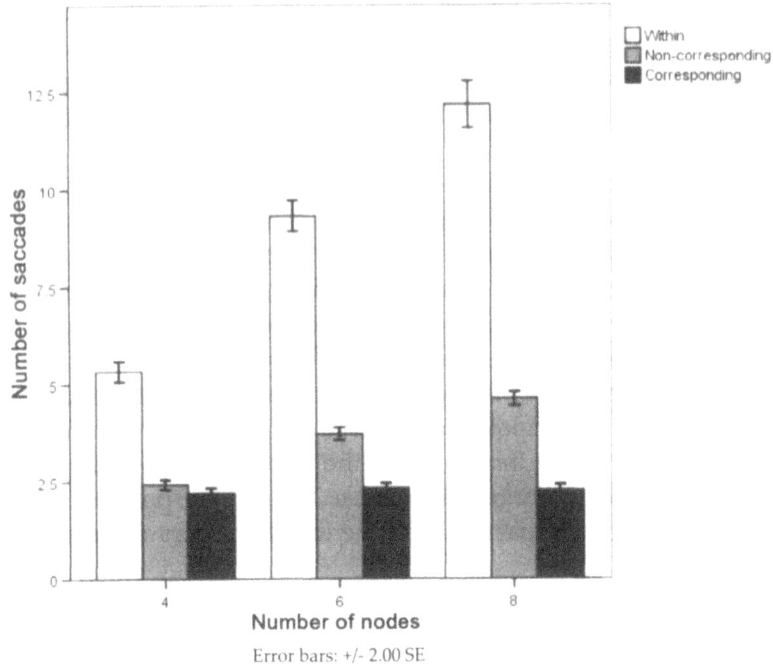

Figure 7.5 The mean number of within, corresponding, and non-corresponding cross saccades as a function of the number of nodes within each pattern

suggest that subjects were not engaged in a systematic region-by-region comparison of the pairs of stimuli. One challenge that we faced in interpreting these data is that we had no clear idea what the eye movements would look like in the absence of a cognitive goal to rate the similarity of the structures. In other words, were those corresponding saccades reflective of meaningful cognitive strategy on the part of the subjects, or were they the result of fairly random eye movements?

To address this question, we ran a simple computer simulation to estimate the pattern of fixations that would emerge at random, in the absence of information from any particular stimulus pair. Determining chance behavior requires some understanding of the probability distribution of fixations over the entire visual display. We chose to estimate this distribution by creating a bivariate histogram of the x and y locations of all subjects' fixations across all probe trials. This approach deliberately ignores information about the stimulus as well as any individual differences that might exist. We then sampled simulated fixations from the resulting probability distribution; a simulated trial for 4 node stimuli included 11 locations sampled from the distribution, a number approximately equal to the average number of fixations for displays of that size. Simulations of stimuli with more nodes included a greater number of sampled locations. These randomly chosen "fixations" were then analyzed for the number of corresponding saccades; our expectation was that the real data would show more corresponding saccades than the simulations of chance behavior.

The simulation led to two informative results. First, the simulation produced 1-2 corresponding saccades on an average trial, just about the same number as our subjects produced. We found this result quite surprising, considering that the simulated fixations ignored all stimulus information. Second, the simulation exhibited a peculiar rotational asymmetry that had also been observed in the human data. In both the human and simulation data, 4- and 6-node graphs yielded the smallest number of corresponding saccades when they differed by 120 degrees of rotation. This result indicates that a significant feature of the rotational variation in corresponding saccades was due to the global spatial distribution of the fixations (concentrated towards the upper middle of the screen) rather than properties of the stimulus graphs themselves.

This simple model lacks any mechanism for identifying corresponding locations across the two patterns, yet it produces a pattern of corresponding saccades that is similar to the patterns produced by our subjects. Given the simulation results, we conclude that the number of corresponding saccades that we find in the human data does not indicate a concerted effort to link corresponding parts of the two regions with a single saccade.

Other factors affecting eye movements and response times

The results summarized so far do not reveal a well-orchestrated strategy that is targeting fixations to precise locations. Nonetheless, the fixations are affected by a number of stimulus properties.

Number of nodes

Each pattern could have 4, 6, or 8 nodes, and the two patterns in a pair always had the same number of nodes. Response times were longer for patterns that have more nodes and are thus more complex. When there were more nodes in the display, there were more fixations and less time spent on each fixation, as shown in Figures 7.6 and 7.7.

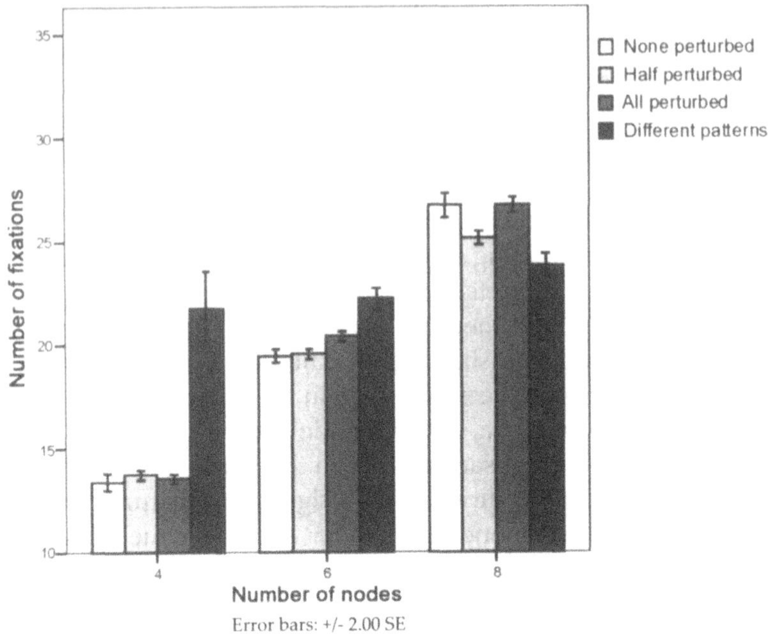

Figure 7.6 The number of fixations per stimulus pair as a function of the number of nodes and amount of perturbation

Perturbation

Recall that, for the non-random stimulus pairs, none, half, or all of the nodes were perturbed on each trial. Those pairs with half the nodes perturbed produced longer response times, more fixations, and longer fixation durations than those with no perturbation. However, as can be seen in Figures 7.6 and 7.7, perturbing all the nodes did not have much more consequence than perturbing half of them. Making local changes within a pattern does make the task more difficult, but there is little difference between moving half the nodes and moving all of them.

Interestingly, perturbation increases the number of within saccades more than the number of cross saccades, as shown in Figure 7.8. Apparently perturbation does not increase the number of required comparisons, but it does increase the degree to which a single pattern is scrutinized. Although perturbation does not affect the number of corresponding cross saccades, it does substantially increase the time necessary to complete a trial once the first corresponding saccade has been made, and has a weaker effect on the time to make the first corresponding saccade once the trial has begun (see Figure 7.9.)

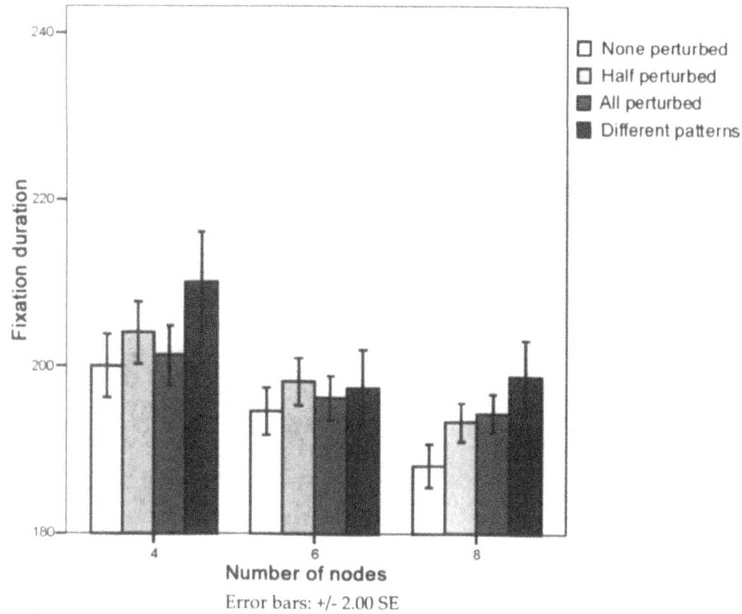

Figure 7.7 Average fixation duration as a function of the number of nodes and amount of perturbation

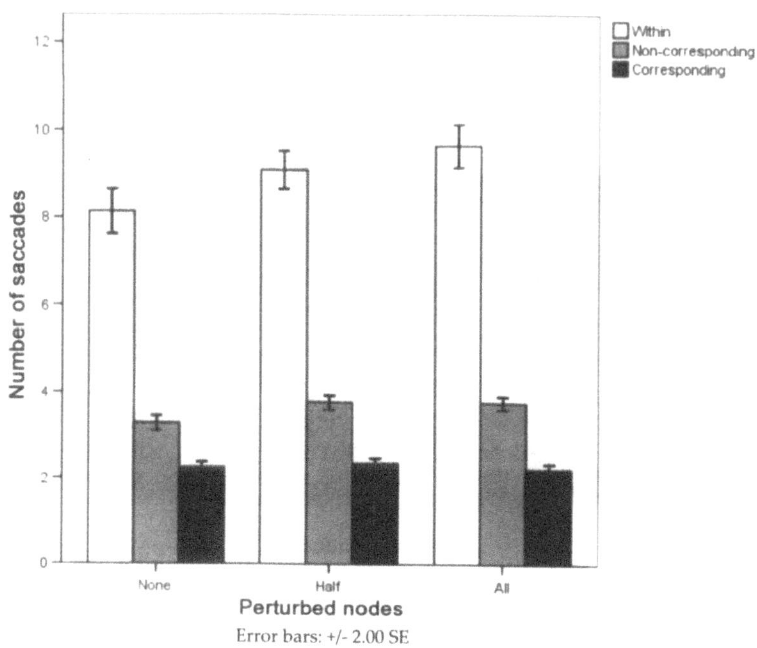

Figure 7.8 Mean number of within, corresponding, and cross saccades as a function of the amount of perturbation

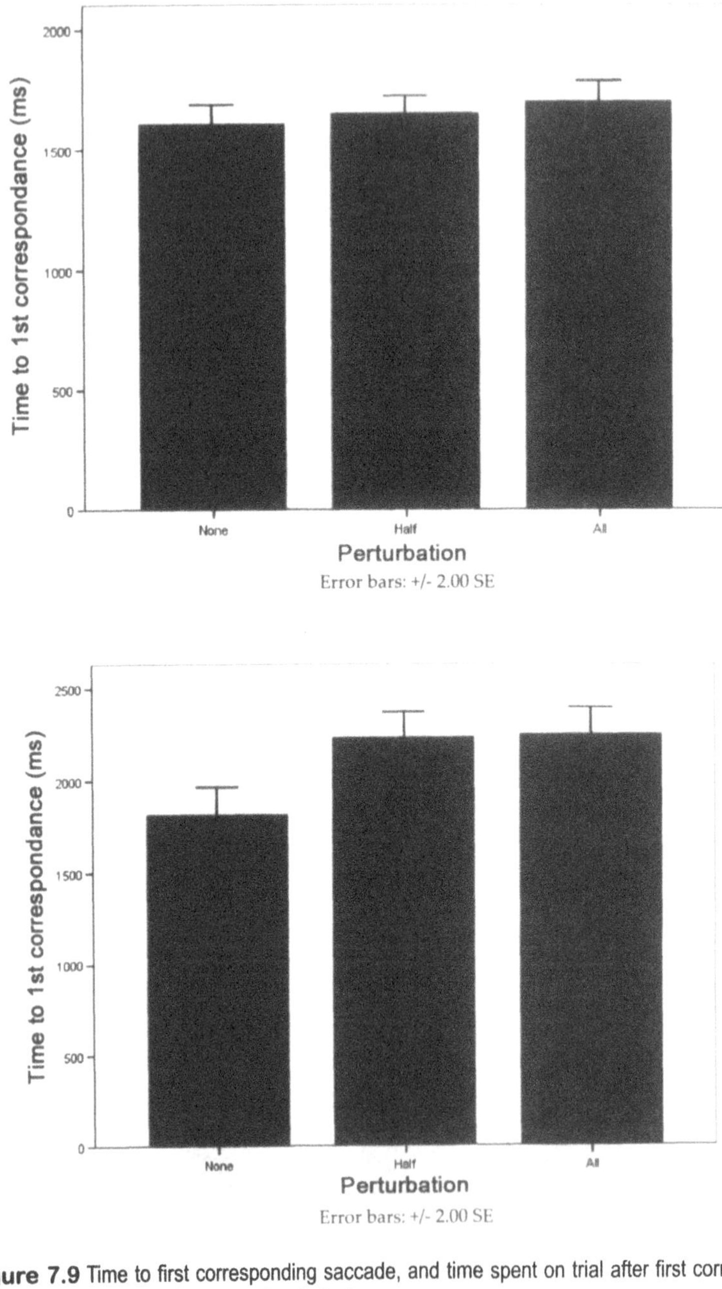

Figure 7.9 Time to first corresponding saccade, and time spent on trial after first corresponding saccade, as a function of amount of perturbation

Rotation

As might be expected, rotating one pattern increased response time, number of fixations, and average fixation duration. In some cases, these effects depended on the complexity of the patterns. In the simplest patterns, with only four nodes, the rotation effect diminished considerably across the hundreds of test trials, and the effect of rotation on the number of fixations also increased with pattern complexity (see Figure 7.10). The fixation duration increased for all orientation differences above 0°, but there were only minor differences between the different nonzero rotations (see Figure 7.11).

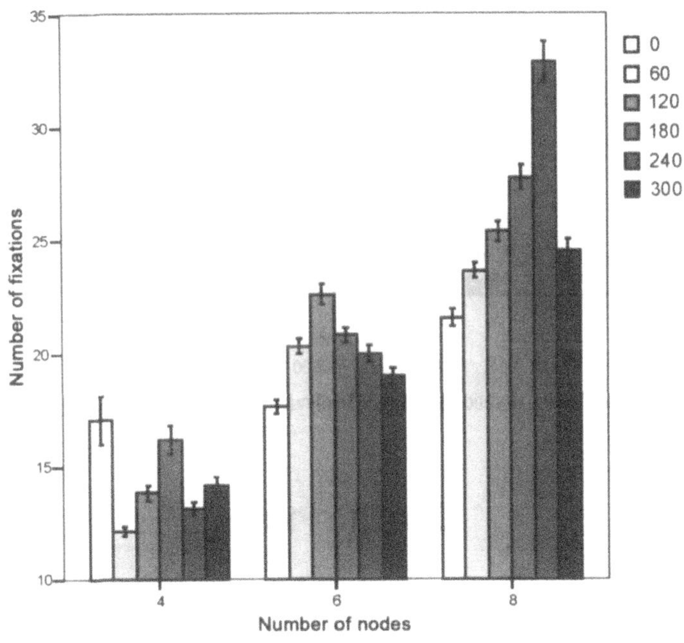

Figure 7.10 Mean number of fixations as a function of number of nodes and degree of rotation

Fixation durations

It is worth noting that the average fixation durations in the task were in the range of approximately 200 ms. Given the complexity of the task, it might be expected that average fixations would be much longer than this (see Castelhano & Rayner, this volume). That is, it is generally assumed that as task difficulty increases, fixation durations also increase. However, the fixation durations for this search task (see Figures 7.7 and 7.11) tended to be relatively short, perhaps because only a small number of different shapes appeared and they were all easily distinguishable once they were attended.

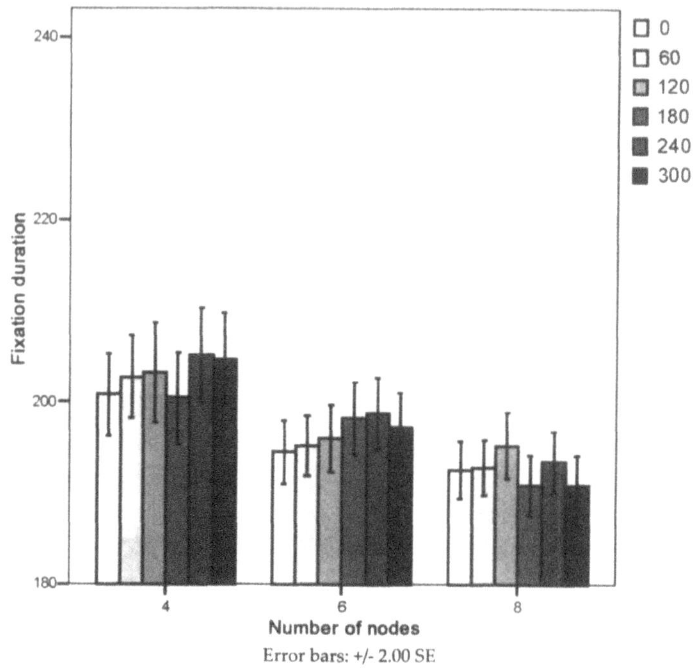

Figure 7.11 Mean fixation duration as a function of number of nodes and degree of rotation

Conclusions

Were the two patterns compared holistically, as two complete units, or were they compared part-by-part or region-by-region in separate steps? At the extreme, a purely holistic comparison would have required only one cross saccade, starting on one side and ending on the other. Instead, the mean number of cross saccades on a trial is close to the number of nodes in each pattern, arguing against holistic comparison. Even for the simple patterns with just four nodes, one fixation is not sufficient to allow all the information from the pattern to be encoded and stored so that it can be compared against the other side. The high number of cross-saccades suggests that the comparison is done one part at a time.

If the comparison is done in parts, then we might expect that a match is found between corresponding parts of the two patterns, and that this first correspondence is then used as a reference point to match up other corresponding parts between the two patterns. However, the evidence in the eye movement data for such a systematic part-by-part matching scheme is limited at best. A piecemeal matching strategy predicts that at any one moment, the part of a pattern being encoded or compared will be fixated, so that eye position is used to select that part of the pattern over other parts. However, on many trials, multiple fixations are clustered in one part of a pattern, and large portions are never fixated at all. Furthermore, there is a preference for fixating in the upper part of the pattern, and a preference for the side that is nearer the other pattern, both of which suggest that the exact position of the fixation within the pattern is not that important. It is possible, of course, that individual regions within a pattern are being selected at different times, but that much of this selection is done with covert attention rather than by targeting fixations.

A piecemeal matching strategy also predicts that there should be a number of corresponding cross saccades, in which the eyes move from one part of one of the objects to the corresponding part of the other object. We were able to identify a number of corresponding cross saccades, but the eye movement data do not suggest that the corresponding saccades played a major role in the matching task. If different regions are matched in separate fixations, then increasing the number of nodes in the patterns would presumably increase the number of regions, and therefore increase the number of corresponding saccades. Instead, our data show that the number of corresponding saccades is unaffected by the number of nodes. Perturbing some or all of the nodes makes the matching task more difficult but does not increase the number of corresponding saccades. More importantly, our computer simulation indicates that the number of corresponding saccades is no higher than what would be expected from random eye-movement patterns. Therefore, the eye-movements do not reveal a systematic region-by-region comparison of the two patterns.

The eye movements from this experiment lead to one of two different conclusions. The two patterns might be compared in a piecemeal approach, in which only one aspect of the patterns is compared within any one fixation, but the comparisons might involve global properties of the entire pattern rather than the configuration in one specific region. For these global comparisons, fixations would not need to be very selective, and would not need to be targeted to specific parts of the configurations. The global properties that are used might include the presence and absence of closure, the number of closed regions, the number of angles around the outer perimeter, or the number of nodes on the edge with only a single connection.

Alternatively, the piecemeal comparison could still be spatially organized, with different regions compared in different fixations, but only if the selection of each region is done more with covert attention than with eye position. If this is true, however, then subjects are not bothering to target their fixations carefully, even though they can do so in other tasks such as reading and visual search. Such a lack of effort in the comparison task but not in the other tasks would be surprising, and thus we conclude that the comparison in this task in done in multiple steps, but that most of the steps are devoted to a comparison of global properties of the stimulus patterns.

Acknowledgments

This work was supported by a grant from the Department of the Interior (NBCH1050007) to CMR, ALC, and KRC.

References

Diwadkar, V. A., & McNamara, T. P. (1997). Viewpoint dependence in scene recognition. *Psychological Science, 8*, 302-307.

Just, M. A., & Carpenter, P. A. (1976). Eye fixations and cognitive processes. *Cognitive Psychology, 8*, 441-480.

Nakatani, C., & Pollatsek, A. (2004). An eye movement analysis of "mental rotation" of simple scenes. *Perception & Psychophysics, 66*, 1227-1245.

Nakatani, C., Pollatsek, A., & Johnson, S. H. (2002). Viewpoint-dependent recognition of scenes. *Quarterly Journal of Experimental Psychology, 55A*, 115-139.

Shepard, R. N., & Metzler, J. (1971). Mental rotation of three-dimensional objects. *Science, 171*, 701-703.

Chapter 8

Using eye movements to study and improve driving safety

Alexander Pollatsek, Donald L. Fisher, and Anuj Pradhan

In the United States (Williams, 2003) and other countries the crash rate for newly licensed drivers is many times higher than for experienced drivers between the ages of 30-50. Studies have shown that there are large differences between these newly licensed drivers and more experienced drivers in the amount of searching done both while driving on the road (Crundall & Underwood, 1998; Mourant & Rockwell, 1972) and while driving in a driving simulator (Chapman & Underwood, 1998). In the studies on the road, searching was indexed by the variability of the fixation location in the Y-axis (i.e., in the horizontal direction); presumably, such variability reflects the number of eye movements that are directed away from looking directly in front and are directed to other lanes of traffic, the side of the road, the rear view mirror, etc. Moreover, these studies also found that this difference between the beginning and more experienced drivers essentially disappeared when the driving was "easy" (i.e., a straight road with little traffic and in rural areas with no side streets, pedestrians, or anything else to look after).

Of course, these studies of drivers' scanning patterns were not gathered during actual crashes. Perhaps the closest thing we currently have to naturalistic studies is analyses of police accident reports. McKnight and McKnight (2003) recently analyzed the records of almost 1,000 automobile crashes in which drivers 16 and 17 years old were involved. They found that failures to search ahead, to the side, and to the rear, were implicated in 42.7% of the crashes. Unfortunately, we do not know whether the pattern of scanning would change for much more experienced drivers since such drivers were not included in the study.

There are two related explanations for why novice drivers might scan the roadway less effectively for information than do experienced drivers. First, part of the problem in the failure to search the driving environment adequately may be that novice drivers think that they are processing more of the visual field than they are. That is, because in general people can get the overall gist of a scene quite quickly from a single fixation (Potter, 1976), this may lead the novice drivers into thinking they are actually processing the details far out into the periphery. However, work on scene processing has shown that in order for an object to be recognized and remembered even a few seconds later with a high probability, it has to be fixated (Hollingworth & Henderson, 2002). Thus, at least part of the problem in searching the roadway adequately may be that novice drivers are unaware of the need to do so because they have not experienced situations where the failure to look has led to negative consequences. The failure here is a general one. However, another part of the problem may be that drivers do not know where to look in the periphery for risks that might materialize, even though they are generally aware of the need to do so. The failure here is a more specific one.

What have more experienced drivers learned?

Although the evidence is correlational, it strongly implicates failure to search adequately as a major contributor to vehicle crashes, and in particular, to the much higher crash rate for beginning drivers. However, as we noted above, this raises the question of what has been learned by more experienced drivers. Do they simply know that they should move their eyes more when the driving situation is not easy (i.e., they have learned a general strategy) or do they know where to look in specific situations to anticipate upcoming potential risks (i.e., they have acquired specific knowledge)? Similarly, if one is attempting to reduce the number of crashes for the beginning drivers, should one merely train people to look around more or should one give them specific knowledge about where and when to look?

Our research, that will be the central focus of this chapter, will not provide definitive answers to these questions. However, it will first demonstrate that beginning drivers fail to look at specific locations that provide information about upcoming risks; in these situations, failure to fixate these locations certainly would contribute to a higher accident rate. Then it will demonstrate that a simple training program that merely provides the knowledge that one should attend to these locations improves the performance of the beginning drivers to a level about equal to that of the experienced drivers. We should emphasize that this training does not involve driving in either the road or the simulator and does not require the trainee to make rapid eye movements to these locations; it merely explains why processing these locations is important and implicitly teaches that they should actually be fixated.

The key to our studies is that the test drives on the simulator contain specific situations—that we call *scenarios*—in which there is a potential danger. Each test drive (which takes about 45 minutes) contains about 12-16 of these scenarios. One example of a scenario is the *truck blocking crosswalk* scenario, which is illustrated in Figure 8.1 by a (top-down) *plan view* in our training program (the red circles and yellow ovals will be explained later in the text, when we explain our training program) and in Figure 8.2 by a frame of what the drivers actually saw in the driving simulator. In this scenario, there is a parked truck which is blocking the view of the driver (the participant driver's vehicle is gray), and pedestrians or bicyclists could emerge from behind the truck onto the roadway in front of the driver with little or no warning. When approaching the parked truck and the crosswalk, a good driver should attend to the left edge of the truck so as to get the earliest indication that a pedestrian or bicyclist is emerging from behind it. Although there is some controversy about whether it is strictly necessary to fixate an area such as this to adequately perceive what is happening, there is no doubt that: (a) fixating the area is a reliable indicator that this information is being attended and (b) perception will be improved if it is fixated. Moreover, as mentioned above, research by Hollingsworth & Henderson (2002) has shown that details of scenes are not likely to be processed if they are not fixated: If an object is not fixated, memory of whether it was present in the scene several seconds later is about at chance.

As indicated above, all of these scenarios are embedded in a larger test drive that goes through both urban and more rural roadways. It is important to note that the scenarios are in no way marked to the participant; they are merely part of the drive. On the driving simulator, there is a *lead car* that the participant is asked to follow; the lead car thus indicates where the driver is to turn and thereby ensures that the same route is driven by all participants. An important point that we should

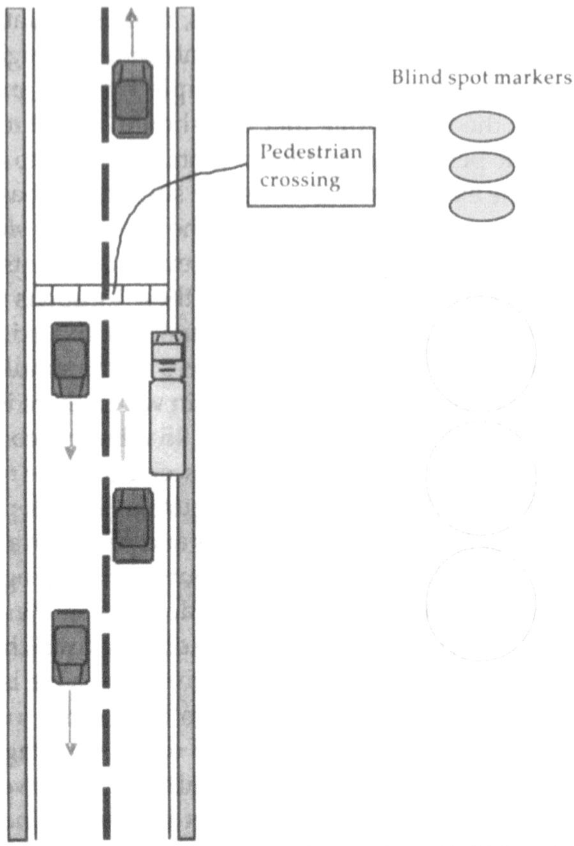

Figure 8.1 Plan view of truck crosswalk scenario used in PC-based training

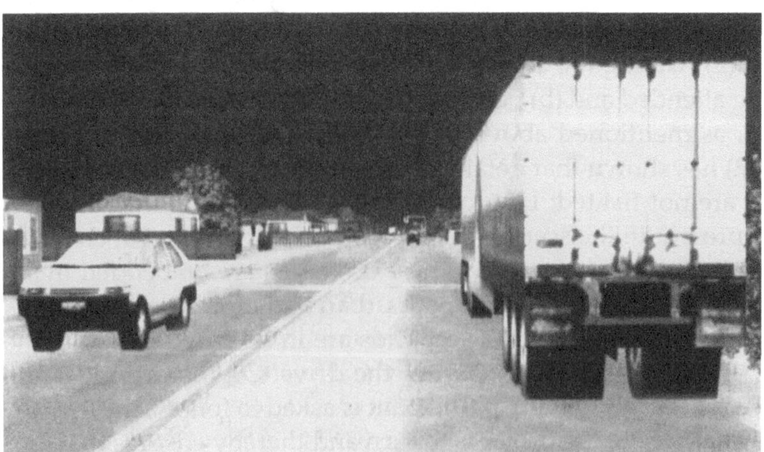

Figure 8.2 Perspective view in driving simulator: truck crosswalk scenario (*See Plate 3.*)

mention about the design is that the risk never actually materializes in any of the scenarios. For example, a pedestrian or cyclist never actually appears from behind the parked truck. This was done to ensure that the drivers would not get unduly cautious.

Obviously, the key question (and the data upon which we have focused) is how often different groups of drivers fixate appropriately in the various scenarios. Scoring these data by an algorithm is close to impossible because the visual scene is constantly changing so that the meaning of an absolute point of fixation changes. Fortunately, the software allows us to replay the drive as seen by a participant with the computed fixation point superimposed on the image by cross-hairs. As a result, our primary data analysis relies on scorers looking at the scenarios in these videotapes and judging whether the person fixated appropriately. The videotapes are scored "blind" (i.e., the scorer does not know which group the participant was in). Moreover, these judgments are usually easy. For example, in the previously discussed *truck blocking crosswalk* scenario, an appropriate fixation sequence would be to start fixating the front left edge of the truck well before coming to the crosswalk and to actually start to look around it as one gets into the crosswalk. Such a sequence would be scored '1' (i.e., correct), and is easily distinguishable from the typical incorrect behavior which is to fixate directly in front for the entire scenario. Typically, fixations which indicate that the driver has looked in the direction of the risk that might materialize are well over 5 degrees of visual angle apart from the fixations which indicate that the driver has not processed the risk and thus are easy to judge from the position of the crosshair on the videotapes.

Simulator study 1: Evaluation of novice, younger and older drivers

The goal of our first study examining eye movements was to determine whether beginning drivers exhibited different (and inferior) scanning behavior in these scenarios than more experienced drivers. Clearly, if the answer was no, then this paradigm would have no clear relevance to the traffic safety issue stated at the onset of this chapter. That is, if there is no difference between beginning drivers and more experienced drivers in this kind of scanning pattern, then there would be no reason to think that differences in such scanning patterns are a cause of the much higher crash rate for the beginning drivers. Our study (Pradhan, Hammel, DeRamus, Pollatsek, Noyce, & Fisher, 2005), examined three groups of drivers (24 participants per group): *older* (60-75 years old), *younger* (18-26 years old) and *novice* (16-17 years old). There were indeed large differences in scanning patterns as a function of the experience of the drivers. In the test drives, the older drivers fixated appropriately in a scenario 66% of the time, the younger drivers fixated appropriately 51% of the time, whereas the novice drivers fixated appropriately only 36% of the time (all pairwise differences were significant). These data thus indicate that it is plausible that these differences in scanning patterns could be an important contributor to the increased crash rates for inexperienced drivers. Needless to say, fixating appropriately does not guarantee that the driver will respond to a risk appropriately if it appears; however, fixating inappropriately will just about guarantee that the driver will not respond appropriately if the risk appears.

Can instruction about dangers change driving behavior?

The above study showed that the scanning patterns of beginning drivers in scenarios that contained potential risks were much worse than those of experienced drivers. We next wanted to know whether a training program that merely imparted knowledge about hidden risks would improve performance. We should emphasize that this training program requires only the manipulating of a mouse on a PC without any game controls (no steering, braking, etc.). No recording of eye movements is done in the PC-based training program nor is there any actual driving through a simulated environment in addition to the training that takes place in our PC-based program. Thus, the PC-based program is not actually training either control of the vehicle or training people to make eye movements more efficiently by capturing those eye movements and providing relevant feedback. The training program is based on scenarios like the ones in the test drive described above (one training scenario is displayed in Figure 8.1). However, the training involves only about half the scenarios that are in the test drive on the simulator. Below, we call the scenarios in the simulator test drive that are very similar to the ones seen in training the *near transfer* scenarios, and the scenarios that have virtually none of the same surface features as any of the scenarios seen in training the *far transfer* scenarios.

The details of our PC-based training program have changed, but in all versions, the instruction involved seeing plan views such as the one of *the truck blocking crosswalk* scenario in Figure 8.1. The essential idea in all of the different versions is that the trainee is told to indicate areas of the scenario to which attention should be directed because some hidden danger might appear. In the earlier versions of the training program, plan views, such as in Figure 8.1, were the primary vehicle for instruction. In later versions, we have also used sequences of (still) photographic images of the same scenario (one in a sequence of photographs is displayed in Figure 8.3; circle number 1 is where the driver should move the mouse, indicating that he or she recognizes that a pedestrian or bicyclist might emerge from behind the line of bushes). However, in all versions of the training program, the major task for the person in training was to mark a location that should be attended (on either the plan view or the photographic image, depending on the version of the training program).

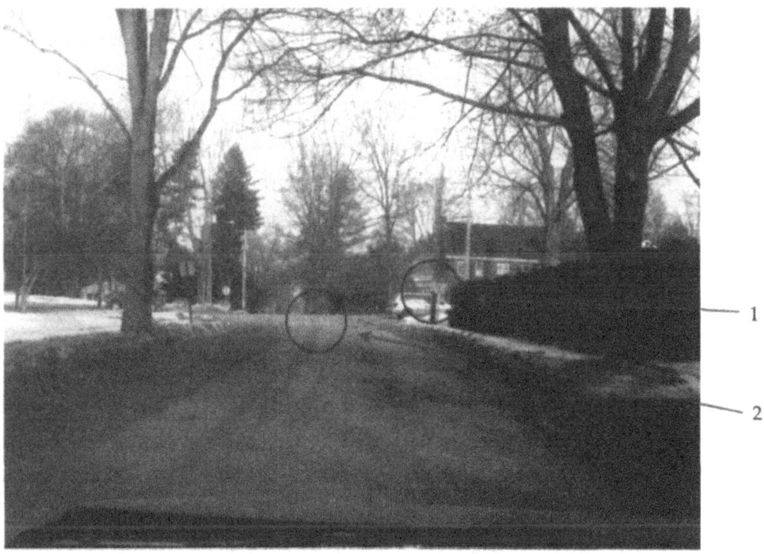

Figure 8.3 Still photograph used In PC-based training (*See Plate 4.*)

Our training programs have three phases. First, there is a pre-test, in which trainees get the sequence of 8-10 scenarios in turn. For each, they are asked to mark on the image (either a plan view or a photographic image depending on the version of the training program) the areas that should be attended to because they contain information about a potential risk. For example, as indicated in the truck blocking crosswalk scenario in Figure 8.1, they are supposed both to drag a yellow oval in front of the truck (indicating that a potential threat to the driver could be obscured from view at the location) and to drag a red circle to the left side of the front of the truck (indicating that this is where they should attend if the potential risk were to materialize). They then go through the training phase, in which they go through the scenarios one at a time and it is explained why it is important to focus on certain areas. In the training phase, they are again asked to mark the relevant areas that should be attended. After the training phase, they are then given a post-test which is identical to the pretest. The training lasts roughly 45 minutes.

Needless to say, given that the PC-based training is quite straightforward, they learn the correct answers and do much better on the post-test than the pre-test. In our first training study, for example, the mean score on the pre-test was 32% correct and it was 90% on the post-test (Pollatsek, Naranayaan, Pradhan, & Fisher, 2006). Thus, it is clear that the knowledge about where to look in such situations was transmitted. However, there is obviously no guarantee that this knowledge will be applied when people actually drive. Thus, the main focus in our experiments is to determine whether people actually do look at such critical areas when they are driving. For practical reasons, most of our experiments have tested this on a driving simulator. However, we have done a test in an actual driving situation (described below) and got virtually the same data as in the driving simulator. Thus, we feel reasonably confident that our results on the simulator do apply to actual driving situations.

Training study 1: Immediate simulator evaluation

In our first training study (Pollatsek et al., 2006) we had two groups of beginning drivers: A trained group and an untrained group. The trained group came to the driving laboratory, went through the training on the PC and then went through the test drive on the driving simulator. The untrained group came to the driving laboratory and was given the same test drive on the driving simulator as the trained group. The results were quite clear and dramatic: The trained group fixated the appropriate areas in the scenarios 58% of the time, whereas the untrained group fixated the appropriate areas only 35% of the time $F(1, 46) = 21.2$, $p < 0.001$. Moreover, the training effect (i.e., the difference between the trained and untrained group) was just about the same for the far transfer scenarios (20%) as for the near transfer scenarios (25%). Thus, training that imparts the knowledge about where risks were likely to be produced a large improvement in the beginning drivers. Moreover, their performance on the test was not that much worse than that observed for the safest group of drivers on the original study (66%; Pradhan et al., 2005). We should point out that there were no significant gender differences here or in any of our other studies.

Training study 2: Delayed simulator evaluation

In this first training study, the driving simulator test was on the same day as training. Although this indicates that appropriate fixation behavior in driving can be trained, it is unclear whether the effects of training rely on such an immediate test. If so, the results of the above experiment would still indicate that it is likely that the inexperienced drivers suffer from a knowledge deficit; however, it would indicate that such a training program is of little practical interest. To assess this, we ran a follow-up study that used the same training program and the same basic design, but in which the test was administered 3-5 days after training (Pradhan, Fisher, & Pollatsek, 2006). (There were only some relatively minor changes in the training module.) The data indicated that the effectiveness of the training was as good as when the test was immediate. Overall, the trained group fixated the appropriate regions 52% of the time compared to 28% percent of the time for the control group, $t(30) = 3.32$, $p < 0.005$. As with the immediate test, the training effect was about equal for far- and near-transfer (26% and 23%, respectively). Thus, our PC-based risk awareness training is effective, at least on a driving simulator, both when evaluated immediately after training and 3-5 days after training.

Training study 3: Field evaluation

In our next study (Pradhan, Fisher, Knodler, Pollatsek and Langone, 2006), we wanted to determine whether what we observed in the driving simulator was merely an artifact of this somewhat artificial driving situation or whether it was a phenomenon that could be observed in actual driving on the road. The drive that we set up as the test went through Amherst, Massachusetts (a town of about 40,000 people) and the surrounding area. It included driving through downtown areas and more rural stretches. The drive included many scenarios that were similar to those on the driving simulator. For example, another scenario that was used on the driving simulator involved a crosswalk at an intersection where the pedestrian entry to the crosswalk was hidden by hedges. This scenario on the simulator, however, was modeled to be similar to an actual intersection in Amherst and this scenario was part of the test drive on the road (see Figure 8.3). Many of the other scenarios on the simulator were also modeled after actual places in the Amherst area and these were used in the test drive. In addition, we staged one or two scenarios.

The test drive took place in an automobile provided by a local driving school and an instructor from the driving school sat in the front passenger seat. There was a second brake pedal available to the instructor, which could be used in the event of an emergency. An experimenter sat in the rear of the vehicle and ensured that the eye movement apparatus was calibrated; he also gave the driver instructions about when to turn. Other than the fact that the test was on the road, the design of the experiment was the same as the first training study described above, including the fact that the (field) test was immediate. However, we should add that this was the point at which the training module was changed somewhat, and the training used photographic images on which the trainee indicated the areas that should be attended. Thus, it is not strictly comparable to the initial training study. (The complete set of slides used in field training is available on the web, www.ecs.umass.edu/hpl. Click on "Younger Drivers".) The results indicated that our training effects we had previously observed on the simulator were not an artifact of the simulator. Overall, the size of the training effect, 27%, (64% for the trained group vs. 37% for the untrained group), $t(22) = 4.96$, $p < 0.001$, was similar to that on the driving simulator. The test drive on the road, like the one in the simulator, had both near and far transfer scenarios. For both, the training effect was significant: 39% for the near transfer scenarios, and 20% for the far-transfer scenarios, $t(22) = 5.57$, $p < 0.001$, $t(22) = 2.87$, $p < 0.01$, respectively. However, unlike the earlier studies, the near-transfer effect was greater than the far transfer effect, $t(22) = 2.32$, $p < 0.05$. This is likely due to the greater similarity between the photographic images used during training and the situations actually tested. However, it is important to note that the difference is merely that the size of the near transfer effect in the field study was bigger than the one observed on the driving simulator; the size of the far transfer effects was about the same in the two studies. Thus, if anything, the driving simulator environment is underestimating the size of the near-transfer training effect.

Simulator study 2: Evaluation of pre-cueing

As mentioned above, a key aspect of all the simulator studies is that the actual risk never appeared. (Obviously, we could not control that in the field study, but it rarely appeared there either.) This raises the question of whether the environment in which our test drives occurred was too uneventful, and whether, if there were signals of potential dangers, beginning drivers would do better at attending to the critical locations in our scenarios. To test that hypothesis, we introduced a *foreshadowing* manipulation to a few of our scenarios (Garay-Vega, Fisher, & Pollatsek, 2008). (This was not a training study.) För example, in the truck crosswalk scenario, we introduced a pedestrian that crossed the crosswalk and reached the other side of the roadway well in advance of the participant driver entering the crosswalk (Figure 8.4, left panel). Thus, there was no need for the participant driver to take any action with respect to this pedestrian. However, the sight of the pedestrian should clearly be a cue to the driver that pedestrians are using the crosswalk and that the driver should anticipate this as best they can (looking to the right as the driver crosses over the sidewalk; Figure 8.4; right panel). As in all the other scenarios, however, a pedestrian never appeared as the participant driver was going through the crosswalk.

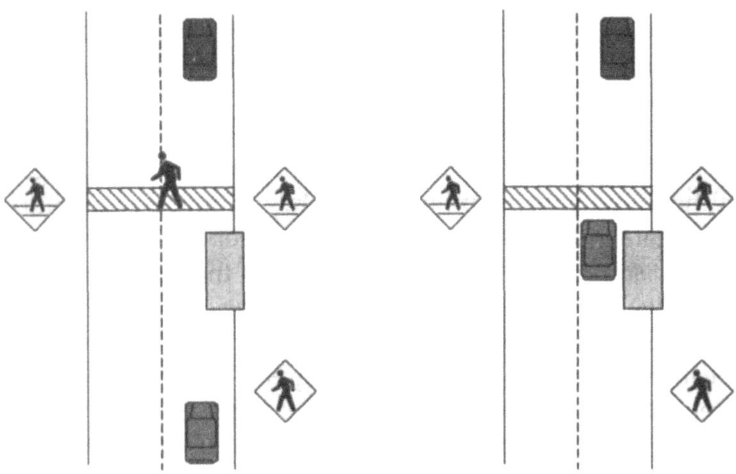

Figure 8.4 Pre-cueing risk (Left panel: pedestrian in sidewalk well ahead of driver; right panel: pedestrian crossed sidewalk before driver navigates over sidewalk.) (*See Plate 5.*)

Again, the key questions were: (a) whether this foreshadowing would increase the chances that people would fixate appropriately when entering the scenario and (b) whether the foreshadowing would decrease the difference in performance between the experienced and beginning drivers. When there was no foreshadowing element in the scenario, the data fairly closely replicated our earlier data: 61% of the experienced drivers scanned the critical area (to the right of the parked truck) but only 34% of the beginning drivers scanned the critical area, a 27% difference. We assessed the foreshadowing trials several ways. First, we examined the difference between experienced and beginning drivers on all the foreshadowing trials. In fact, the 26% difference between the two groups (79% vs. 53%) was virtually the same as on the trials with no foreshadowing, $t(46) = 3.09$, $p<0.005$. However, we thought the most relevant analysis was to examine only those trials in which the participant fixated the foreshadowing element. That is, it is only on these trials that one can be reasonably sure that the participants perceived the foreshadowing element adequately. On these trials, there was even a larger difference (37%) between the experienced and beginning drivers (85% vs. 48%), $t(46) = 4.00$, $p<0.001$. Thus, the answer to the first question above is "yes": In those trials where the foreshadowing element was present, participants fixated the appropriate region of the scenario more often than when there was no foreshadowing element. However, the answer to the second question is "no": The foreshadowing element did not decrease the difference in performance between the experienced and beginning drivers, and actually increased the difference if the foreshadowing element was perceived.

These data thus indicate that the problem with the beginning drivers can not be eliminated by giving them a hint that something might happen in the immediate future to which they should pay attention. Instead, the data indicate that the problem is deeper and that beginning drivers lack some overall knowledge that: (a) there is a class of situations (that we have illustrated with our scenarios) in which there are hidden potential risks and (b) these situations require attention to a specific location. Moreover, the somewhat greater effect of the foreshadowing element for the experienced drivers suggests that such cues are actually better for more experienced drivers because they resonate with the knowledge that these drivers have accumulated during their driving.

Discussion

We introduced this chapter by discussing the very high crash rate for beginning drivers and arguing that police accident reports indicated that it was due, in part, to failures to scan the environment appropriately. Our work, and the work of others, has shown that the eye movement patterns of beginning drivers and experienced drivers on driving simulators differ in a way consistent with these accident reports. However, as indicated earlier, the focus of our experiments and the types of analyses we have done differ from the other studies (Fisher, Pollatsek, and Pradhan, 2006). That is, much of the work, especially the work from the laboratory of Underwood (e.g., Chapman & Underwood, 1998; Crundall & Underwood, 1998), has focused on global patterns of eye movements, especially the amount of variation in the Y (horizontal) direction of eye gaze. (How much drivers move their eyes up and down was considered to be largely irrelevant to safety issues.) In contrast, of course, we have focused on specific points in the drive in which safe driving virtually requires eye movements of a certain type and have examined the data to see whether drivers make these eye movements.

For the most part, the studies using the two paradigms have come up with similar data. The experiments using the more global measures have shown: (a) that more experienced drivers make more of these horizontal eye movements than beginning drivers and (b) that beginning drivers can be trained to make more horizontal eye movements (their training program was in many ways similar to ours at it trained drivers to identify hazardous situations in videotapes of driving). Similarly, we have shown that there are large differences in whether beginning and experienced drivers look at appropriate places in a risky scenario and that beginning drivers can be trained to perform almost as well as the safest group of drivers. It thus appears that both programs of research are studying a phenomenon related to increased crash rates and have developed training programs that have some chance of ameliorating the problem of high crash rates for beginning drivers. This raises the question, however, of which level of analysis is best: A global one or a local one.

We think that our local level of analysis is more likely to be fruitful. First, on some level, it has a higher "face validity". That is, by examining specific scenarios, we have demonstrated that both experienced and trained beginning drivers are looking more at the regions that would reveal potential risks. As we said earlier, although there is no guarantee that drivers will execute the appropriate driving behaviors if and when the potential risk actually appears, there is a very high likelihood that they will do something fairly dangerous if the risk appears and they haven't attended to that region. In contrast, the research demonstrating more global changes in eye movements is more circumstantial. That is, if drivers are making more horizontal eye movements away from the road directly ahead, there is an increased probability that they will make an appropriate eye movement in a risky scenario. Thus, because the training program of Chapman, Underwood, and Roberts (2002) produced more horizontal eye movements in beginning drivers, it probably caused them to make more fixations on the right place in potentially hazardous scenarios. However, one can't be sure. Moreover, making eye movements away from the roadway in front has a cost. That is, the roadway ahead is clearly something that needs to be attended a large fraction of the time. Moreover, there is evidence (Klauer, Dingus, Neale, Sudweeks, & Ramsey, 2006) that another cause of accidents for beginning drivers is that—just before the accident—the driver has looked away from the roadway in front of them for an extended period that is too long. In fact, Chapman et al. also observed more horizontal eye movements in their trained drivers in easy stretches of driving where such eye movements were not required; moreover, their experienced drivers did not do so suggesting that such eye movements were unnecessary and perhaps counterproductive. Thus, their training may have produced costs as well as benefits.

In conclusion, we think that our research indicates that examining people's eye movements while they are driving is a very fruitful paradigm. Although it is logically possible that the differences in fixation patterns for the beginning and experienced drivers have nothing to do with the differences in their crash rates, it seems very unlikely. Moreover, we have shown that a fairly simple training program that we have developed (which is accessible on the web) markedly improves the fixation patterns of the beginning drivers. Clearly, this is just a beginning. First, we need to determine whether the effects of our training last more than 3-5 days, and if not, determine how to expand on the training so it does so. However, given that the period where beginning drivers have markedly elevated crash rates is their first six months on the road after they receive their full license, if we can insure that the effects last for six months, we would have a real chance of markedly reducing crash rates. Second, we need to assess whether our training does have an effect on the crash rates of our trainees. We are currently planning a large-scale study that will assess this. We are also hoping to develop other training programs as well, including one that trains drivers to guard against long period of non-attention to the road while driving—caused by events such as reading signs or looking for something in the car or getting involved in a cell-phone conversation. In all of this research, assessing eye movement behavior is critical to understanding what is going on.

References

Chapman, P. R., & Underwood, G. (1998). Visual search of driving situations: Danger and experience. *Perception, 27,* 951-964.

Chapman, P., Underwood, G., & Roberts, K. (2002). Visual search patterns in trained and untrained novice drivers. *Transportation Research Part F, 5,* 157-167.

Crundall, D. E., & Underwood, G. (1998). Effects of experience and processing demands on visual information acquisition in drivers. *Ergonomics, 41,* 448-458.

Garay-Vega, L., Fisher, D. L., & Pollatsek, A. (2008). Hazard anticipation of novice and experienced drivers: Empirical evaluation on a driving simulator in daytime and nighttime conditions. *Transportation Research Record,* 1-7.

Fisher, D. L., Pollatsek, A., & Pradhan, A. (2006). Can novice drivers be trained to scan for information that will reduce their likelihood of a crash? *Injury Prevention,12, Supplement 1,* i25-i29.

Hollingworth, A., & Henderson, J. M. (2002). Accurate visual memory for previously attended objects in natural scenes. *Journal of Experimental Psychology: Human Perception and Performance, 28,* 113-136.

Klauer, S. G., Dingus, T. A., Neale, V. L., Sudweeks, J. D., & Ramsey, D. J. (2006). *The impact of driver inattention on near-crash/crash risk: An analysis using the 100-car naturalistic driving study data* (Report No. DOT HS 810 594). Washington, D.C.: National Highway Traffic Safety Administration.

McKnight, J. A., & McKnight, S. A. (2003) Young novice drivers: Careless or clueless. *Accident Analysis and Prevention, 35,* 921-925.

Mourant, R. R., & Rockwell, T. R. (1972). Strategies of visual search by novice drivers and experienced drivers. *Human Factors, 14,* 325-335.

Potter, M. C. (1976). Short-term conceptual memory for pictures. *Journal of Experimental Psychology: Human Language and Memory, 2,* 509-522.

Pollatsek, A., Narayanaan, V., Pradhan, A., & Fisher, D. L. (2006). The use of eye movements to evaluate the effect of PC-based risk awareness training on an advanced driving simulator. *Human Factors, 48,* 447-464.

Pradhan, A. K., Fisher, D. L., & Pollatsek, A. (2006). Risk perception training for novice drivers: Evaluating duration of effects on a driving simulator. *Transportation Research Record*, 58-64.

Pradhan, A. K., Fisher, D. L., Pollatsek, A., Knodler, M., & Langone, M. (October, 2006). Field evaluation of a risk awareness and perception training program for younger drivers. *Proceedings of the Human Factors and Ergonomics Society 50th Annual Meeting*, San Francisco, 2388-2391.

Pradhan, A. K., Hammel, K. R., DeRamus, R., Pollatsek, A., Noyce, D. A., & Fisher, D. L. (2005). The use of eye movements to evaluate the effects of driver age on risk perception in an advanced driving simulator. *Human Factors, 47*, 840-852.

Williams, A. F. (2003). Teenage drivers: Patterns of risk. *Journal of Safety Research, 34*, 5-15.

Section 4

Eye movements during scene perception, search, and mental rotation

Chapter 9

Do emotional scenes catch the eye?

Lauri Nummenmaa, Jukka Hyönä and Manuel G. Calvo

To cope with the information processing limitations of the cognitive system, the attentional system ensures that the brain prioritizes the processing of highly salient and unexpected stimuli at the expense of other ongoing neural activity and behavior (Corbetta & Shulman, 2002). Emotional processes assess the importance of sensory events to our well-being and adjust our physiological, behavioral and cognitive responses to cope with encountered challenges by governing approach-avoidance behavior (Frijda, 1986; Lazarus, 1991; Scherer, 1999). Thus, emotion and attention are related as they both manage information processing priorities in the human brain (Oatley & Johnson-Laird, 1987) based on the perceived visual and phylogenetic salience of events occurring in the environment.

Both neuropsychological and behavioral studies suggest that affective stimuli are highly salient and consequently are especially likely to capture attention (for reviews, see Compton, 2003; Vuilleumier, 2005). Effective visual perception relies on the visual system's ability to acquire detailed information from the environment. Visual acuity is highest around the fovea. As the diameter of the foveal field of vision is small (2.5 degrees, see Wandell, 1995), the attentional system must be complemented by a perceptual mechanism that governs where the fovea is positioned from moment to moment (i.e., where to position the center of an eye fixation).

There has been some debate about what factors guide the eyes during scene perception. Although it is widely agreed that overall the eyes spend more time fixating informative regions of a visual scene than less informative regions (see Castelhano & Rayner, this volume; also Buswell, 1935; Henderson, Weeks, & Hollingworth, 1999; Loftus & Mackworth, 1978; Mackworth & Morandi, 1967; Yarbus, 1967; for a review, see Henderson & Hollingworth, 1999), there is some disagreement about the features of the scene that drive the eyes initially. In other words, the debated question is what determines where the eyes land initially on a scene. A seminal study of Loftus and Mackworth (1978) provided evidence supporting semantic guidance (for a review, see Henderson & Hollingworth, 1999). Surprising objects that did not fit in the scene (e.g., a lawnmower in the kitchen) were more likely to be fixated following the first saccade within the scene than scene-consistent objects (e.g., a toaster on the kitchen table). However, more recent studies of Henderson et al. (1999) and De Graef, Christiaens and d'Ydewalle (1990) could not replicate this early inconsistency effect. According to these studies, observers were not more likely to launch the initial saccade to an inconsistent than to a consistent object. Yet, the most recent studies of Underwood (2005) and de Graef (2005) have obtained evidence consistent with the early study of Loftus and Mackworth (see also Gordon, 2004, who showed, using a probe recognition paradigm, that attention is very rapidly and automatically drawn toward an inconsistent object). In sum, based on the available evidence it is not clear whether the initial eye fixation on a visual scene is primarily guided by low-level visual factors or by knowledge-based (semantic) guidance.

In the present chapter, we review studies that investigate whether the affective content of visual scenes is capable of automatically engaging the oculomotor system. More specifically, we examine whether participants are more likely to make an initial fixation on an emotional than neutral picture when an emotional and a neutral picture are presented simultaneously. We also examine whether saccadic trajectory is affected by parafoveally presented emotional pictures. In the final section we discuss the implications of our findings to the models of eye movement guidance during scene perception.

Prioritized processing of emotional content in the human brain

Four lines of evidence suggest that the brain prioritizes the processing of emotional information. Firstly, event-related-potentials (ERPs) recorded from the visual cortices demonstrate differences between schematic emotional and neutral faces as early as 80-90 ms from stimulus onset (Eger, Jedynak, Iwaki, & Skrandies, 2003) and around 250 ms from stimulus onset of complex emotional scenes (Junghöfer, Bradley, Elbert, & Lang, 2001). This suggests that discrimination between emotional and neutral visual information occurs early during visual processing. Secondly, even unattended emotional facial expressions produce enhanced responses in the fusiform face area when compared to unattended neutral facial expressions (Vuilleumier, Armony, Driver, & Dolan, 2001; see also Vuilleumier, Armony, & Dolan, 2003, for a recent review), though allocation of attention to another, resource-consuming task can interfere with the processing of task-irrelevant emotional information (Pessoa, McKenna, Gutierrez, & Ungerleider, 2002; Pessoa, 2005). Thus, the high saliency of emotional stimuli could result from an enhanced sensory response to them, rendering them more—but not completely—resistant to suppressive interference (Vuilleumier, 2005). Thirdly, although visual acuity decreases rapidly outside foveal vision, both brain imaging and behavioral studies show that at least gross emotional information can readily be extracted even from the parafovea. Vuilleumier et al. (2001) demonstrated that fearful faces presented outside participants' foveal vision and visual attention can increase amygdala activity—a response traditionally attributed to processing of fear (see Adolphs, 2002). Similarly, when emotional visual scenes exceeding the area of foveal vision were presented 1.3° away from the fixation point, Keil, Moratti, Sabatinelli, Bradley, and Lang (2005) found enhanced cortical activation in the occipito-temporal and parietal regions in comparison with neutral scenes. These results suggest that the perceptual span may be wider for emotional than neutral scenes. This finding is corroborated by Calvo and Lang (2005). Employing a recognition priming paradigm, they presented two prime pictures (one neutral, one emotional) simultaneously to the left / right parafoveal visual field for 150 ms, followed first by a mask and then by a probe picture. Emotional probes were more likely to be recognized than neutral probes when primed by a picture of identical semantic content but different in size, orientation, and color, thus suggesting a parafoveal processing advantage for emotional over neutral content. The prioritized processing of emotional information is likely to be related to the amygdalar processing of emotional information and the amplified processing of emotional information in the visual cortex (VC) resulting from the thalamo-amygdalar projections to the visual cortex (see LeDoux, 1995; Vuilleumier, 2005, for reviews). Fourthly, as processing of emotional information is prioritized in the visual system, it logically follows from this that perception of emotional content brings about a reflexive shift of visual attention and an accompanying saccade to the emotional picture. Below we review in more detail our studies bearing on this final point.

Attentional capture by emotional pictures

Although a strong behavioral (Henderson, 2003) and neuropsychological (Awh, Armstrong, & Moore, 2006) relationship has been established between covert and overt orienting, only recently have the eye movement recording techniques been applied to the study of attentional capture by emotional content. Studies employing manual response latency paradigms have provided support for an attentional bias at different phases of attention orienting described by Posner's (1980) three-stage cycle of attention orienting: (1) disengagement of attentional resources from the currently attended objects, (2) shift of attention towards a new object, and (3) engagement of attention on the new object.

Studies using a modified version of Posner's cueing task with emotional pictures as cues have mainly demonstrated a bias in attentional engagement for emotional content, such as angry faces (Fox, Russo, Bowles, & Dutton, 2001; Fox, Russo, & Dutton, 2002), or complex pictures of threat-related scenes (Yiend & Mathews, 2001). The dot probe variant of the cuing task involves simultaneous presentation of two pictures, one emotional and one neutral, prior to the target dot probe that appears at the location of either of the pictures. The underlying assumption in this paradigm is that if an emotional picture captures attention, the dot probe that replaces this picture will be responded to faster than a dot probe that replaces a neutral picture. Anxious individuals have been found to react particularly quickly when the dot replaces an angry face (Bradley, Mogg, Falla, & Hamilton, 1998; Mogg & Bradley, 1999). Armony and Dolan (2002) found with aversively conditioned angry faces that all participants were faster to respond to the probe that replaced an angry face in comparison with a neutral face. Similarly, when the stimuli depict highly threatening scenes rather than emotional faces, all individuals tend to show a bias towards them (Mogg, McNamara et al., 2000).

Studies employing variants of the visual search task have provided corroborative evidence. In such tasks participants are required to search for a pre-specified target stimulus or for a non-prespecified discrepant object, for example, a spider, embedded in an array of non-target stimuli such as flowers. Studies have consistently demonstrated that a discrepant schematic angry face is detected faster among other faces than a friendly or sad face (Calvo, Avero, & Lundqvist, 2006; Fox et al., 2000; Öhman, Lundqvist, & Esteves, 2001; Tipples, Atkinson, & Young, 2002). Studies employing more complex stimuli such as pictures of animals have demonstrated search time advantages for fear-relevant animals amongst fear-irrelevant stimuli (Öhman, Flykt, & Esteves (2001). Moreover, a search advantage has also been observed for pictures of both threatening and pleasant animals (Tipples, Young, Quinlan, Broks, & Ellis, 2002), phylogenetically non-significant but nevertheless unpleasant stimuli such as guns and syringes (Blanchette, 2006), and for any animal irrespective of its fear relevance (Lipp, Derakshan, Waters, & Logies, 2004).

Eye movement studies on attentional capture by emotional pictures

The experimental paradigms reviewed above are limited in the sense that they only enable the assessment of one or two attentional components at a time. The visual search and dot probe tasks do not allow us to distinguish between the biases in orienting versus engagement of attention. In theory, a modified Posner's cueing task could enable this, but demonstrating attentional bias in orienting as a function of the emotional meaning of the cue is probably very difficult, as the mere onset of the cue singleton consists of a highly visually salient event which might override the more subtle effects arising from the picture content. However, by employing eye movement recordings in a variety of experimental paradigms we feel that we have successfully avoided these limitations.

General methodology of the studies

In all the studies reviewed below, the participants were university students; the majority of them were females. The basic setup in most studies (Calvo & Nummenmaa, 2007, is the exception) was one where emotional-neutral picture pairs were simultaneously presented, one in the right and another in the left visual field. The possibility for an overt attentional bias toward emotional content was studied by recording the viewers' eye movements when they were examining the scenes. Depending on the experiment, the pictures were presented either parafoveally or peripherally. Different task instructions were used (see the respective experiments for details) in order to study both automatic and controlled orienting of attention. The stimuli were selected from the International Affective Picture System (IAPS; see Lang, Bradley & Cuthbert, 2005). Stimulus displays consisted of two scenes. On each trial, an unpleasant, neutral, or pleasant target scene depicting people was presented with a neutral control scene (Nummenmaa, Hyönä & Calvo, 2006), which all depicted inanimate objects (see Figure 9.1 for stimulus examples). The unpleasant target scenes depicted people exposed to threat or suffering from a serious harm, the neutral target scenes involved people in daily non-emotional activities, and the pleasant target scenes involved people enjoying themselves or showing positive affect. Unpleasant and pleasant target pictures were matched for their perceived arousal level; moreover, unpleasant, neutral, and pleasant target pictures as well as control pictures were matched for low-level visual features such as luminosity, contrast density, color channel saturation and complexity.

Stimuli were presented on a 20-inch 200 Hz ViewSonic monitor with a 2 GHz Pentium III computer. Participants' eye movements were recorded with an EyeLink II eye tracker connected to a 2 GHz Pentium III computer. The sampling rate was 500 Hz, and the spatial resolution was better than 0.5 degrees.

Emotional content influences saccade target selection

In Experiment 1 of Nummenmaa et al. (2006) participants were presented with emotional and neutral pictures (involving humans) paired with neutral control pictures (involving objects). The pictures were lo-

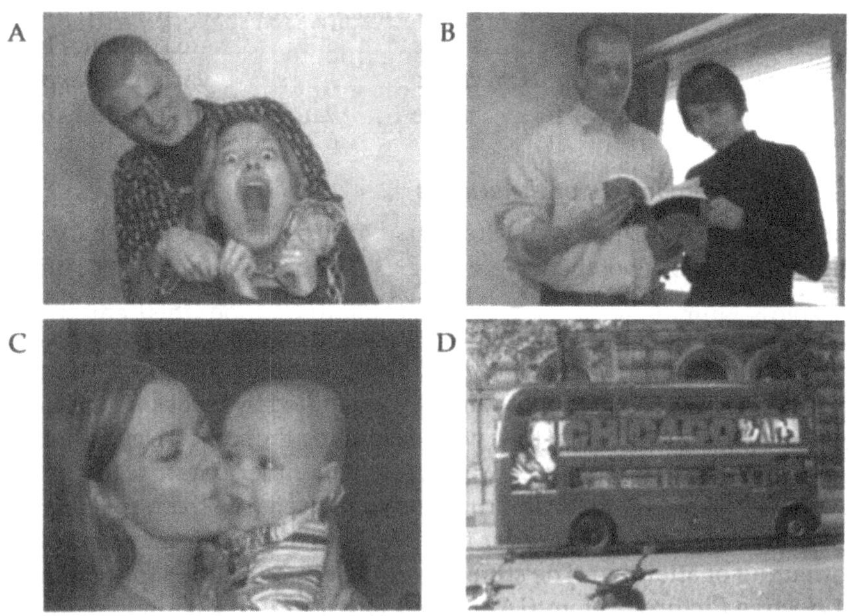

Figure 9.1 Illustration of unpleasant (A), neutral (B), pleasant (C), and control (D) stimuli used in the studies. Note that these example pictures were not among the experimental stimuli. (*See Plate 6.*)

cated at opposing corners of the screen, and the distance between the initial fixation and the innermost edge of the pictures was 4 degrees of visual angle. Pictures were presented for 3 s with the instruction to compare whether they are equally pleasant (neutral-neutral trials) or not (emotional-neutral trials). This bogus task ensured that participants had to look at both pictures. However, the task did not constrain the order in which the two pictures were looked at. The picture pairs were shown twice in two separate blocks to assess potential effects of the novelty of the emotional scenes. The probability of the first fixation landing on different types of target scenes was used as an index of bias in overt orienting of attention, and the number of first pass fixations was used to index the bias in attentional engagement.

The probability of first fixation was influenced by emotional valence (see Figure 9.2(A)). More specifically, both unpleasant and pleasant pictures received the first fixation with a greater likelihood than neutral pictures, suggesting a bias in attentional orienting towards emotional

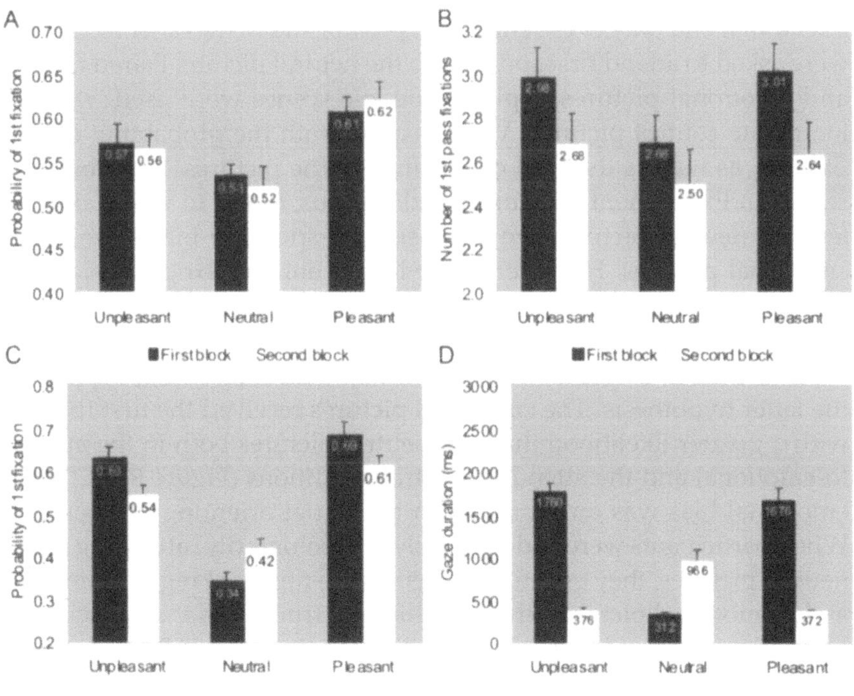

Figure 9.2 Probability of first fixation (A) and number of first pass fixations (B) as a function picture valence and block in Experiment 1, and probability of first fixation (C) and gaze duration (D) as a function of picture valence and attentional condition in Experiment 2.

content. The number of first pass fixations was influenced both by emotional valence and block, with both unpleasant and pleasant pictures receiving more first pass fixations than neutral ones, and with less overall first pass fixations in the second than in the first block. However, valence and block did not interact with each other. The main effect of valence implies here that emotional content biases engagement of attention, and the main effect of block reflects the fact that participants pay less attention to the familiar pictures.

In sum, the above results suggest that both initial saccade target selection and subsequent engagement of attention are biased towards emotional content present in complex visual scenes. However, the results do not necessarily reflect the fact that the bias is purely exogenous (stimulus-driven, automatic) in nature. It may as well be the case that the participants were deliberately paying more attention to the emotional than neutral pictures. Experiment 2 was conducted to test this possibility. It was a replication of Experiment 1 with an addition of two new task instructions. In one block the participants were instructed to attend first and only to the emotional picture and in the other block they were asked to attend first and only to the neutral picture. Paired neutral and emotional pictures depicting people scenes were used, with no inanimate control pictures. We measured both the probability of first fixation, as well as the total dwell time on the pictures. If the bias observed in Experiment 1 is purely endogenous, trying to voluntarily attend to neutral pictures would easily override the bias toward the emotional pictures. However, if the bias is entirely exogenous, trying to voluntarily attend to neutral pictures would not diminish the tendency to fixate the emotional picture first.

The results of Experiment 2 of Nummenmaa et al. (2006) supported the latter hypothesis. The emotional pictures received the first fixation with a greater likelihood than the neutral pictures both in the attend-to-emotional and the attend-to-neutral conditions (Figure 9.2(C)). The emotional bias was only present in the initial orienting of attention. When participants were endogenously (i.e. voluntarily) attending to the neutral pictures, they eventually spent more time looking at them than at the emotional pictures (the opposite was true when the participants were asked to attend to the emotional pictures) (Figure 9.2(D)). In other words, participants were able to devote the fixation time according to the task instructions. However, they could not inhibit first overtly attending to an emotional picture when the instruction was to attend to the neutral picture. All in all, Experiment 2 confirmed that the bias towards emotional pictorial content is at least partly exogenous. However, the bias was not purely exogenous in nature as it was slightly diminished in the attend-to-neutral condition.

Emotional content biases saccade initiation

The above results lend support to the view that the content of parafoveally or peripherally presented visual scenes can exert a relatively automatic influence on saccade target selection. Even though the emotional pictures were completely comparable to the neutral pictures in their low-level visual features in both Experiment 1 and 2 of Nummenmaa et al. (2006), they still attracted initial saccades with a greater likelihood. However, these studies are limited in the sense that they are only capable of demonstrating an emotional bias in attentional selection. The question arises whether a similar bias is also observed, when the task does not require the participants to deliberately attend to the picture contents. Thus, our current work is aimed at determining whether the bias extends to saccade programming when the triggering of saccades is not based on the picture contents. We have recently run variants of the study reviewed above with important modifications in the saccade task. More specifically, paired emotional and neutral pictures were presented horizontally to the opposite visual fields, and participants performed saccades towards one of the pictures according to an imperative signal that had nothing to do with the picture contents. In order to produce voluntary saccades, in one experiment the imperative signal was a change in color of the initial fixation cross; in another experiment reflexive saccades were produced by an abrupt luminosity onset (the white border surrounding the pictures changed color). The imperative signal cued either the emotional or the neutral picture. In other words, in the voluntary saccade experiment, participants were asked to look at the left picture when the fixation cross turned green and to the right picture when the cross turned orange (for half of the participants it was reversed: green-right, orange-left). Analogous instructions were employed in the reflexive saccade experiment.

If emotional pictures exert an influence on the saccade generation system, we should expect shorter saccadic reaction times and less misdirected saccades when the imperative signal cued the emotional than the neutral picture. Our results generally support this hypothesis. For voluntary saccades, significantly shorter latencies were observed for saccades made towards unpleasant or pleasant pictures than toward neutral pictures, when the imperative signal was presented 150 ms before (RTs 345, 347, and 353 ms) or 150 ms after (RTs 316, 319, and 325 ms) the onset of the target pictures. For reflexive saccades, similar results were observed when the imperative signal was presented simultaneously (RTs 258, 259, and 268 ms) or 150 ms after (RTs 249, 239, and 253 ms) the onset of the target pictures. The fact that we found a significant emotional effect also for the exogenous (i.e. reflexive) saccades suggests that the effect does not need voluntary control to be materialized, and it is in that sense automatic.

Another follow-up experiment implementing the oculomotor inhibition paradigm provided even more convincing evidence for the view that emotional content is capable of affecting automatic saccade programming. In this experiment, the emotional-neutral picture pairs were presented as in the previous experiments (i.e., one to the left and one to the right of the center fixation point), but now participants did not initiate a saccade to one of the pictures but to a cross that was presented orthogonally (up or down) to the picture locations. A cross appearing at the visual periphery aligned with the central vertical axis served as the imperative signal and the saccade target. In other words, participants made vertical saccades in the presence of horizontally and parafoveally presented visual scenes that now served as distracters. Thus, the emotional and neural pictures did not share a spatial or response compatibility with the demanded saccade response. The participants were told to ignore the pictures and perform vertical saccades according to the imperative signal (i.e. to the cross appearing up or down).

The premotor theory of attention (Rizzolatti, Riggio, Dascola, & Umilta, 1987) posits that shifts of covert attention involve programming (but not executing) an eye movement. This theory has been supported by data showing that saccades deviate away from a location that has recently been attended to (for a review, see Van der Stigchel, Meeter, & Theeuwes, 2006). This is explained by the notion that competition takes place between the stimuli in the neural map that specifies the saccade goal (e.g. Godjin & Theeuwes, 2004). Competing stimuli that can potentially serve as a saccade target activate separate populations of neurons. If a distracter is presented simultaneously with or before the task-relevant saccade target, and this distracter competes for a candidacy for a saccadic target, the inhibition of the saccadic response to the spatial location of the distracter will reduce the activity of neurons responsible for programming a saccadic response to the distracter below the baseline level. This causes the task-relevant saccade to curve away from the distracter. Thus, a measure of saccadic curvature and saccadic error (i.e. deviation of the saccade endpoint from the designated target) can be used to study whether a saccade has been initially programmed (and soon inhibited) towards the location of the distracter. Figure 9.3 illustrates how to compute these two measures, saccadic curvature and endpoint deviation. Saccadic curvature is the maximum curvature away from a distracter that is observed in the saccadic trajectory. Endpoint deviation refers to the size of the saccadic error: how much the observed landing position deviates from the intended location.

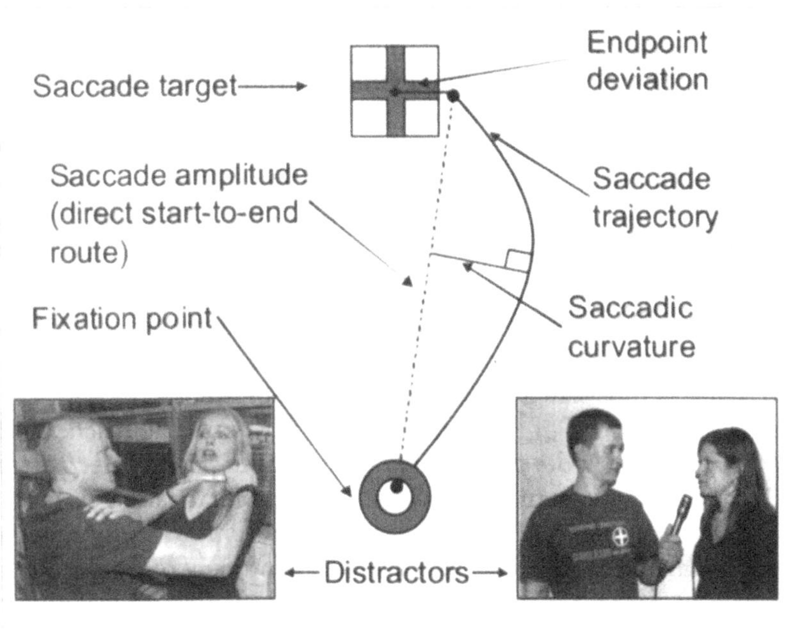

Figure 9.3 An illustration of the measure of saccadic curvature and saccade endpoint deviation. An emotional distracter appears on the left and a neutral distracter on the right. (*See Plate 7.*)

Based on the findings reviewed above, we predicted emotional pictures to automatically attract an eye movement. In the present task, such an eye movement would be inappropriate and thus be inhibited. If so, the actually performed saccade should deviate away from the emotional picture that is now a distracter. This in turn would give us reason to argue that the emotionality of an unattended stimulus is encoded and subsequently influences saccade programming. This was exactly what we observed in our experiment. The saccades deviated away from the location occupied by the emotional pictures. In other words, when an emotional picture was located to the left of the center fixation point, the endpoint of the vertical saccade (up or down) was shifted away from the visual field where the emotional picture was presented. Similarly, the saccadic trajectory curved away from the emotional picture. These findings provide strong support for the notion that (1) emotional content can be readily detected from the parafovea and (2) that perception of emotional content brings with it an automatic saccade towards the location occupied by the emotional scene.

What information is extracted from parafoveally or peripherally presented emotional pictures?

Given the results discussed above, the question arises whether specific emotional content can be readily extracted from peripheral vision. In other words, can observers detect that there is a pleasant or an unpleasant picture in the parafovea (or periphery)? If this is not possible, it would mean that the eyes are captured by the stimulus merely being emotionally arousing, without any discrimination of affective valence (i.e. pleasant or unpleasant content). If so, this would suggest that high-arousal pictorial materials in general possess "magnetizing power".

Previous studies on object recognition have demonstrated that rapid object categorization is indeed possible from the visual periphery, provided that stimulus size exceeds the spatial resolution of the peripheral retina (e.g. Thorpe, Gegenfurtner, Fabre-Thorpe, & Heinrich, 2001). Moreover, there is evidence that emotional valence can be detected very fast from foveally presented stimuli (e.g. Junghöfer, Bradley, Elbert, & Lang, 2001). Calvo and Nummenmaa (2007) set out to study whether emotional valence can be detected and even genuinely recognized from parafoveally presented pictures. It is possible that parafoveal vision only allows detection of previously familiar emotional material. That is, pictures that have previously been perceived under foveal vision might be quickly detected from the parafovea, but the emotional valence of totally novel pictures might not be encoded parafoveally. Such an argument has recently been put forth by Cave and Batty (2006) and Storbeck, Robinson and McCourt (2006). The idea is that emotional valence cannot be encoded pre-attentively, but object or scene features need to be first attentively identified before genuine affective analysis of the scene as a whole is possible.

In order to test whether encoding of emotional valence is possible for novel stimuli, Calvo and Nummenmaa (2007) conducted a set of experiments by using the affective priming paradigm. Also the gaze-contingent masking paradigm was implemented in a subset of the experiments. In the affective priming experiments a pleasant or unpleasant prime picture was presented parafoveally for 150 ms, followed by a 150 ms blank screen and a centrally presented probe picture that was either congruent (e.g. pleasant-pleasant) or incongruent (e.g. pleasant-unpleasant) with respect to the affective valence of the prime. By pressing a designated key in the computer keyboard, participants were asked to respond as fast as possible whether the probe picture was pleasant or unpleasant. In the gaze-contingent masking paradigm, a visual mask covering the foveal area moves along with the participant's eyes. Thus, even if the participant makes an eye movement to a parafoveally presented picture, its foveal inspection is rendered impossible by the visual mask. In their Experiment 5, the foveal masking paradigm was employed to directly study (i.e. not via priming) the valence identification (via subjective report) of parafoveally presented emotional pictures.

The initial experiment assessed whether foveal pre-exposure is necessary for the affective priming effect to occur. Half of the participants were presented foveally with the prime stimuli before the experiment proper, whereas the other half of the participants were presented with a set of unrelated pictures. As expected, the priming effects were only observed in the foveal pre-exposure group (see Figure 9.4(A)) but not in the no-preview group. This suggests that the encoding of emotional valence is possible for unattended, parafoveally presented scenes only when they have been previously processed, but not for novel stimuli. Interestingly, the significant affective priming effect was only observed when the primes were presented in the left visual field. Subsequent experiments of Calvo and Nummenmaa (2007) further confirmed this left visual field advantage and demonstrated that valence discrimination can be undertaken for parafoveally presented pictures, but only when they are presented repeatedly to the parafovea. A crucial demonstration of this effect was Experiment 4 in which the parafoveal primes were presented four times, once in each block under gaze-contingent foveal masking that strictly prevented the foveal inspection of the primes. In this experiment (see Figure 9.4(B)) the priming effects emerged only in the fourth block (i.e. when the prime was presented to the parafovea for the fourth time). Importantly, the priming effect was again observed only when the primes were presented to the left visual field.

Experiment 5 of Calvo and Nummenmaa (2007) tested directly the processing of parafoveally presented pictures. Participants' task was to evaluate the affective valence of the pictures. They responded whether the single picture presented for 150 ms to the parafovea was pleasant or unpleasant. To make sure that foveal inspection of the pictures was not

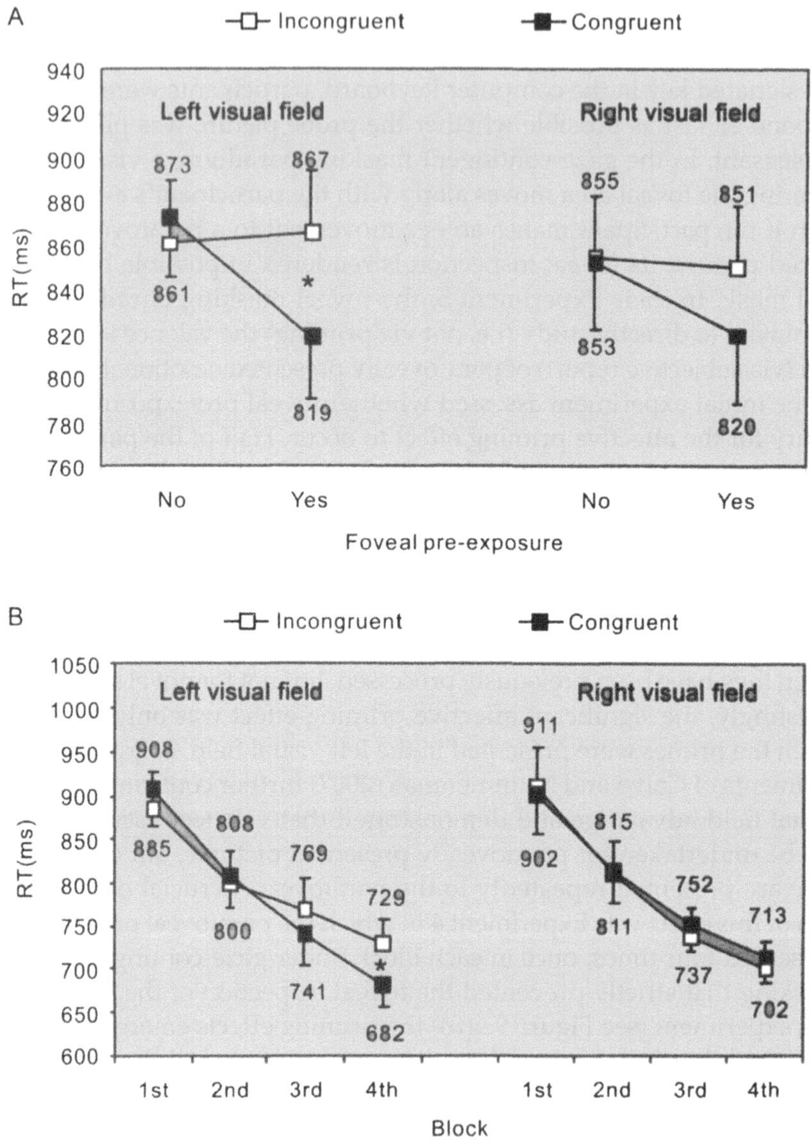

Figure 9.4 Reaction times as a function of prime-probe congruency, the visual field of the prime, and foveal preview in Experiment 1 (A), and as a function of prime-probe congruency, the visual field of the prime, and block in Experiment 4 (B) of Calvo and Nummenmaa (2007).

possible a gaze-contingent foveal mask was used. The presentation of the picture set was repeated three times. Experiment 5 confirmed the results of the priming studies by demonstrating that the recognition of affective valence improved with repeated exposure to the same pictures and was better for the pictures presented to the left visual field. Interestingly, the recognition was above chance even during the first exposure to the pictures, which suggests that observers are able to pick up from the parafovea affectively relevant information.

The general conclusion derived from the priming experiments of Calvo and Nummenmaa (2007) is that emotional valence may be detected parafoveally, but only when they have pre-exposed to the picture either foveally or parafoveally. In other words, no affective priming was observed when the prime picture was presented for the first time; the effect only appeared when the observers had a chance to see the picture a few times. This is consistent with the view (Cave & Batty, 2006) that a repeated parafoveal exposure leads to a sufficient recognition of the scene to render possible its affective evaluation. Experiment 5 provided evidence in support of the view that emotional valence may be recognized even for novel stimuli. This suggests that, although affective valence of overtly unattended scenes is quickly detected and encoded, affective priming requires stronger activation that is accrued through repeated exposure. In any case, the effects only emerged or were greater, both for affective encoding and priming, when the pictures were presented in the left than right visual field. This supports a right hemispheric specialization in visual emotional processing.

General discussion

Reflexive attentional capture by emotional pictures

Dual-process theories of attention (see Barrett, Tugade, & Engle, 2004; Corbetta & Shulman, 2002; Egeth & Yantis, 1997) distinguish between a reflexive and a voluntary mechanism of attention orienting. In the former case attention is captured exogenously, preattentively, by the stimulus properties, whereas in the latter case the allocation of attention is controlled endogenously by the individual's goals and interests. The findings presented in this chapter consistently suggest that there is a genuinely exogenous attentional capture by emotional stimuli. Further, the results lend support to the notion that not only covert attention but also the saccade generation system is automatically recruited to orient the organism towards events that are pertinent to the organism's well being (i.e. events that entail threat or potential for positive affect). The model of saccade generation by Findlay and Walker (1999) suggests that peripheral visual events, such as remote luminosity onsets, can trigger automatic saccades. Our results lend support to the notion that emotional pictures having high intrinsic salience can also trigger a reflexive saccade. The data presented in this chapter suggest that both the saccade target selection and the saccade initiating system are automatically influenced by emotional picture content.

The role of parafoveal perception in eye movement guidance during picture viewing

We have shown that emotional valence can be detected (Calvo & Lang, 2004, 2005; Nummenmaa et al., 2006) and even discriminated (e.g. pleasant vs. unpleasant, Calvo & Nummenmaa, 2007) from the parafovea. The eye-tracking studies reviewed above have also systematically demonstrated both a voluntary and involuntary attentional bias towards emotional pictures of both pleasant and unpleasant valence. Therefore, it is useful to discuss the implications of these findings on the models of eye movement guidance during high-level scene perception.

It is generally accepted that salient low-level visual features, such as contrast, color, and intensity, attract the eyes during picture viewing. However, as reviewed in the Introduction, the evidence for a higher-level semantic guidance is less clear. While some studies (De Graef, 2005; Loftus & Mackworth, 1978; Mackworth & Morandi, 1967; Underwood, 2005) have provided evidence for semantic guidance (observers fixate a scene-incongruous object earlier than a scene-congruous object), other studies (De Graef et al., 1990; Henderson et al., 1999) have failed to do so. The present set of experiments demonstrates that emotional content is capable of governing the eyes in a reflexive fashion. This implies that some aspect of the picture content is readily perceived in the parafovea or periphery, which then captures the eyes. As our stimulus pictures were controlled for differences in low-level visual features, we are left with the argument that emotional valence is extracted of the visual scenes. It should be noted, however, that we do not argue that specific semantic content is necessarily picked up from the emotional pictures. Instead, our contention is that observers can readily perceive whether or not a scene contains emotionally arousing material. We feel that such a conclusion can be made relatively safely on the basis of the evidence reviewed above. It is generally consistent with the findings of Calvo and Nummenmaa (2007) who found no affective priming for novel pictures. However, that study contains evidence (their Experiment 5) suggesting that even the recognition of emotional valence may be possible in the parafoveal vision.

This conclusion bears some similarity to findings demonstrating that the gist of a visual scene (e.g. that the picture depicts a traffic situation or a football game) can be perceived very rapidly (in about 100 ms; e.g. Biederman, 1972; Boyce & Pollatsek, 1992; for a review, see Underwood, 2005). However, these two findings differ in that the "gist effect" implies that global, non-specific semantic information is readily perceived of a scene, whereas our emotional effect suggests that stimulus features that give rise to emotional arousal (regardless of their specific emotional content) can be readily picked up from the periphery.

References

Adolphs, R. (2002). Neural systems for recognizing emotion. *Current Opinion in Neurobiology, 12*, 169-177.

Armony, J. L., & Dolan, R. J. (2002). Modulating of spatial attention by fear-conditioned stimuli: An event-related fMRI study. *Neuropsychologia*, 40, 817-826.

Awh, E., Armstrong, K. M., & Moore, T. (2006). Visual and oculomotor selection: Links, causes and implications for spatial attention. *Trends in Cognitive Sciences, 10*, 124-130.

Barrett, L. F., Tugade, M., & Engle, R. W. (2004). Individual differences in working memory capacity and dual-process theories of mind. *Psychological Bulletin, 130*, 553-573.

Biederman, I. (1972). Perceiving real-world scenes. *Science, 177*, 77-80.

Blanchette, I. (2006). Snakes, spiders, guns, and syringes: How specific are evolutionary constraints on the detection of threatening stimuli? *Quarterly Journal of Experimental Psychology, 59*, 1484-1504.

Boyce, S. J., & Pollatsek, A. (1992). Identification of objects in scenes: The role of scene background in object naming. *Journal of Experimental Psychology: Human Perception and Performance, 18*, 531-543.

Bradley, B. P., Mogg, K., Falla, S., & Hamilton, L. R. (1998). Attentional bias for threatening facial expressions in anxiety: Manipulations of stimulus duration. *Cognition and Emotion, 12*, 737-753.

Buswell, G. T. (1935). *How people look at pictures*. Chicago: University of

Chicago Press.

Calvo, M. G., Avero, P., & Lundqvist, D. (2006). Facilitated detection of angry faces: Initial orienting vs. processing efficiency. *Cognition and Emotion, 20,* 785-811.

Calvo, M. G., & Lang, P. J. (2004). Gaze patterns when looking at emotional pictures: Motivationally biased attention. *Motivation and Emotion, 28,* 221-243.

Calvo, M. G., & Lang, P. J. (2005). Parafoveal semantic processing of emotional visual scenes. *Journal of Experimental Psychology: Human Perception and Performance, 31,* 502-519.

Calvo, M. G., & Nummenmaa, L. (2007). Processing of "unattended" emotional visual scenes. *Journal of Experimental Psychology: General, 136,* 347-369.

Cave, K., & Batty, M. (2006). From searching for features to searching for threat: Drawing the boundary between preattentive and attentive vision. *Visual Cognition, 14,* 1-18.

Compton, R. J. (2003). The interface between emotion and attention: A review of evidence from psychology and neuroscience. *Behavioral and Cognitive Neuroscience Reviews, 2,* 115-129.

Corbetta, M., & Shulman, G. L. (2002). Control of goal-directed and stimulus-driven attention in the brain. *Nature Reviews Neuroscience, 3,* 201-215.

De Graef, P. (2005). Semantic effects on object selection in real-world scene perception. In G. Underwood (Ed.), *Cognitive processes in eye guidance* (pp. 189-211). Oxford: Oxford University Press.

De Graef, P., Christiaens, D., & d'Ydewalle, G. (1990). Perceptual effects of scene content on object identification. *Psychological Research, 52,* 317-329.

Eger, E., Jedynak, A., Iwaki, T., & Skrandies, W. (2003). Rapid extraction of emotional expression: Evidence from evoked potential fields during brief presentation of face stimuli. *Neuropsychologia, 41,* 808-817.

Egeth, H. E., & Yantis, S. (1997). Visual attention: Control, representation and time course. *Annual Review of Psychology, 48,* 269-297.

Findlay, J. M., & Walker, R. (1999). A model of saccade generation based on parallel processing and competitive inhibition. *Behavioral and Brain Sciences, 22,* 661-721.

Frijda, N. H. (1986). *The emotions.* New York: Cambridge University Press.

Fox, E., Lester, V., Russo, R., Bowles, R. J., Pichler, A., & Dutton, K.

(2000). Facial expressions of emotion: Are angry faces detected more efficiently? *Cognition and Emotion, 14,* 61-92.

Fox, E., Russo, R., Bowles, R., & Dutton, K. (2001). Do threatening stimuli draw or hold visual attention in subclinical anxiety? *Journal of Experimental Psychology: General, 130,* 681-700.

Fox, E., Russo, R., & Dutton, K. (2002). Attentional bias for threat: Evidence for delayed disengagement from emotional cues. *Cognition and Emotion, 16,* 335-379.

Godjin, R., & Theeuwes, J. (2004). The relationship between inhibition of return and saccade trajectory deviations. *Journal of Experimental Psychology: Human Perception and Performance, 30,* 538-554.

Gordon, R. D. (2004). Attentional allocation during the perception of scenes. *Journal of Experimental Psychology: Human Perception and Performance, 30,* 760-777.

Henderson, J. M. (2003). Human gaze control during real-world scene perception. *Trends in Cognitive Sciences, 7,* 498-504.

Henderson, J. M., & Hollingworth, A. (1999). High-level scene perception. *Annual Review of Psychology, 50,* 243-271.

Henderson, J. M., Weeks, P. A., Jr., & Hollingworth, A. (1999). Effects of semantic consistency on eye movements during scene viewing. *Journal of Experimental Psychology: Human Perception and Performance, 25,* 210-228.

Junghöfer, M., Bradley, M. M., Elbert, T., & Lang, P. J. (2001). Fleeting images: A new look at early emotion discrimination. *Psychophysiology, 38,* 175-178.

Keil, A., Moratti, S., Sabatinelli, D., Bradley, M. M., & Lang, P. J. (2005). Additive effects of emotional content and spatial selective attention on electrocortical facilitation. *Cerebral Cortex, 15,* 1187-1197.

Lang, P. J., Bradley, M. M., & Cuthbert, B. N. (2005). *International affective picture system (IAPS): Digitized photographs, instruction manual and affective ratings.* (Tech. Rep. A-6). Gainesville: University of Florida, The Center for Research in Psychophysiology.

Lazarus, R. S. (1991). *Emotion and adaptation.* London: Oxford University Press.

LeDoux, J. E. (1995). Emotion: Clues from the brain. *Annual Review of Psychology, 46,* 209-235.

Lipp, O. V., Derakshan, N., Waters, A. M., & Logies, S. (2004). Snakes and cats in the flower bed: Fast detection is not specific to pictures of fear-relevant animals. *Emotion, 4,* 233-250.

Loftus, G. R., & Mackworth, N. H. (1978). Cognitive determinants of fixation location during picture viewing. *Journal of Experimental Psychology: Human Perception and Performance, 4*, 565-572.

Mackworth, N. H., & Morandi, A. J. (1967). The gaze selects informative details within pictures. *Perception & Psychophysics, 2*, 547-552.

Mogg, K., & Bradley, B. P. (1999). Orienting of attention to threatening facial expressions presented under conditions of restricted awareness. *Cognition and Emotion, 13*, 713-740.

Mogg, K., McNamara, J., Powys, M., Rawlinson, H., Seiffer, A., & Bradley, B. P. (2000). Selective attention to threat: A test of two cognitive models of anxiety. *Cognition and Emotion, 14*, 375-399.

Nummenmaa, L., Hyönä, J., & Calvo, M. G. (2006). Eye movement assessment of selective attentional capture by emotional pictures. *Emotion, 6*, 257-268.

Oatley, K., & Johnson-Laird, P. N. (1987). Towards a cognitive theory of emotions. *Cognition and Emotion, 1*, 29-50.

Öhman, A., Flykt, A., & Esteves, F. (2001). Emotion drives attention: Detecting the snake in the grass. *Journal of Experimental Psychology: General, 130*, 466-378.

Öhman, A., Lundqvist, D., & Esteves, F. (2001). The face in the crowd revisited: A threat advantage with schematic stimuli. *Journal of Personality and Social Psychology, 80*, 381-396.

Pessoa, L., McKenna, M., Gutierrez, E., & Ungerleider, L. G. (2002). Neural processing of emotional faces requires attention. *Proceedings of the National Academy of Sciences, 99*, 11458-11463.

Pessoa, L. (2005). To what extent are emotional visual stimuli processed without attention and awareness? *Current Opinion in Neurobiology, 15*, 188-196.

Posner, M. I. (1980). Orienting of attention. *Quarterly Journal of Experimental Psychology, 32*, 3-25.

Rizzolatti, G., Riggio, L., Dascola, I., & Umilta, C. (1987). Reorienting attention across the horizontal and vertical meridians: Evidence in favor of a premotor theory of attention. *Neuropsychologia, 25*, 31-40.

Scherer, K. R. (1999). Appraisal theory. In T. Dalgleish, & M.J. Power (Eds.), *Handbook of cognition and emotion* (pp.637-663). New York: John Wiley & Sons.

Storbeck, J., Robinson, M. D., & McCourt, M. E. (2006). Semantic processing precedes affective retrieval: The neurological case for cognitive primacy in visual processing. *Review of General Psychology, 10*, 41-55.

Thorpe, S. J., Gegenfurtner, K. R., Fabre-Thorpe, M., & Bülthoff, H. H.

(2001). Detection of animals in natural images using far peripheral vision. *European Journal of Neurosciences, 14*, 869-876.

Tipples, J., Atkinson, A. P., & Young, A. W. (2002). The eyebrow frown: A salient social signal. *Emotion, 2*, 288-296.

Tipples, J., Young, A. W., Quinlan, P., Broks, P., & Ellis, A. (2002). Searching for threat. *Quarterly Journal of Experimental Psychology, 55A*, 1007-1026.

Torralba, A., Oliva, A., Castelhano, M. S., & Henderson, J. M. (2006). Contextual guidance of eye movements and attention in real-world scenes: The role of global features on object search. *Psychological Review, 113*, 766-786.

Underwood, G. (2005). Eye fixations on pictures of natural scenes: Getting the gist and identifying the components. In G. Underwood (Ed.), *Cognitive processes in eye guidance* (pp.163-187). Oxford: Oxford University Press.

Van der Stigchel, S., Meeter, M., & Theeuwes, J. (2006). Eye movement trajectories and what they tell us. *Neuroscience and Biobehavioral Reviews, 30*, 666-679.

Vuilleumier, P. (2005). How brains beware: Neural mechanisms of emotional attention. *Trends in Cognitive Sciences, 9*, 585-594.

Vuilleumier, P., Armony, J. L., Driver, J., & Dolan, R. J. (2001). Effects of attention and emotion on face processing in the human brain: An event-related fMRI study. *Neuron, 30*, 829-841.

Vuilleumier, P., Armony, J. L., & Dolan, R. J. (2003). Reciprocal links between emotion and attention. In K. J. Friston, C. D. Frith, R. J. Dolan, C. Price, J. Ashburner, W. Penny, S. Zeki, & R. S. J. Frackowiak (Eds.), *Human brain function* (pp. 419-444). New York: Academic Press.

Wandell, B. A. (1995). *Foundations of vision*. Sunderland, MA: Sinauer.

Yarbus, A. L. (1967). *Eye movements and vision*. New York: Plenum.

Yiend, J., & Mathews, A. (2001). Anxiety and attention to threatening pictures. *Quarterly Journal of Experimental Psychology, 54A*, 665-681.

Chapter 10

Eye movements in search for multiple targets

Tamaryn Menneer, Michael J. Stroud, Kyle R. Cave, Nick Donnelly, and Keith Rayner

Visual search for a complex object in a cluttered array of distractor objects requires some mental representation of the target object or target features to be found (Duncan & Humphreys, 1989; Cave & Wolfe, 1990; Desimone & Duncan, 1995). In some situations it is necessary to search for two or more targets simultaneously. Simultaneous search presents an additional challenge for the attentional system, because the target representation or template must be broad enough to include all of the possible targets. Representing multiple targets and searching for them simultaneously could potentially lower search performance, and the performance drop could provide new insights into how search targets are specified and how search is accomplished. In this chapter we consider whether search for two targets results in a lower level of performance than that achieved by conducting two independent single-target searches.

There are three possible scenarios for target representations when search is conducted for two targets. First, the representation(s) for two targets could be the same as the two representations in single-target searches, therefore resulting in dual-target search that selects the same items as those selected in the single-target searches, while rejecting the same distractors. In this case, accuracy and search time will be equal across single-target and dual-target search. A second possibility arises if there is some overlap between the features of the two targets, so that the target representation can be based at least in part on those shared features. This situation could produce efficient dual-target search, and dual-target performance might even be better than the summed performance across single-target searches. The third possibility is that the two target representations interfere with one another. The attentional system may not be able to represent two very different objects or two very different features within the same dimension simultaneously. For instance, if one target is red and another is green, it may only be possible to represent red and green by specifying a broad range of colors that includes both red and green. In this case attention will probably also be directed to distractors within the entire range, and thus search time would be wasted attending to distractors that are not similar to either target.

In earlier experiments, search for two targets has been efficient provided that each of the targets was defined exclusively in different feature dimensions (Treisman & Gelade, 1980; Quinlan & Humphreys, 1987; Treisman, 1988), or the features specifying the targets were linearly separable from distractors in feature space (D'Zmura, 1991; Barrett, Menneer, Phillips, Cave, & Donnelly, 2003). In both cases, there should be little interference between target feature values, in the first case because there is only one target value in each feature dimension, and in the other because a single-target category can be specified that does not include distractor values. In contrast to this previous research, this chapter reviews a large body of research in which search for two targets displays a performance cost over two independent single-target searches. This dual-target cost is demonstrated by comparing the joint performance across two independent single-target searches with the performance in a simultaneous search for the same two targets. The dual-target cost arises when targets are defined within the same feature dimension, and distractor values fall between the target values in stimulus feature space. The cost is exhibited in the time required to search the display, in the accuracy, or in both, depending on the type of stimuli used.

Targets defined within a single dimension: Color, shape, and orientation

The first set of experiments investigated search for two simple targets defined within the same feature dimension. Separate experiments tested search for target pairs defined by color, shape and orientation. In each experiment, a cost in performance was revealed for simultaneous search for two dissimilar targets compared with two independent single-target searches (Menneer, Barrett, Phillips, Donnelly, & Cave, 2007). A staircase procedure was used to determine the exposure time necessary to achieve a predetermined level of accuracy in search of eight-item displays. Ideally this exposure time would give us a single measure that could then be used to compare search performance across the single-target and dual-target conditions. However, fluctuations in accuracy did occur and therefore, in addition to our analyses of exposure times, we also analyzed a measure that adjusted each exposure time by the log of probability of error responses (Mean Exposure Threshould / log[P(error)], J. Townsend, personal communication). The times reported here are the adjusted values, although the conclusions are similar with or without the adjustment.

With color-defined targets, stimuli were squares of 3.0° by 2.9° visual angle that were colored according to one of 16 evenly spaced colors in a ring in CIE color space (see Figure 10.1). The two targets were selected from positions opposite each other in the color ring in order to maximize the difference between the two and the number of distractor values between the target feature values. The results showed that it was twice as efficient to combine two independent searches as it was to perform a single dual-target search (1237 ms versus 2694 ms: $t(25) = 4.39$, $p<0.01$). In dual-target search each participant primarily searched for one target in preference to the other and the accuracy on this less-preferred target was lower in the dual-target condition than on the less-preferred target across single-target searches ($t(25) = 2.65$, $p<0.01$).

In the search for complex shapes, the stimuli were 14 abstract black shapes constructed by pair-wise combination of six simple components. Targets were paired such that they each had a different number of minima of curvature and were composed from different components (see Figure 10.2). In contrast to the results with color stimuli, the summed single-target search time was equivalent to the dual-target search time. However, accuracy was again lower in dual-target search, to the extent that the less-preferred target was only detected at chance-level accuracy. Each participant was effectively only searching for one target. Thus the shape search also exhibits a severe dual-target cost, although the nature of the cost is very different from that in the color search.

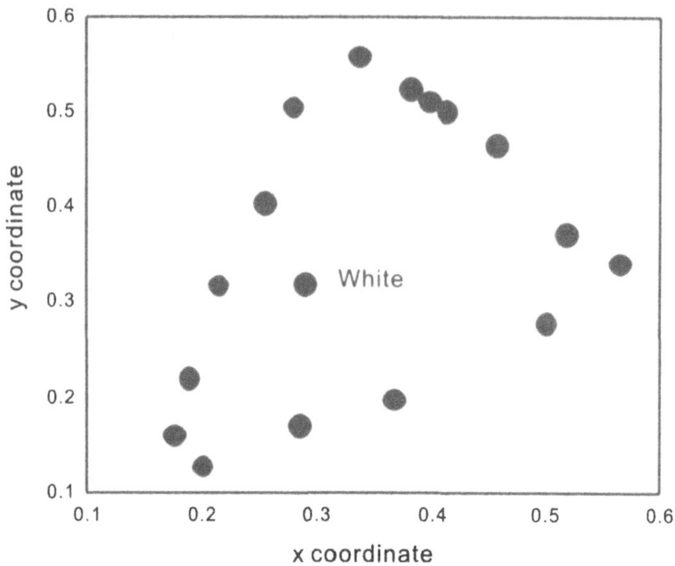

Figure 10.1 CIE (x, y) coordinates of the colors for color-defined stimuli

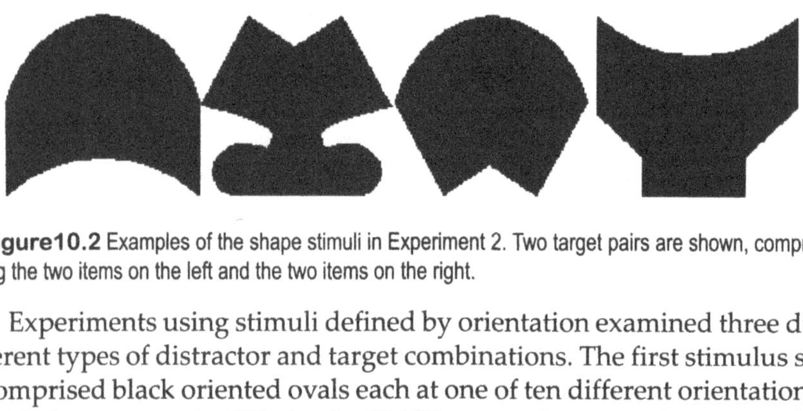

Figure10.2 Examples of the shape stimuli in Experiment 2. Two target pairs are shown, comprising the two items on the left and the two items on the right.

Experiments using stimuli defined by orientation examined three different types of distractor and target combinations. The first stimulus set comprised black oriented ovals each at one of ten different orientations, with the two targets differing by 90°. The second set was the same as the first except that the ovals were colored using the colors in Figure 10.1. The two targets again differed by 90° and the color variation was irrelevant to the task. The third set was the same as the second, but the task was to search for one color target and one orientation target. In search for two black orientations and in search for one color and one orientation, the total time for both single-target searches was the same as that required for the dual-target search, indicating no dual-target time cost. In search for two orientations when stimuli were irrelevantly colored, there was a dual-target time cost ($t(19)=2.88$, $p<0.01$). In all three conditions, the search time data are compromised by the accuracy: Dual-target accuracy was lower than the mean of single-target search accuracies (Orientation: $t(19)=3.79$, $p<0.01$; Orientation with irrelevant color: $t(19)=2.48$, $p<0.05$; Orientation and color: $t(19)=2.20$, $p<0.05$), and participants again biased search towards one of the two targets. Thus, even when targets are defined by different feature dimensions (color and orientation) and when the time measures indicate efficient search, there is an accuracy cost in dual-target search indicating that both features cannot be simultaneously maintained. Such a cost may not have been discovered in previous research demonstrating efficient search with between-dimension targets (Treisman et al., 1980; Quinlan et al., 1987; Treisman, 1988) because the accuracy data for each target was not examined.

In summary, there is a dual-target cost in search for targets defined by color, shape or orientation, although in the latter two cases the cost manifests solely as a reduction of accuracy in detecting the non-preferred target rather than an increase in the time needed to accurately discriminate its appearance in the display. This pattern indicates that in the dual-target condition, participants found it impossible to sustain attention across both targets and made strategic decisions to attend to one target or the other.

Conjunction targets: Color and shape

The second study tested more complex searches. The stimuli were abstract colored shapes, and targets were defined by a color-shape conjunction. The stimuli were designed to be representative of x-ray images of guns and improvised explosive devices (IEDs), while controlling for area and color, in order to make the results applicable to security search of baggage x-rays. In x-ray images, guns are typically blue and IEDs typically consist of orange explosives with blue wires, and thus the main part of each type of target is very different in color to the other. This difference was mirrored in the abstract stimuli: For each subject, the main colors for the two targets were taken from opposite sides of the color circle in Figure 10.1. Each stimulus was constructed using a combination of a small rectangle and a large rectangle, providing three types of stimuli: corresponding to a gun, an IED, and a plain rectangle, as illustrated in Figure 10.3. Target pairs of gun and IED targets were colored such that the stripe of the IED was the same color as the gun, and the main color of the IED was maximally different to the color of the gun. Distractors were all three types of object colored with a randomly selected color from the set of 16. The stripes of distractor rectangles were always the same color as the target IED stripe.

A dual-target cost was demonstrated in both time and accuracy in two separate experimental procedures. The first was a staircase procedure and the second was a set-size manipulation in which the number of items in the display was varied to provide a slope indicating the response time per item. Further investigation with response time slopes showed that the time cost is eliminated with practice, with the summed slopes for single-target searches being the same as the slope for dual-target search. However, even after extensive practice (4800 trials) there remained a cost in accuracy, with mean accuracy for single-target searches being higher than the accuracy in dual-target search ($t(23)=4.01$, $p<0.01$).

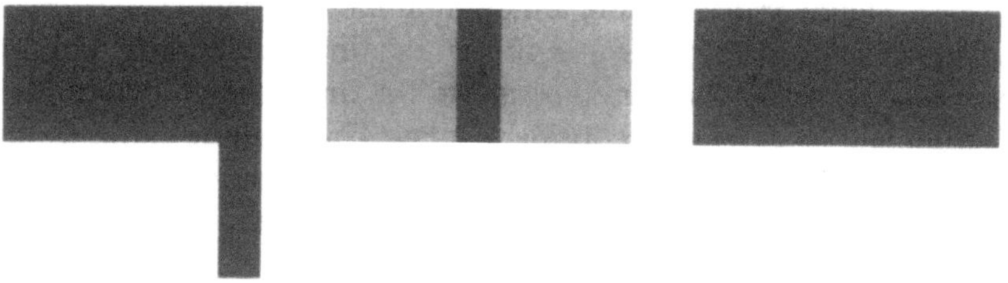

Figure 10.3 Examples of the three types of stimuli use: gun, IED and plain rectangle. The gun and the IED shown here comprise a target pair for dual-target search. (*See Plate 8.*)

Manipulating target similarity: Color and orientation

It is apparent that simultaneous search for two targets is compromised when the defining features conflict with each other and allow distractor feature values to fall between the target values. Therefore in the third study (Barrett et al., 2003) the effect of featural similarity between the targets on dual-target search efficiency was investigated. Similarity between two targets is measured here in terms of the number of distractors that fall between the targets in feature space together with the absolute distance between the target features in feature space. Results with both color-defined targets and orientation-defined targets, within the stimulus sets previous described, clearly showed that when the two targets were adjacent in stimulus space, search was efficient in terms of time and accuracy. However, when the targets were not adjacent in stimulus space, search performance was significantly reduced.

Understanding the dual target cost: Eye movements

The studies described up to this point demonstrate that dual-target costs arise in a wide variety of different search tasks, and raise questions about specifically how the introduction of a second target causes search performance to break down. The final study uses information on eye movements during search to understand more about the attentional limitations that produce dual-target costs (Stroud, Menneer, Cave, Donnelly, & Rayner, 2008). Eye movements were recorded during search for two targets that in the first experiment shared the same color and in the second experiment did not. These experiments were run using the same color-shape conjunctions as previously described (Figure 10.3) with the addition of a fourth shape resembling a knife (see Figure 10.4), which was used in conjunction with all 16 colors (Figure 10.1). Target pairs either comprised a gun and IED that were of maximally different dominant colors, or a gun and knife of the same color.

In both of these search tasks, there are large color differences across the elements within a search array. We can expect that these color differences can be identified preattentively and used to guide attention to-

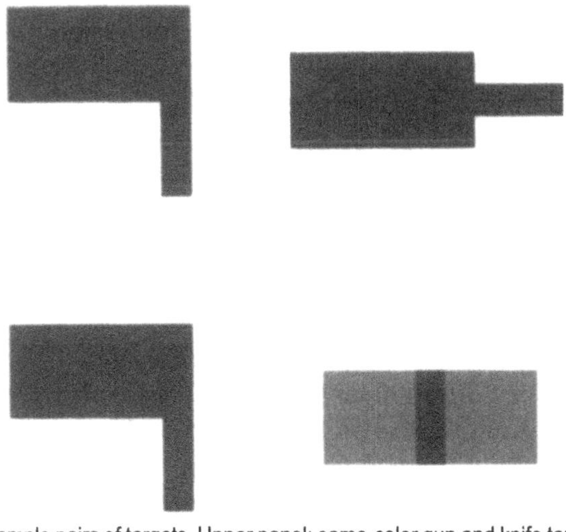

Figure 10.4 Example pairs of targets. Upper panel: same-color gun and knife targets. Lower panel: different-color gun and IED targets. (*See Plate 9.*)

ward items with the target color and away from distractors with very different colors. On the other hand, the shape discriminations necessary in this task are more difficult. When a single stimulus item is attended, its shape is easily discriminated from the other possible shapes used in these experiments. However, because the shapes consist of different configurations of the same two component rectangles, distinguishing them preattentively is difficult, and the shape information may not be very helpful in directing attention to potential targets. Thus, color is likely to be very helpful in search, while shape is likely to be much less helpful. Within this framework of wide color variation and more narrow shape variation, the two experiments measured dual-target search costs when the two targets shared the same color and when they were primarily of different colors. The results demonstrated that the probability of fixating given distractors differs across the two types of dual-target search, thereby revealing the source of the dual-target cost when targets are distant from each other.

When the two targets shared color, single-target search results revealed that the distractor colors that are likely to be fixated are within two color-steps of the target color. The graphs in Figure 10.5 illustrate this very effective color selectivity. In these graphs, the X-axis represents the color of each item, with the target color on the left, the color most dissimilar to the target color on the right, and the other colors arranged along the X-axis according to their similarity to the target color. The data for dual-target search in Figure 10.5 show that fixations are generally limited to items with colors similar to the target color, demonstrating color selectivity similar to that observed in the single-target searches. Such color selectivity allows search for two targets to be very efficient, providing both targets are the same color. Although it is not shown in the graphs, shape selectivity was very poor, with approximately the same number of fixations to each of the different shape types. The combination of effective color selectivity and ineffective shape selectivity avoids any dual-target cost and instead produces a large advantage for dual-target search over single-target search, provided targets have the same color.

When the two targets are separated in color space, the pattern of eye movements is very different, as shown in Figure 10.6. In these graphs, the color of the gun target is on the left end of the X-axis, and the color of the IED is on the right end. Color selectivity is again high for single-target searches, with participants limiting their fixations primarily to those elements with colors similar to the target color. However, color se-

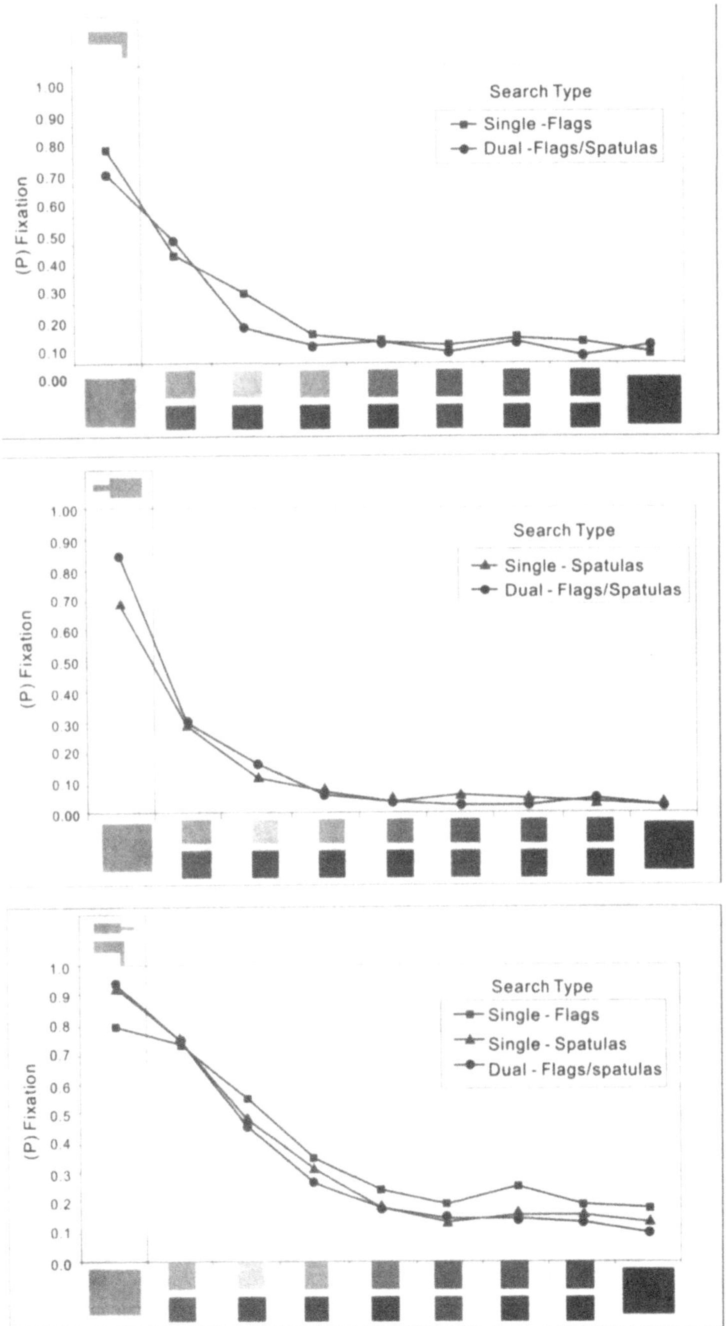

Figure 10.5 Probability of fixating a target of a given color when targets share the same color on gun present trials, knife present trials and absent trials. (*See Plate 10.*)

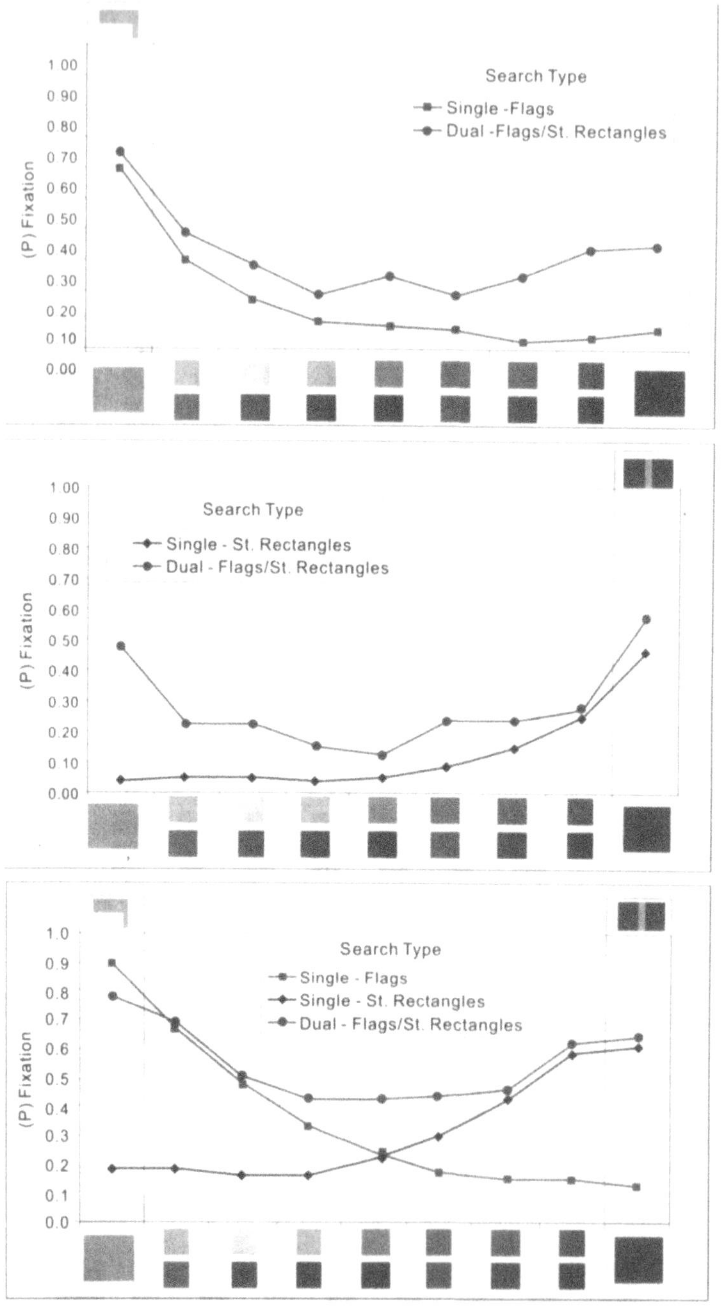

Figure 10.6 Probability of fixating a target of a given color when targets have different colors on gun present trials, IED present trials, and absent trials. (*See Plate 11.*)

lectivity breaks down in the dual-target search, in which there are more fixations across all colors compared with single-target search. The most surprising results are revealed for distractors that are not similar to either target color, represented in the middle region of each graph. These distractors are fixated much more often in dual-target search than in either of the single-target searches. The gap between the dual-target search line (more fixations) and the two single-target search lines (fewer fixations) represents the distractor fixations that only occur in the dual-target searches. This gap is the dual-target cost, and it demonstrates that the ability to guide fixations by color breaks down when the searcher attempts to specify two different target colors simultaneously. Two distinct target feature values cannot be simultaneously represented for guided search without also incorporating many distractors that would otherwise be excluded.

When color can be used effectively to guide search to both target types while eliminating differently colored distractors, dual-target search can be as effective as single-target search. However, when the color of the targets is in conflict, a single feature value cannot be used to guide search for both target classes. Additional experiments have shown that practice gives rise to an overall improvement in efficiency and accuracy, and can eliminate any time cost, but a dual-target cost in accuracy remains. Thus there is no evidence that multiple distinct target representations can be simultaneously maintained. The dual-target cost found in these studies suggests that dual-target search is often guided by a single representation of shared target features. When distractor values lie between target values within a given feature dimension (here, color), this representation will often misguide searches such that resources are wasted attending to these distractors. Direct evidence for this misguidance comes from the eye-movement experiments described above. This finding illustrates that even though there are attentional mechanisms that can guide attention and eye movements according to any of a number of different features, there are fundamental limitations to how search targets can be represented, and these limitations can prevent efficient searches from occurring in complex situations.

Acknowledgments

This work was supported by the Human Factors Program of the U.S. Department of Homeland Security's Transportation Security Laboratory. Thanks to Doug Barrett, Luke Phillips, Mark Auckland, Xingshan Li, and the UMass Eyetracking Laboratory for their contributions to the series of experiments described here.

References

Barrett, D. J. K., Menneer, T., Phillips, L., Cave, K. R., & Donnelly, N. (2003, April). *The breakdown of efficient feature search for multiple, same dimension targets.* Paper presented at the meeting of the Experimental Psychology Society, University of Exeter, UK.

Cave, K. R., & Wolfe, J. M. (1990). Modeling the role of parallel processing in visual search. *Cognitive Psychology, 22,* 225-271.

D'Zmura, M. (1991). Color in visual search. *Vision Research, 31,* 951-966.

Desimone, R., & Duncan, J. (1995). Neural mechanisms of selective visual attention. *Annual Review of Neuroscience, 18,* 193-222.

Duncan, J., & Humphreys, G. W. (1989). Visual search and stimulus similarity. *Psychological Review, 96,* 433-458.

Menneer, T., Barrett, D. J. K., Phillips, L., Donnelly, N., & Cave, K. R. (2007). Costs in searching for two targets: Dividing search across target types could improve airport security screening. *Applied Cognitive Psychology, 21,* 915-932.

Quinlan, P. T., & Humphreys, G. W. (1987). Visual search for targets defined by combinations of color, shape, and size: An examination of the task constraints on feature and conjunction searches. *Perception & Psychophysics, 41,* 455-472.

Stroud, M. J., Menneer, T., Cave, K. R., Donnelly, N., & Rayner, K. (2008). The reduction of color selectivity in search for multiple targets: Evidence from eye movements. Revision submitted for publication.

Treisman, A. (1988). Features and objects: The fourteenth Bartlett memorial lecture. *Quarterly Journal of Experimental Psychology A, 40,* 201-237.

Treisman, A. M., & Gelade, G. (1980). A feature-integration theory of attention. *Cognitive Psychology, 12,* 97-136.

Chapter 11

Eye movements and individual differences in mental rotation

Ibrahim Dahlstrom-Hakki, Alexander Pollatsek, Donald L. Fisher, Brett Miller, and Keith Rayner

The issue of mental imagery has long been of interest to cognitive psychologists. Originally, the debate centered on what it meant to form such images and, if so, what form the mental representations were in (i.e., 2-dimensional images like photographs or representations containing 3-dimensional information). The seminal work by Shepard and colleagues (e.g., Shepard & Metzler, 1971; Shepard & Cooper, 1986; Finke & Shepard, 1986) indicated that, in at least some circumstances, such mental images had 3-dimensional properties. The chief paradigm in which it was shown that people could create and manipulate images with 3-dimensional properties was the *mental rotation* task.

In the basic experimental paradigm used by Shepard and colleagues, line drawings of two 3-dimensional objects are presented sequentially and participants decide whether they are representations of the same 3-dimensional object, even though they may be oriented differently with respect to the viewer. (In many of the experiments, the objects were abstract 3-dimensional forms, which were often formed as if about 5-10 identical cubical building blocks were glued together.) Typically, participants were allowed to examine the representation of the first object for as long as they wanted. Then, the comparison stimulus was presented and their response time to judge whether it was the same as or different from the first stimulus was measured.

The finding that led people to conclude that the task was solved by an analogue process of mental rotation was that response time was a linear function of the angular disparity between the two representations of the objects (e.g., Shepard & Metzler, 1971). Although it is logically possible that this linear function could result from a non-analogue process, the most compelling explanation for such a linear function is that there is a mental rotation process in which the rotation speed is constant and the slope of the linear function is the velocity of the mental rotation process. Logically, the process could either be one in which a mental representation of the initial stimulus was mentally rotated to match the representation of the second stimulus or one in which the second stimulus was mentally rotated to match the memory representation of the first. However, the first alternative seems more plausible. Another interesting finding was that the time for trials where the rotation was 2-dimensional (i.e., around an axis parallel to the line of sight and hence in the plane in which the image was being presented) did not differ from that taken to perform the rotation in depth (i.e. around an axis perpendicular to the line of sight).

These experiments raise the question of whether there are limits to what can be mentally rotated. The answer is that people have great difficulty with mental rotation when the axes of rotation are oblique with respect to the viewer and the object (Pani, 1993). For example, it is quite difficult to form a mental image of a cube when two opposite corners of it are on an axis parallel with the line of sight. (Its projection is a hexagon divided in three equal parts.) One possible reason that mental rotation tasks in the standard paradigm are easier than tasks that ask one to imagine a familiar object rotated into a non-standard orientation is that the paradigm developed by Shepard merely asks whether the objects depicted in two images would match (and the differences don't depend on subtle differences between the objects), whereas the paradigm developed by Pani and others requires people to form a complete mental representation of the 2-dimensional projection of a 3-dimensional object in order to perform the task correctly. However, in a task similar to the standard mental rotation task involving simple scenes containing three objects on a desktop (Nakatani & Pollatsek, 2004), it was found that the comparison process was more complex than a simple rotation process and involved separate processes of rotating the scene framework and rotating individual objects. We will return to discuss these experiments later.

Individual differences in mental rotation

Just and Carpenter (1985; see also Carpenter & Just, 1978) attempted a finer analysis of the processes used in mentally rotating a 3-dimensional object by examining the pattern of eye movements while people performed a simple variant of Shepard's task. Given that eye-movement data have provided valuable insights into various aspects of cognitive processing (Rayner, 1998), it is surprising that more studies utilizing eye movements to examine mental rotation have not been reported (see de'Sperati, 2003). In addition to examining eye movements in a mental rotation task, Just and Carpenter (1985) were also interested in determining whether there were qualitative differences between groups of people when they were solving such mental rotation tasks. Their stimuli were somewhat different from those employed by Shepard and Metzler in that they used single cubes (shown in an isometric projection) that had an alphanumeric character in the center of each visible face (see Figure 11.1). The task was the same at a general level: to judge whether the two 2-dimensional drawings could be representations of the same object. However, at a more detailed level the task was somewhat different than the Shepard and Metzler task because, geometrically, the stimuli were always identical cubes, so that the judgment depended on whether the characters on the faces would "line up" when the cube was rotated. Because the use of the characters as significant features made it plausible that the pattern of scanning the faces of the cube would reveal details of the judgment process, Just and Carpenter examined eye movements as well as response times. They also asked participants to verbally report what they had done after every trial.

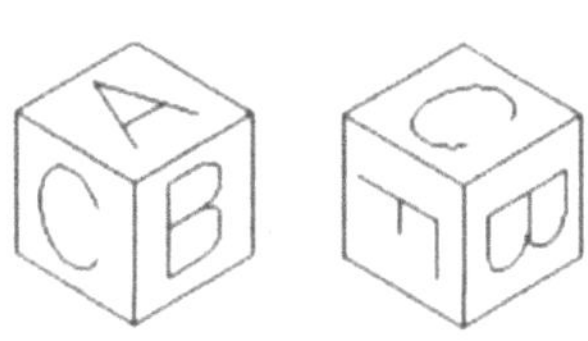

Figure 11.1 An example of the type of judgment involved in the Just and Carpenter rotation task. This is an example of a 90-degree rotation in which the two cubes match. (The actual representation of the cubes was somewhat different in the Just and Carpenter study; in their figures, there was a front face, which was a square and the top and side faces were parallelograms).

Just and Carpenter outlined four strategies that they believed could be used to perform the task, but reported that their participants only used three of them. Two were variants of analogue mental rotation. In the first, the *standard axis* strategy, one of the cubes is rotated along one of the standard axes (i.e., the three axes that are perpendicular to the faces of the cube and go through the centers of two opposite faces); if a task can not be solved by a single rotation around one of these standard axes (which we refer to as X, Y, and Z), the desired rotation is achieved by concatenating these standard rotations, such as first rotating the cube about the X-axis by 90 degrees and then around the Y-axis by 90 degrees. In the second, the *direct rotation* strategy, participants first find the axis that allows them to achieve the desired orientation using a single direct rotation (logically, there is always an axis that will allow such a rotation to take place), and then they rotate it along that axis to see whether there is a match. For both of these strategies (as well as Shepard and Metzler's task) there is the question of how the viewer either knows the appropriate direction of rotation or knows how much rotation to apply to one of the objects. The most likely hypothesis for the mental processing used to perform the cube rotation task is that there is a preliminary stage in which two matching characters are found (there was always at least one pair of matching characters on every trial), and the angular discrepancy between these matching characters is computed and used to rotate one of the cubes. For Shepard and Metzler's task there are no characters, but there are well defined ends of the stimuli for which a similar computation of the appropriate rotation can plausibly be done.

In the third strategy proposed by Just and Carpenter, the *orientation-free* strategy, the method of solving the mental rotation task is essentially symbolic recoding, involving abstracting spatial relations among the characters on the faces (e.g, "the top of the *A* is pointing to the 6 on the adjacent face") and checking to see whether these relations are consistent across the two figures. Although such a strategy can plausibly be used to solve this task, it is less clear whether it could be used to solve mental rotation problems for fairly complex objects with features that may not be easily coded in this manner (such as the Shepard and Metzler types of figures). In the final strategy that Just and Carpenter posited, the *perspective shift* strategy, participants mentally change their perspective, or imagine what the object would look like if viewed from a different position. So instead of rotating the object, they imagine themselves moving around a static object. However, Just and Carpenter reported that no one reported using this strategy. It is also not clear how one could tell the difference between such a strategy and either of the first two strategies by behavioral measures.

Just and Carpenter reported three experiments, but only one involved eye-movement data in the cube-rotation task. In this experiment, they selected four participants who scored high on a spatial relations test and four who had scored low on the test. Perhaps unsurprisingly, they found that the groups differed in their response times. They also found roughly linear increases in response time for both groups with increasing angle of disparity between the two stimuli. What may be a bit more surprising is the size of the effect. The slope for the low spatial group was over twice that of the high spatial group. They also claimed that the groups used different strategies: They classified the entire low spatial group as using the standard axis strategy, three of the four participants in the high spatial group as using the direct rotation strategy, and the other high spatial participant as using an orientation-free strategy. However, evidence for these strategies came from verbal reports, and it is unclear that there was anything in the response-time data or eye-movement data to support these claims.

Just and Carpenter used the eye-movement data to partition the trial into phases. The first phase, the *search* stage, appeared to correspond to the process of finding two matching faces. The second stage, the *initial rotation* phase, was defined by the first successive gazes on two matching faces. Most of the rest of the trial was deemed the *confirmation* phase, although there was also a last phase that appeared to be a double-checking stage. They found that the groups differed hardly at all in the search phase, a bit in the initial rotation phase, but that most of the difference between groups in the response times was in the confirmation phase. Largely on the basis of the verbal reports, they claimed that people use quite straightforward techniques for performing the task and they presented computer simulations that seemed to fit the response-time data reasonably well. However, the requirement of verbalizing their strategies after performing each trial may have constrained the participants to use a strategy that they could comfortably verbalize. Even so, it is unclear how Just and Carpenter generated predictions from their models of how participants would execute these strategies or what their criteria were for fitting the response-time data or the eye-movement data.

In particular, several aspects of the data suggested some disconnect between the verbal reports and the actual processing. First, Just and Carpenter asserted that all four of the low spatial group participants used the standard axis rotational strategy (i.e., sequential rotations around standard coordinate axes), whereas three of the four high spatial group participants used the direct rotational strategy (i.e., a single rotation around a non-standard axis). However, there was little in the response-time or eye-movement data that corroborated this. For example, a test could have been constructed using their three 180-degree rotation conditions because all of these conditions were 180-degree rotations using the standard axis rotation strategy, but only the 1-dimensional rotation condition would involve a 180-degree rotation using the direct rotational strategy—the other two 180-degree conditions would involve smaller rotations (120 degrees) using a direct strategy. To illustrate, in the second column of Figure 11.2 (an illustration of the stimuli in our experiment described below), the rotation needed to align the cube in the '180-degree rotation across 1 axis' condition with the 'standard' is a 180-degree rotation around an axis going through the face with a '*B*' on it; however, a direct rotation for the cube in the '180-degree rotation across 2 axes' condition to align the two faces containing '*A*'s would be a 120-degree rotation around a non-standard axis. Thus, one would expect the low spatial group to perform equivalently in the three conditions, but the high spatial group to take longer in the 1-dimensional condition than in the other two 180-degree rotation conditions. Instead, the response-time data indicated a similar response-time pattern for the high and low spatial groups across the three conditions, with one of the two multidimensional conditions taking less time than the other two conditions for both groups. (In fact, this difference was actually more pronounced for the low spatial group.)

Second, it is not clear that the labels assigned to some of Just and Carpenter's posited stages plausibly represent actual processing activities. The characterization of the search stage seems appropriate, but the division into later processing stages seems less so. Their initial rotation stage did not look much like a rotation stage as there was no consistent effect of rotation angle on its duration in their data; instead, the duration of this stage was shorter in the no-rotation condition than the other conditions, but there was no consistent difference among the other rotation angles. Thus, as virtually all of the rotation effect was contained in their confirmation phase, this stage also seems mislabeled.

As a result of the above analysis of Just and Carpenter's study, we had misgivings both about whether (a) the need to verbalize a strategy affected the response time and eye movement behavior in this task, and (b) a clean separation into phases could be made on the basis of the eye-

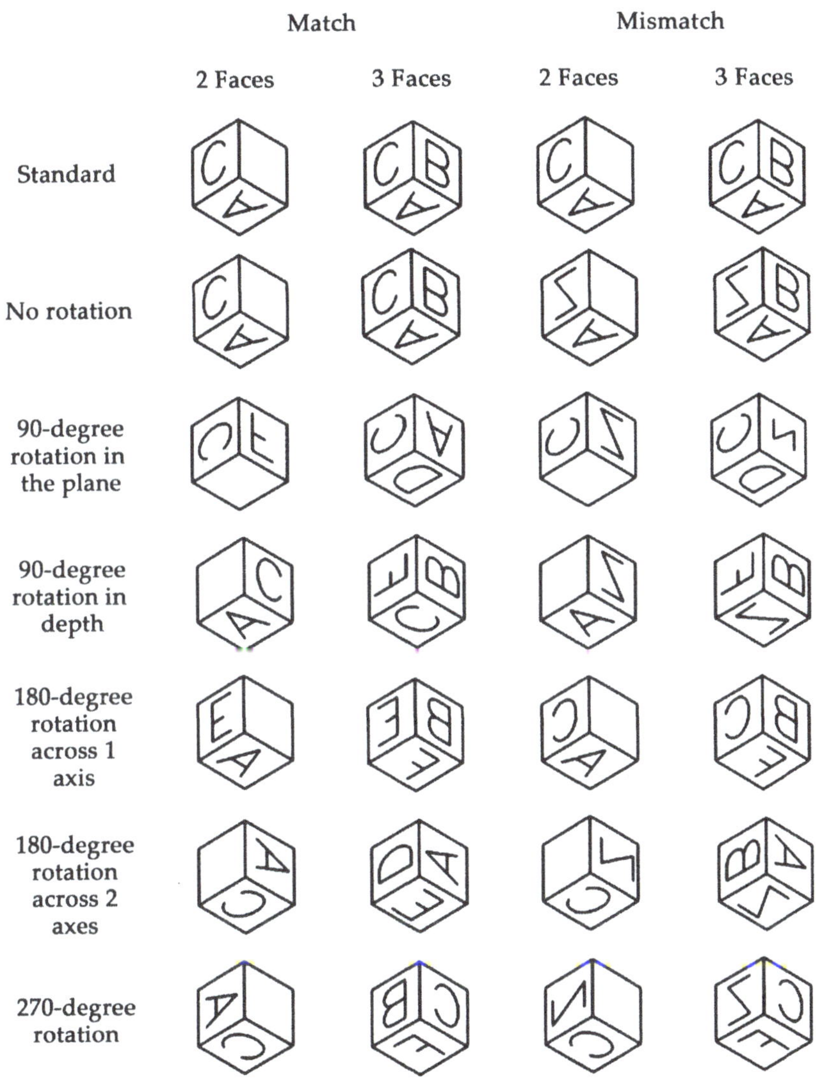

Figure 11.2 An illustration of the conditions in the current experiment. The top two cubes are each meant to illustrate one of the cubes presented on a trial (in the two-face and three-face conditions, respectively), and the cubes below them illustrate the other cube that would be presented on the same trial. The first six cubes below each of the first two "standard" cubes illustrate match trials in the six rotation conditions: the 0 degree condition, the two 90-degree conditions, the 180-degree 1-dimension condition, the 180-degree 2-dimensional condition, and the 270-degree condition, respectively. The six cubes below each of the last two standard cubes illustrate mismatch trials in the respective rotation conditions.

movement data. As a result, we ran a pilot study using a cube-rotation task quite similar to that used by Just and Carpenter, but one in which the participants solved a block of experimental trials without verbalizing the technique they used. (They were given a few trials after this block, in which they attempted to verbalize how they were solving the task.) As with Just and Carpenter, we selected high spatial and low spatial group participants in a gender-blind manner. We came away from the pilot study with two major realizations. First, the majority of our participants' eye movements were not obviously diagnostic of which of the models presented by Just and Carpenter a participant was employing. Second, the majority of our high spatial group participants were male and all of our low spatial group participants were female so that gender is likely to be significantly confounded with spatial ability.

Our study

These findings prompted us to carefully examine the eye movements of participants as they attempted to solve the cube-rotation task when gender and spatial ability (as measured by a standard test) were factorially varied. As will be seen, this is important, as males and females appear to have somewhat different patterns of data, even when equated for spatial ability. Our study employed twenty participants (10 men and 10 women) from the University of Massachusetts community with normal or corrected-to-normal vision. Half the participants in each gender group, who had a score of 100 or more on the Purdue Spatial Visualization Test (Guay, 1977), were classified into a high spatial group; while the other half, who had a score of 60 or less on the test, were classified into a low spatial[1] group. The stimuli were images containing two side-by-side orthographic views of simple blue cubes (each subtending 8.6 degrees vertically and 7.3 degrees horizontally) set against a black background containing characters at the centers of the faces (see Figure 11.2). Participants were asked to decide whether one of the cubes could be rotated to match the other cube. They were also told that a given character would only appear once on any given cube and that, on each trial,

1 However, because the accuracy for one of the males in the low spatial group was only slightly better than chance (52%) and his response times were both very fast and unaffected by rotation condition, we assumed he wasn't taking the task seriously; thus he was removed from the analyses below.

the two cubes would share at least one character.

Half of the trials were match trials, on which one of the cubes could be rotated so that the two cubes would match. The other half were mismatch trials, on which no rotation could be performed on one of the cubes to have it match the other cube. One difference between our study and that of Just and Carpenter was that we manipulated the number of characters on the visible faces: On half of the trials, both cubes had characters on all three of their visible faces, and on the other half, both cubes had characters on only two faces (see Figure 11.2). (All of Just and Carpenter's stimuli had characters on all three visible faces.) This manipulation of number was included in the hope that trials containing only two populated cube faces would be easier for participants to solve and simpler for us to analyze[2]. Participants were told to respond based on whether or not a match was possible given the three faces that were visible, consistent with the assumption that a character could appear only once on a cube. They were also told to assume that there could be multiple blank faces on a cube and that hidden faces could be assumed either to be blank or contain any character that was not already visible on the cube.

There were six rotation conditions (see Figure 11.2). In the no-rotation condition, on match trials, the two cubes were identical, and on mismatch trials, two faces were identical and the characters on the other face did not match. All the other rotation conditions are best described by a single rotation around one of the standard orthogonal axes or as a combination of such rotations. There were two different 90-degree rotation conditions, which represented two different rotations in depth. There were also two 180-degree rotation conditions: (a) one 180-degree rotation around a single axis, and (b) two separate 90-degree rotations along two of the orthogonal axes (Figure 11.2). All 180-degree "one axis rotations" and some 180-degree "two axis rotations" left the two cubes with only a single character shared between the two. We therefore excluded any 180-degree rotations across two axes that would leave only one shared character in the creation of mismatch trials for that condition. For the 180-degree one-axis mismatch trials, the stimuli maintained two of the original characters in their original positions on the cubes, but each character underwent a 180-degree rotation, so that regardless of which matching face one started with, the rotation required to match its

2 Participants were faster to respond when there were only two faces, but this variable had no other sizeable effect and did not interact with other manipulations. Hence, we will not discuss it.

corresponding face would be a single 180-degree rotation (and in both cases a single face would mismatch). Finally there was a 270-degree condition, consisting of one 180-degree rotation along one of the standard axes, and a 90-degree rotation along one of the other axes.

In sum, there were three within-participant variables in a factorial design: (1) six rotation conditions, (2) match vs. mismatch, and (3) cubes with either 2 or 3 populated faces. Each of these conditions appeared twice for a total of 48 experimental trials. Eye movements were recorded with the Eyelink I head-mounted eyetracking system, which was attached to a lightweight helmet. The eyetracking system samples at the rate of 250 Hertz. Although the Eyelink I system is able to compensate for some head movements, participants were encouraged to minimize their head movements during the experimental trials. Manual responses were collected using two marked keys on a keyboard.

Overall performance: Response times and accuracy

The first question is whether performance on the visualization task predicted how well participants would do in the cube-rotation task. The answer was yes, as high spatial group participants had much shorter response times than low spatial group participants (6.13 s versus 13.50 s), $F(1, 15) = 7.51$, $p < 0.025$, and were somewhat more accurate (92.1% versus 83.6% correct), $F(1, 15) = 4.34$, $p < 0.10$. Overall, there was a suggestion of gender differences even when spatial ability was controlled, as men were slightly faster than women (9.63 s versus 10.00 s), and more accurate (90.1% versus 85.6%), though neither difference was close to significant. This overall pattern was a bit hard to interpret because of large variability in the low spatial groups, but when high spatial group men and women were analyzed separately, there was an interesting difference between them: The women in the high spatial group were significantly faster than the men in the high spatial group, $t(8) = 3.92$, $p < 0.01$, but the men in the high spatial group were significantly more accurate than the women in the high spatial group, $t(8) = 4.93$, $p < 0.001$. In fact, all of the men in the high spatial group were slower and more accurate than all of the women in the high spatial group. Although most of the differences among the high spatial group participants may be due to a speed/accuracy trade-off (and thus not to any fundamental differences in how they performed the task), there appear to be differences that may be more fundamental. For example, two of the men in the high spatial group not only had the fastest times among the men in that group, they were also the most accurate.

Of chief interest, of course, is what could be inferred about the par-

Table 11.1 Mean response time (and standard error) as a function of spatial ability and gender

Gender	Spatial ability	
	Low	High
Women	15.29 s (4.58 s)	4.70 s (0.19 s)
Men	11.71 s (4.28 s)	7.56 s (0.79 s)

Table 11.2 Mean accuracy (and standard error) as a function of spatial ability and gender

Gender	Spatial ability	
	Low	High
Women	85.4% (7.1%)	85.9% (2.7%)
Men	81.8% (5.1%)	98.3% (0.9%)

ticipants' rotation strategies. Our focus is on the high spatial groups for two reasons. First, the data in the low spatial groups are quite difficult to interpret because of (a) the variability between participants, (b) the men in the low spatial group had high error rates which makes their response times and eye movement patterns difficult to interpret, and (c) the women in the low spatial group had very long response times, which suggests that they did lots of double-checking. However, perhaps of greater importance is that the patterns of the high spatial group participants are of greater theoretical interest because Just and Carpenter (1985) reported that all of their high spatial group participants employed non-standard rotation strategies.

The first thing to notice is that the effects of rotation (see Figures 11.3 & 11.4) were fairly linear with respect to rotation angle (especially for response times). Thus, for the most part, we present rotation effects as the slopes of best fitting straight lines (expressed in ms/degree and percent/degree for the response time and accuracy data, respectively). A slope, for response time, can be interpreted as the velocity of the mental rotation. These analyses, however, tacitly assume the standard axis strategy, as they are collapsed over the two 90-degree and two 180-degree conditions. Averaged over the four groups, the slope of the rotation effect on response times was 32.4 ms/degree, $F(1, 15) = 45.0$, $p < 0.001$ (see Figure 11.3). Group differences in slopes mirrored the group differences in response times. First, the low-spatial group had over double the slope of the high spatial group (44.6 ms/degree versus 21.2 ms/de-

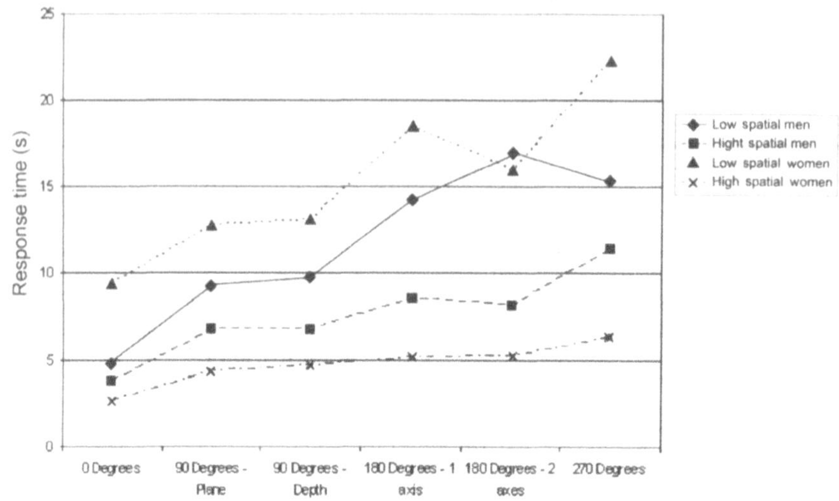

Figure 11.3 Mean response times for the four groups of participants as a function of rotation condition

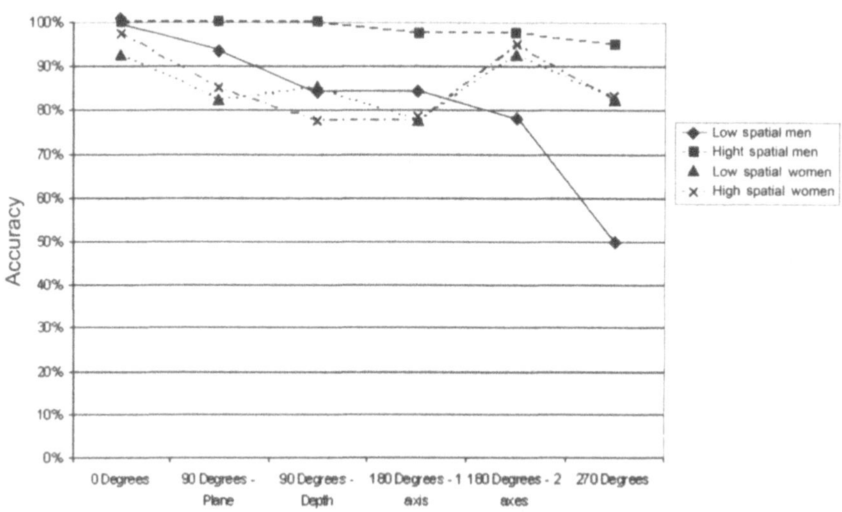

Figure 11.4 Mean accuracy for the four groups of participants as a function of rotation condition

gree), $F(1, 15) = 6.41$, $p < 0.05$. Second, the slope for women in the high spatial group was significantly less than for the men in that group (12.9 ms/degree versus 27.4 ms/degree), $t(8) = 2.42$, $p < 0.05$. (There was little difference in the slopes between men and women in the low spatial group.) However, there appeared to be more variability in slopes among the high spatial group participants. In particular, one of the women had an appreciably smaller slope (3.8 ms/degree) than any of the other high spatial group participants. Indeed, a slope of 3.8 ms/degree is so small as to cast doubt on whether she was performing any kind of analogue rotation in order to perform the task.

The more interesting theoretical issue is whether there was any evidence for participants using a direct-rotation strategy, as Just and Carpenter claimed. The above analysis of slopes tacitly assumes that the participants were following the standard-axis strategy, as the angle of rotation assumed in the analysis is the rotation angle if they are using that strategy for rotating the cube. However, as we indicated earlier, if one follows a direct-rotation strategy (i.e., rotating around a non-standard axis), the two-dimensional "180-degree rotation" condition only involves a 120-degree rotation. Moreover, the (2-dimensional) "270 degree rotation" condition involves a direct rotation of only 180 degrees. (This would be around the axis going through the lower left corner and upper right corner of the cube depicted at the bottom of the second column in Figure 11.2.) This provides us with two tests of the use of a direct-rotation strategy. First, a direct-rotation strategy predicts that responses in the 2-dimensional 180-degree condition should be faster than in the 1-dimensional 180-degree rotation condition because, as argued above, the latter requires a rotation of 180 degrees. However, over all participants, mean response times in the one-dimensional and two-dimensional 180-degree rotation conditions were 11.56 s and 11.55 s, respectively, $t < 1$, consistent with the hypothesis that all were using the standard-axis strategy. The pattern for the high spatial group participants (when analyzed separately) was similar: Mean response times in the single-axis and double-axis 180-degree rotation conditions were 6.85 s and 6.68 s, $F < 1$. Thus, from these data, there is little evidence that any participant was using a direct-rotation strategy any significant fraction of the time. Second, contrary to the prediction of a direct-rotation strategy, there was a large difference (2.25 s) in the mean response times for the 270-degree and 180-degree single axis rotation conditions, $t(15) = 2.95$, $p < 0.01$, and this difference was not much smaller than the difference between the single-axis 180-degree rotation condition and the 90-degree rotation conditions (2.89 s), consistent with the standard-axis strategy. The difference between the 270 degree and 180-degree single axis rotation conditions for the high-spatial participants was also quite substantial, 8.85 s and 6.85 s, respectively, $t(8) = 2.08$, $p < 0.10$. Thus, there is little evidence from the response-time data that any participant was using a direct rotational strategy.

Another finding of interest casts doubt on a classic mental-rotation analysis for this task. That is, the usual analysis of mental-rotation tasks basically assumes that there are three stages: (a) a preliminary encoding of the second stimulus and a decision about how to rotate (presumably based on finding two matching faces); (b) doing the rotation; (c) then comparing the rotated image with the other stimulus. However, such a model of the task assumes that all the rotation goes on before the comparison stage and thus it would predict that the rotation function for match trials should be the same as the rotation function for mismatch trials. Contrary to that prediction, the slope of the rotation function for match trials (36.4 ms/degree) was significantly greater than that for mismatch trials (28.4 ms/degree), $F(1, 15) = 5.83$, $p < 0.05$.

A possible alternative model that can explain these data is that, rather than there being one rotation process for the entire cube, the faces are rotated one at a time, and after each face is rotated, it is compared with the face on the other cube that should match. If a mismatch is found, a response can be made. However, if a match is found, then the next face is rotated. Thus, for match trials, all faces must be compared, whereas for mismatch trials, the process often does not require all faces to be matched. If we assume that the first pair of matching faces is found in the preliminary stage and doesn't require explicit rotation, then this model would assume that there are two rotation operations required for match trials. On the other hand, for mismatch trials, the mismatching face would, on average be encountered half the time after the first rotation and half the time after the second rotation, so that, on average, 1.5 rotations would be required on mismatch trials. This model thus predicts that the slopes for match trials and for mismatch trials would be 2:1.5 or 1.33. This is quite close to our observed ratio of 1.28. We should point out that, the ratio of the slopes in the match and mismatch responses appeared to differ somewhat across groups; however, neither the main effect of spatial ability or gender on this difference nor the interaction between the two was close to significant ($Fs < 1.1$).

Accuracy also decreased as rotation angle increased. Over all participants, the size of the rotation effect on the percentage of correct responses was -0.068%/degree, $F(1, 15) = 40.3$, $p < 0.001$, and the (negative) slopes were larger for the low spatial groups than for the high spatial groups, $F(1,15) = 11.3$, $p < 0.01$. There was a significant gender by spatial ability interaction, $F(1,15) = 15.5$, $p < 0.01$, that was the opposite of that in the response-time data: The slope for women in the high spatial group was greater than that for the men in the high spatial group

(-0.044%/degree versus -0.0194%/degree), whereas the slope was less for women in the low spatial group than that for men in the low spatial group (-0.032%/degree versus -0.175%/degree).

Eye-movement analyses

We examined the eye-movement data to get some more detail on how participants made their judgments, and in particular to determine whether they could provide any information about stages of processing. Each fixation (except the first and last) was assigned to one of the six visible faces; the face that a fixation was attributed to was the one whose center point was closest to the fixation. (The mean distance of a fixation from the center of a face was 1.2 degrees.) Gaze duration on a face was the sum of the fixations on that face before another face was fixated. We initially attempted an analysis similar to that reported by Just and Carpenter: The initial search phase included all fixations prior to two successive gazes on the same face, the initial rotation phase was the sum of these two gazes, and the confirmation phase was the rest of the trial. However, such an analysis did not seem to work because (a) participants often appeared to fixate two matching faces within the first second by pure chance and (b) in 33.1% of the trials, two matching faces were never fixated in serieo. However, there was a general trend in the fixation duration data among all participants for there to be a series of fixations at the beginning of each trial that were markedly shorter than the fixations during the remainder of the trial. These fixations appeared to mark an initial phase of processing that was plausibly an encoding stage for the two cubes prior to active rotation and comparison. We quantified the boundary between the initial stage and the later stages as follows. Two running averages were computed for every six consecutive fixations (starting with an average of the 2nd, 3rd, and 4th compared to the average of the 5th, 6th, and 7th fixations). When the ratio between the average fixation duration of one set of three consecutive fixations and the following set of three was greater than 1.2, the initial scan was deemed to be terminated with the end of the first fixation of the later set of three. (The initial fixation in each trial was excluded because that fixation started before the stimulus was displayed.) Thus, the initial scan, as computed above, would last at minimum from the stimulus onset time to the end of the fifth fixation. In a few cases (5.6% of trials), when no such increase in average fixation duration was observed across sets of three consecutive fixations, scan times were assumed to terminate at the end of the fourth fixation. On the other 94.4% of the trials, the mean fixation time during the scan period was 194 ms and the mean fixation time for the next three fixations was 277 ms, a highly significant difference $t(878) = 35.14$, $p < 0.001$.

The mean scan time across participants was 1.29 s. It was virtually identical for men and women ($F < 1$) and there was only a suggestion that it differed between high- and low-spatial participants (1.36 s versus 1.22 s), $F(1, 15) = 2.94$, $p < 0.20$ (see Table 11.3), and it did not differ across rotation-angle conditions, $F < 1$. These data indicate that the initial scan time is indexing a stage of processing prior to any rotation and comparison. Thus, our scan period seems quite similar, in overall characteristics, to the initial search phase of Just and Carpenter and is probably a search for two matching letters.

Table 11.3 Mean scan time, gaze duration, and number of gazes for the four groups (Standard errors are in parentheses)

Measure	Group			
	High-spatial men	High-spatial women	Low-spatial men	Low-spatial women
Scan time	1.27 s (0.08 s)	1.18 s (0.08 s)	1.30 s (0.09 s)	1.42 s (0.08 s)
Gaze duration	357 ms (21 ms)	314 ms (21 ms)	388 ms (24 ms)	390 ms (21 ms)
Number of gazes*	15.1 (5.4)	9.4 (5.4)	23.3 (6.0)	27.3 (5.4)

Note: The number of gazes and mean gaze duration excluded fixations from the scan.

Our primary measures in the later processing stages were the durations of *individual* gazes (time spent on a single cube face before moving onto a different face), and the number of total gazes (excluding the scan period). (Note that there can be several gazes on any given face in a trial.) There were substantial spatial-ability differences on both these measures. The mean gaze duration was 64 ms greater for the low spatial group than for the high spatial group, $F(1, 15) = 6.18$, $p < 0.05$, and the low spatial group had over twice as many gazes as the high spatial group, $F(1, 15) = 5.52$, $p < 0.05$, but neither the gender main effect nor the spatial by gender interaction was significant on either measure, $Fs < 1.1$ (see Table 11.3).

Of central interest was how these measures were influenced by rotation angle. That is, one theoretical rationale for creating these two measures is that it is plausible that mental rotation goes on during a gaze on a face. This is particularly plausible given the above model of sequential rotation of faces. If so, then such a model suggests that it is the slope of the rotation function for gaze duration that is the true speed of a mental-rotation operation and that effects on the number of gazes may reflect how many mental operations take place. That is, an increasing rotation effect on number of gazes may reflect more rotation operations because more double-checking is needed for larger rotations. In fact, both gaze durations and number of gazes significantly increased as rotation angle increased: The slopes (averaged over the four groups) were 0.41 ms/degree for gaze duration, $F(1, 15) = 49.4$, $p < 0.001$, and 0.059 gazes/degree for number of gazes, $F(1, 15) = 35.5$, $p < 0.001$, (see Figures 11.5 & 11.6). Moreover, there was a large difference in slope between low and high spatial groups for number of gazes, (0.082 gazes/degree versus 0.037 gazes/degree), $F(1,15) = 5.23$, $p < 0.05$, whereas there was little difference between low and high spatial group participants in their gaze-duration slopes, 0.40 ms/degrees versus 0.37 ms/degree, respectively ($F < 1$). The main effect of gender for the slope for number of gazes was not significant (*Fs* < 1), but the slope for gaze duration was marginally significant, $F(1, 15) = 3.22$, $p < 0.10$. Neither difference in spatial ability by gender interaction was significant (*Fs* < 1). As with the slope data from the response times, the women in the high spatial group appeared to be faster than the men in that group on both of these measures (0.50 ms/degree versus 0.24 ms/degree and 0.047 gazes/degree versus 0.026 gazes/degree); however, neither difference was significant, $t(8) = 1.63$, $p < 0.20$, $t(8) = 1.75$, $p < 0.20$, respectively.

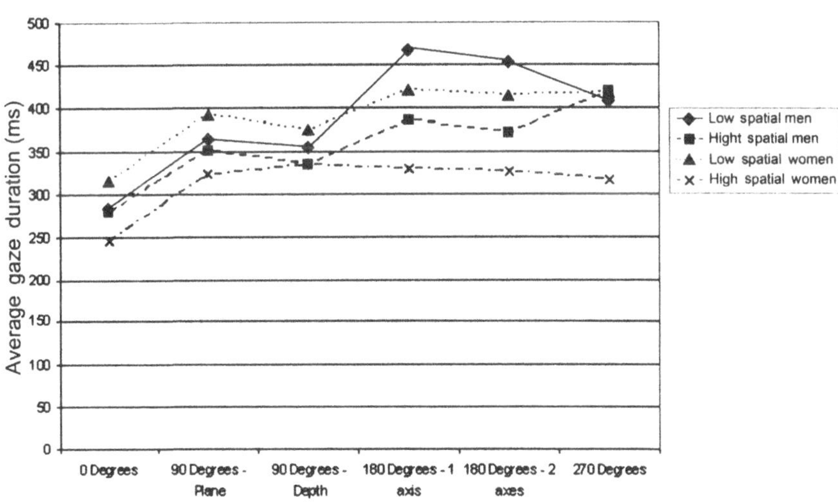

Figure 11.5 Mean gaze durations for the four groups of participants as a function of rotation condition

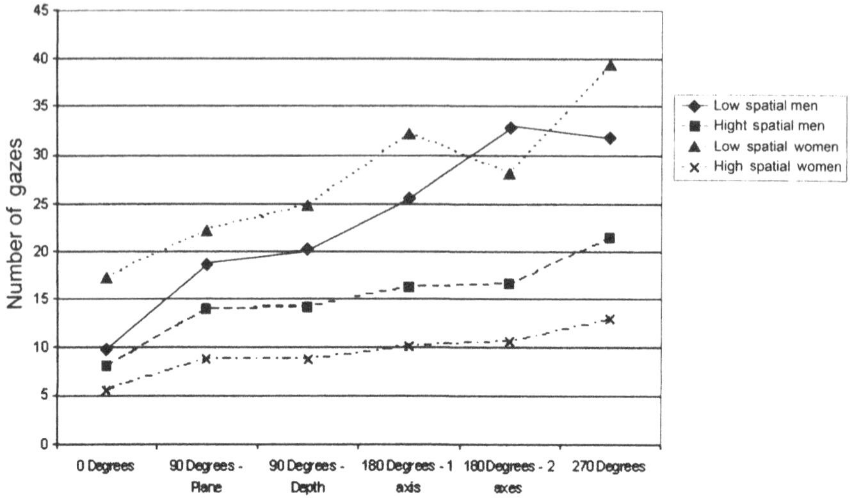

Figure 11.6 Mean numbers of gazes for the four groups of participants as a function of rotation condition

Thus, if one accepts the theoretical distinction we suggested between the mean gaze-duration measure and the number-of-gazes measure, there appears to be little difference between the high spatial and low spatial groups in their speed of mental rotation, and the differences between the groups may be mainly because the low spatial group may do more double-checking for larger rotations. However, this is quite speculative, and another possibility is that, if, as the data suggest, most participants are using some form of the standard-axis strategy (e.g., doing 180-degree rotations as two successive 90-degree rotations around different standard axes) that the low-spatial group may tend to fixate a new face between these 90-degree component rotations whereas the high-spatial group may tend to maintain fixation on a single face during the whole rotation. In any event, we estimated that about three quarters of the difference in rotation effect in response time between low and high spatial groups (44.6 ms/degree versus 21.2 ms/degree) was due to the increase in number of gazes.

Discussion

Our study raises a number of questions regarding the claims made by Just and Carpenter (1985), both with respect to their general analysis for how the task was done and the sources of individual differences among participants. We found little to support their claim that high spatial group participants adopted either a direct-rotation strategy,in which a cube is rotated directly around the axis giving the shortest rotation angle, or a non-rotational strategy in which the relevant information is essentially verbally coded (e.g., "tip of A pointing at left side of C"), whereas the low-spatial participants adopted the standard-axis rotational strategy (in which rotations consisted of concatenations of rotations around the principal axes of the cube). The only support we obtained for this description was the one woman in the high spatial group who showed virtually no "rotation effect" and thus plausibly used a non-rotational strategy. However, there was virtually no evidence in the response time or the eye-movement data for use of the shortest rotation strategy. (There was also no indication of the use of this strategy in the Just and Carpenter data; their identification of a direct rotational strategy was based on verbal reports.) Given this strategy, and a rotation time of at least 20 ms/degree, rotation should have been about 1200 ms faster in the 180-degree rotation conditions that involved rotations around more than one of the standard axes than 180-degree rotations around a single-axis, but there was little or no difference between these conditions. Our data thus indicate that the other nine high spatial group participants were using some form of the standard-axis rotational strategy. Perhaps Just and Carpenter's participants felt the need to come up with a coherent report of what they were doing and reported what they hoped to be doing. We are skeptical that there is much, if any, use of a direct rotation strategy in this task.

There was some indication of differences among the high spatial group participants besides the one woman in the high spatial group who appeared to be using a non-rotational strategy, as the rest of the women were also faster than the men in the high spatial group. Although this may merely be some form of speed/accuracy trade-off, it is curious that there should have been such a gender-based speed/accuracy difference among the high spatial group participants given that the opposite pattern was observed for the low spatial group participants (i.e., for the low spatial group participants, the women, on average were slower but more accurate than the men).

Like Just and Carpenter, we found evidence for a preliminary stage in which participants were presumably looking for two matching faces to begin the rotation process; however, as we could not successfully apply their algorithm to our data, we delineated this stage by the duration of individual fixations: The initial fixations were notably shorter than most of the later ones. There was virtually no rotation effect in this preliminary stage, but there was a clear rotation effect on the remainder of the time in the trial. However, we found no clear stage division in this later processing stage; people seemed to be both attempting to rotate and to compare information throughout the remainder of the trial.

The hypothesis that people were mixing rotation and comparison throughout the rest of the trial was supported by our analysis comparing the slope of the rotation effect on response times on the match and mismatch trials. That is, the fact that the ratio of the slopes was about 4 to 3 was consistent with a model in which individual faces of one of the cube were rotated and compared to the faces of the other cube sequentially. This hypothesis of piecemeal rotation is consistent with the finding of Nakatani and Pollatsek (2004) cited earlier.

Their study employed a standard mental rotation task in which the two stimuli to be compared were presented sequentially, with participants being allowed to examine the first of the two stimuli for as long as they wanted. However, the stimuli were somewhat more complex than a single object: They were simple scenes with three objects placed on a desktop. (The stimuli were placed fairly far apart so that there would be little or no occlusion of one object by another.) Nakatani and Pollatsek found mental-rotation effects in the sense that response times were longer the greater the rotation angle. However, they also found, contrary to the findings in the original experiments by Shepard, that rotations in depth produced greater rotation effects than rotations around the other two rotation axes employed in the experiment. Moreover, the pattern of eye movements indicated a piecemeal rotation process. Of central importance was dividing the total response time into the time elapsed from the beginning of the trial until an object received a second gaze, and the time from the beginning of this second gaze until the end of the trial. For convenience, we will call this latter stage *stage two*. Two findings are of central interest. First, there was no rotation effect for the rotational axes other than the in-depth rotations in stage one, suggesting that all rotational effects for the rotations that were not in-depth rotations were due to double checking. Second, there were two kinds of mismatch trials: *location changes and orientation changes*. Location changes were when the locations of two or all three of the objects were switched, and orientation changes were when one or more of the objects was rotated to face in a different direction with respect to the desktop. The data indicated that most of the mental rotation of individual objects occurred in stage two; whereas much of the mental rotation of the object locations and the desktop frame occurred in stage one.

Unfortunately, the pattern of fixations on individual faces in the current experiment was not as coherent and did not lend itself to a similar stage analysis beyond the division of the trial into the initial scan and the rest of the trial. Instead, we attempted to understand the rotation effect in more detail by accounting for increases in time due to increased rotation angles in terms of increased mean gaze durations and increased numbers of gazes. The most striking finding was that most of the difference between the high spatial and low spatial groups in terms of rotation speed (as estimated from the response times) was due to an increase in the number of gazes rather than to an increase in mean gaze duration. This suggests that the major difference between the high spatial and low spatial group individuals may be the number of partial rotations they had to perform to complete a rotation rather than the speed of the mental-rotation operation. This plausibly could be either because (a) high spatial group individuals were able to rotate more information within a single rotation operation or (b) they had a better memory of the rotations and comparisons they already did and thus engaged in less double-checking and hence fewer rotations (or both).

In sum, we replicated two of the central findings of Just and Carpenter (1985): (a) the time to solve the cube rotation task is a reasonably linear function of the angle between the two cubes and is plausibly an indication of a mental-rotation operation for most participants; and (b) this rotation function as measured by response times differs between groups whose spatial ability has been diagnosed by a standard test. In addition, our data indicate that this distinction is not merely a gender distinction, as there were roughly similar spatial-ability differences for men and women. However, we found little or no support for the hypothesis that the high and low spatial groups used different strategies with the exception of one woman in the high spatial group who appeared to be using a rotation-free strategy. Instead the remaining participants all appeared to be using a principal-axis rotational strategy. In addition, our analyses suggested that the major reason that the rotation speed for the low spatial group was twice as slow as for the high spatial group was that the low spatial group participants needed to do more comparisons (as indexed by a greater number of gazes) rather than that the speed of individual rotations was slower (as indexed by mean gaze duration).

Acknowledgments

This research was supported by Grants HD17246 and HD26765 from the National Institutes of Health, KDI Grant 9980045 from the National Science Foundation, and by a grant from the General Electric Fund. We thank Rebecca Goertz for her help in running the experiment. Brett Miller is now at the National Institute of Child Health and Human Development.

References

Carpenter, P. A., & Just, M. A. (1978). Eye fixations during mental rotation. In J. Senders, R. Monty, & D. Fisher (Eds.), *Eye movements and psychological functions II.* Hillsdale: Erlbaum.

de'Sperati, C. (2003). Precise oculomotor correlates of visuospatial mental rotation and circular motion imagery. *Journal of Cognitive Neuroscience, 15,* 1244-1259.

Guay, R. (1977). *Purdue spatial visualization tests.* Purdue Research Foundation, West Lafayette, Indiana.

Finke, R. A., & Shepard, R. N. (1986). Visual functions of mental imagery. In K. R. Boff, L. Kaufman, & J. P. Thomas (Eds.), *Handbook of perception and human performance* (pp. 37.1-37.55). New York: Wiley.

Just, M. A., & Carpenter, P. A. (1985). Cognitive coordinate systems: Accounts of mental rotation and individual differences in spatial ability. *Psychological Review, 92,* 137-171.

Nakatani, C., & Pollatsek, A. (2004). An eye movement analysis of "mental rotation" of simple scenes. *Perception & Psychophysics, 66,* 1227-1245.

Pani, J. R. (1993). Limits on the comprehension of rotational motion: Mental imagery of rotations with oblique components. *Perception, 22,* 785-808.

Rayner, K. (1998). Eye movements in reading and information processing: 20 years of research. *Psychological Bulletin, 124,* 372-422.

Shepard, R. N., & Cooper, L. A. (1986). *Mental images and their transformations*. Cambridge: MIT Press.

Shepard, S. M., & Metzler, J. (1971). Mental rotation of three-dimensional objects. *Science, 171*, 710-703.

Section 5

Eye movements in reading Chinese

Chapter 12

Eye movements in reading Chinese

Yiu-Kei Tsang and Hsuan-Chih Chen

There are wide varieties of written languages currently used by the people around the world. For example, those in Europe typically adopt an alphabetic system in which the visual symbols are used to represent basic units in speech (i.e., phonemes). The writing system used in China, however, is constructed on the logographic principle in which the orthographic units are made to correspond to the fundamental elements of meaning (i.e., morphemes). The differences between the distinct orthographies have momentous implications for attempts to construct comprehensive theories about reading. This is because it is not self-evident that the same processes are activated and used to encode and comprehend the information written in scripts constructed on exceedingly different principles. Consequently, it is critical to conduct cross-script reading research to reveal both universal and script-specific processes associated with the reading of different orthographies.

Given the way in which texts are presented for conventional reading, executing a series of eye fixations spaced between voluntary eye movements called saccades is the only way to encode textual information for comprehension. Consequently, a substantial amount of research has been conducted monitoring patterns of eye movements and fixation durations during reading. The purpose of this chapter is to review what is known about eye movements in reading Chinese. We chose to focus on this topic not only because written Chinese is perhaps the most persistent and widely used script, but, more importantly, because it differs drastically from alphabetic scripts such as English with which most reading research has been done. There are six parts to the chapter. The first reviews some notable properties of written Chinese. The second summarizes basic eye-movement patterns in reading Chinese with skilled adult readers. The third presents developmental a characteristics of eye movements in reading Chinese. The fourth describes the effective visual field during Chinese reading. The fifth discusses lexical access in reading Chinese. The final section concerns how textual integration is done during reading for comprehension in Chinese.

Some notable properties of written Chinese

Adopting a logographic writing system, Chinese text possesses a number of peculiar properties not found in alphabetic texts such as English (Chen, 1992; 1996; 1999; 2006). This can be demonstrated in the example presented in Figure 12.1. As can be clearly seen from the figure, the most noticeable difference between the two types of written languages is the size and shape of basic units with which the text is constructed. In written English, spaces are used explicitly to mark word boundaries, making words salient "building blocks" of alphabetic text. Moreover, alphabetic words can have various lengths (e.g., "the" VS. "psychology") and shapes (e.g., "man" VS. "bag"), providing a great deal of visual spatial cues to readers in their parafoveal vision (Reichle, Rayner, & Pollatsek, 2003). These cues are crucial in reading alphabetic text such as English. Indeed, when these visual spatial cues are absent, reading rates drop sharply by about 50 percent or more (Rayner, Fischer, & Pollatsek, 1998).

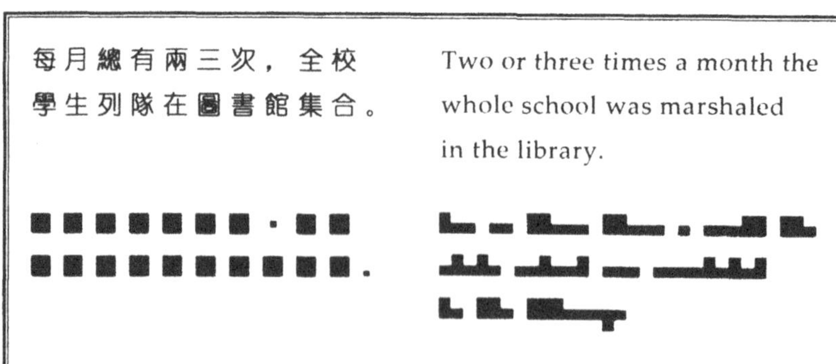

Figure 12.1 A Chinese sentence, its translation equivalent in English, and the quantized versions

On the other hand, text written in Chinese is constructed by arrays of equally spaced boxlike symbols called characters. Although individual characters can be combined to form multi-character words, these words cannot be distinguished physically as they are not marked by extra space. Therefore, not surprisingly, characters are the salient orthographic units in encoding Chinese text, at least among proficient readers (Chen, 1992; Chen, Song, Lau, Wong, & Tang, 2003; Yang & McConkie, 1999). Furthermore, since various characters differ in the number of strokes (from as complex as "籲" to as simple as "乙"), the number of components (e.g., "石" VS. "磊"), and the manner of construction (e.g., the same components "木" and "加" can be arranged horizontally as in "枷" or vertically as in "架"), the visual complexity of the character can be rather high. An obvious consequence of having relatively high constructional complexity and a constant shape is that character recognition relies heavily on visual encoding in the center of vision. Hence, foveal vision may be particularly important in reading Chinese (Chen, 1992).

Another interesting characteristic of written Chinese concerns its direction of scanning. As physical variations extend mainly along the horizontal dimension in alphabetic texts, it is obvious even to naïve readers that the text should be scanned row by row. In contrast, however, as mentioned above, the square-shaped Chinese characters give no clues about how the text is organized. Indeed, written Chinese can be arranged either vertically from top-to-bottom within each column and from right-to-left column by column (i.e., the most popular writing format traditionally) or horizontally as in English. Although the vertical format of printing can still be commonly seen in certain areas such as Taiwan, horizontal printing and writing has been very routinely used especially in Mainland China.

It has been shown that reading experience with a specific format of print is the main determinant of the preferred pattern of directional scanning (Chen & Chen, 1988; Sun, Morita, & Stark, 1985). For instance, having little experience with horizontally printed Chinese text, a vertical over horizontal reading advantage was demonstrated among first graders in Hong Kong. This effect gradually disappeared and finally reversed with increased practice in horizontal reading of Chinese.

Basic eye movement patterns in reading Chinese

Nowadays, most research on reading Chinese involves presenting the text printed horizontally from left to right, both to facilitate comparisons with English (Sun et al., 1985) and to ensure an optimal reading efficiency among college students, who are the major source of participants (Chen & Chen, 1988; Chen & Tang, 1998). For example, in horizontal reading, Sun et al. reported that Chinese readers displayed the stereotypic, qualitative scanning pattern consisting of successive long fixations separated by small and rapid progressive saccades. When the end of a line was reached, a large leftward return sweep with small corrective saccades (if the return was inaccurate) served to bring the eyes to the beginning of the next line. Thus, the overall pattern of scanning from left to right, and from top to bottom, in reading horizontally printed Chinese text is similar to the scanning pattern (Sun & Feng, 1999; Sun et al., 1985) observed in reading English.

Besides the exclusive use of saccadic movements in text reading, Chinese and English readers also produce fixations with similar durations between saccades. Among skilled English readers, fixation durations mainly fall within the range of 180 to 270 ms, with the peak at around 250 ms (Reichle et al., 2003; Schilling, Rayner, & Chumbley, 1998). The eye movement data in reading Chinese reveal somewhat shorter values, from about 180 ms (Inhoff & Liu, 1998) to 230 ms (Chen et al., 2003). Although the similarity in fixation duration across scripts should be interpreted with caution because many factors are left uncontrolled, the consistency across studies suggests that the initial encoding in reading Chinese, despite its high constructional complexity, is as efficient as in reading English.

The uniqueness of Chinese reading and possible effects of the high visual complexity of the characters start to emerge when one inspects the lengths of forward saccades and the subsequent landing locations. In reading English, as measured in letter spaces, forward saccades usually move the eyes about 7-9 letters away from the present fixation (Rayner, 1998). Moreover, the length of the following word is an important factor in saccade planning because English readers appear to have a preferred landing position (Rayner, 1979) which is located about midway between the beginning and the middle of the to-be-fixated word. Such preference is presumably the result of the clear word boundaries in English (Yang & McConkie, 1999) and the readers' tendency to move the eyes toward points with maximum information (but see Rayner, 1998 for the slight discrepancy between preferred and optimal landing locations).

As the letter is not a physical unit in Chinese script, saccade length is typically measured in number of characters. Estimates from different sources are highly consistent, ranging from 2.0 to 3.0 characters (Chen et al., 2003; Inhoff, Liu, & Tang, 1999; Sun et al., 1985). More importantly, two groups of researchers (Inhoff & Liu, 1998; Yang & McConkie, 1999) converged on their findings that, unlike the case in English, the length of the to-be-fixated word does not moderate saccade length. In other words, Chinese readers do not compute a "preferred landing position" in saccadic programming: As a whole, all characters in the words are equally likely to be fixated. This observation is contradictory to what one would expect if saccades are targeting toward words. Can we then say that saccadic planning is made on the basis of the character? Although it is certainly possible, as pointed out by Yang and McConkie (1999), there is no clear evidence at present to confirm this possibility. On the other hand, Rayner, Li, and Pollatsek (2007; see also this volume) have recently extended the E-Z Reader model to Chinese and demonstrated that it does a good job of accounting for the data. This is interesting because the Chinese version of E-Z Reader is word based.

Given an average saccade length of about two characters in reading Chinese, it flows naturally that during forward saccadic movements, about half of the single-character words (Inhoff & Liu, 1998), or at least one character in a two-character word (Yang & McConkie, 1999), will be skipped. In fact, about 42 percent of the characters in a normal Chinese passage with multiple sentences are not fixated in the first pass, though a lower skipping rate may be found if individual sentences are used as stimuli (Chen et al., 2003). Interestingly, the high skipping rate does not seemingly hinder the overall reading efficiency in any significant manner: Skilled Chinese readers are able to read through the text at a remarkable rate of about 600 characters per minute, without an obvious drop in comprehension accuracy (Sun & Feng, 1999; Sun et al., 1985). This ability to maintain performance in spite of the high skipping rate becomes less surprising if one takes into account the size and shape of the perceptual span in Chinese reading, a topic which will be covered soon. Before that, we will first look at the developmental change in eye movement patterns among primary school children as they learn to read Chinese.

Development of eye movements in reading Chinese

Practice makes perfect; it is beyond doubt that reading efficiency increases with more experiences with written Chinese. But how is this improvement realized in various eye movement indices in reading? This question has been investigated by Chen et al. (2003), who recorded the eye movements of about 150 children of different grades during reading of Chinese texts. It turns out that the most salient product of effective practice in reading Chinese appears to be a reduction in the time needed to process a character (given that it is fixated), but not in determining the location of saccade target. Specifically, their results showed that while there were large proportional declines from beginning readers (i.e., second graders) to skilled readers (i.e., undergraduates) in first fixation durations (21%), gaze durations (29%), and total reading times (38%), other reading indices such as regression rates and saccade length were relatively more stable across different grades. This seems to suggest that beginning Chinese readers are equipped with the skills needed to move their eyes along the direction of scanning to take up new information for comprehension. This pattern is indeed unique to Chinese readers, because similar research in English children showed remarkably continuous change in saccade lengths and regression rates throughout primary school (Taylor, 1965). The finding that additional experience does not have much impact on where the eyes are going to land in reading Chinese but not in reading English is presumably due to the physical layout of Chinese text, which requires smaller and less variable saccades for effective visual encoding.

It is also interesting to note the distinctive developmental paths in three eye fixation indices (i.e., first fixation duration, gaze duration, and total reading time) reported in the study of Chen et al. (2003). According to Daneman, Reingold, and Davidson (1995), these indices reflect different stages of processing in reading, with first fixation durations and gaze durations being more sensitive to early lexical access and total reading times having closer links to high-level integration within the text. As mentioned previously, in the study of Chen et al., from beginning to skilled Chinese readers, total reading times in reading Chinese showed the greatest change, and both first fixation durations and gaze durations didn't change as much. Moreover, a relatively large improvement could still be shown between sixth graders and undergraduates for total reading times (i.e., about a 10% decrease), but not for the other two indices (only about 3-4%). This pattern of differential growth suggests relatively easy lexical access in Chinese reading that the kids can master by the end of primary school. In contrast, the ability to perform higher level textual integration needs a longer time to mature, making its development extend into secondary school.

Besides the general quantitative development in reading proficiency from primary school to university, there is also an important qualitative change in the orthographic units the readers most rely on for reading comprehension. Using multiple regression analyses, Chen et al. (2003) examined the unique contributions of different predictors in explaining the variances of a number of eye movement indices in reading Chinese. They included a number of factors which could be organized into character, word, and sentence-level predictors. The most striking finding is that while second graders' eye movement patterns were more readily explainable by the word-level predictors, those factors at the character level began to override word effects among the fourth and the sixth graders.

The developmental shift from relying more on word properties to relying more on character properties during reading in Chinese has two important implications. First, it reinforces our earlier conclusion, which was drawn on the basis of a physical analysis of Chinese text, that characters are the more salient orthographic unit for visual encoding, at least among more experienced readers. Second, even though ultimately, Chinese readers are able to isolate individual characters, which also represent distinct morphemes, they are not born with this skill. Readers of Chinese need practice before they can excel at the task of processing characters in reading.

Note that although words are not explicit frame units in written Chinese and the concept of the word has a considerable degree of fluidity even to highly educated Chinese people (for relevant discussions see, e.g., Chen, 1992; Hoosain, 1991), there is evidence to show that various properties of the word can affect skilled Chinese readers' performance (e.g., Chen, 1999; Rayner, Li, Juhasz, & Yan, 2005; Yan, Tian, Bai, & Rayner, 2006; Yang & McConkie, 1999). For example, Yan et al. found a reliable word frequency effect on fixation times in reading individually presented Chinese sentences. In addition, Rayner et al. manipulated the contextual strength of a sentence to the target words in reading Chinese and found that when the constraint was strong, readers tended to have shorter fixations and more skipping on the target. Thus, although there is a great deal of evidence indicating that characters and morphemes have a prominent role to play in processing Chinese, one should not overlook the importance of words in reading Chinese.

Clearly, characters are the distinct orthographic units well known to Chinese readers. However, as pointed out earlier, Chinese readers do not read every character in an ordinary text. Rather, up to about 40 percent of the characters can be skipped in reading Chinese text (Chen et al., 2003). In fact, a typical finding is that only a single fixation is needed to process a two-character word, which is the most "popular" size of compound word in Chinese (Yang & McConkie, 1999). This phenomenon can be understood by considering the size and shape of the perceptual span in reading Chinese.

Perceptual span in Chinese

The perceptual span (also known as "effective visual field") refers to the region within which readers can obtain useful visual information in a single fixation (Chen & Tang, 1998; Rayner, 1998; 2004; Tang, Au Yeung, & Chen, 1997). Previous research in alphabetic scripts, particularly in English, has demonstrated an asymmetric perceptual span that extends 4 letters to the left and 15 letters to the right, as measured from the point of fixation (McConkie & Rayner, 1975; Rayner, 2004). Interestingly, when people read Hebrew, which is arranged from right to left, the span skews to the left (Pollatsek, Bolozky, Well, & Rayner, 1981). In other words, it seems like that the shape of the perceptual span has been optimized to the text's scanning direction in order to allow readers to gain some previews of the next word and to increase reading efficiency.

What is the size and shape of the perceptual span in reading Chinese, a script with many unique characteristics? Previously, Hoosain (1991), after an analysis of the physical layout of Chinese text similar to the one we offered in the first section, claimed that characters located in the parafoveal region are not too useful in Chinese reading because of the high visual complexity enclosed in the small square areas. According to Hoosian, the size of the effective parafoveal vision in Chinese should be smaller than that in alphabetic languages, which provides extensive low spatial frequency cues along the horizontal scanning direction. Successive investigations have indeed confirmed this prediction (Chen & Tang, 1998; Inhoff & Liu, 1997; 1998; Tang et al., 1997). For example,

Chen and associates (Chen & Tang, 1998; Tang et al., 1997) employed a self-paced, moving window technique to study the perceptual span when proficient Chinese readers read horizontally arranged text from left to right. Their results showed that when viewing was limited to the fixated character, reading performance was relatively poor, and that extending the size of the viewing window on the right (but not on the left) improved reading efficiency, especially when the window contained the fixated character and two characters to its right. These results suggest an effective visual field of about three characters in reading Chinese.

Although the self-paced moving window technique provides valuable insights about the effective visual field of Chinese readers, it is not ideal due to its involvement of a motor control component not present in natural reading. In fact, to investigate various issues related to parafoveal visual processing during reading, including the perceptual span, a better technique to use is the gaze-contingent display-change technique (also called the moving window paradigm) invented by McConkie and Rayner (1975). In this technique, normal text is shown within a pre-determined window around the reader's fixation point, but degraded or masked information is presented outside the window. The effective perceptual span can be determined through increasing the window size systematically and observing under which condition of window size reading performance does not further improve.

Using this gaze-contingent moving window paradigm, Inhoff and Liu (1997, 1998) obtained an estimation of perceptual span as extending one character to the left and three characters to the right of fixation. This result is similar to what was found by Chen and associates (Chen & Tang, 1998; Tang et al., 1997). Thus, the results from Chinese reading studies reveal interesting similarities, as well as differences, compared with those in reading English. Specifically, while the shape of the visual span in reading Chinese is skewed towards the direction of scanning, just as the asymmetry observed in reading alphabetic scripts, the overall span size is much more limited. Specifically, the visual span in reading Chinese covers about 3.2 degrees (Chen & Tang, 1998) to 4.5 degrees (Inhoff & Liu, 1998) of visual angle, while the value in English goes up to about 6.3 degrees of visual angle (McConkie & Rayner, 1975).

There are two additional findings in Inhoff and Liu (1998) that are noteworthy. First, they obtained identical estimation of the span size in reading Chinese "irrespective of the length of the fixated Chinese word" (p. 32), suggesting that visual perceptual factors, rather than linguistic or semantic factors, have a relatively large influence in determining the size of effective visual field. Hence, using the number of characters, rather than the number of words, to determine the visual span in reading Chinese seems more justified. Second, and more importantly, the overlap of visual spans in successive fixations is relatively small, as the average length of forward saccades is very similar to the size of the span. In fact, given that a typical forward saccade ranges from 2 to 3 characters, there is at most an overlapping of 2 characters across saccades. This small overlapping stands in sharp contrast to the 12 letters overlapping in English with an average saccade length of about 7 letters. In other words, there is very little redundancy in successive fixations in reading Chinese, indicating that visual encoding in reading Chinese is a highly efficient process, which may be responsible for the relatively high speed in ordinary Chinese reading (about 600 characters per minute according to Sun et al., 1985).

Eye movements and lexical access in Chinese

The employment of the eye monitoring procedure in studying reading hinges critically on the eye-mind hypothesis (Just & Carpenter, 1980), which stated that readers' eye movements faithfully reflect the ongoing information processing. Therefore, people will fixate on a particular part of the text longer when they encounter difficulties in comprehension. Studies in English have provided an enormous amount of data supporting this assumption (see Rayner, 1998; Reichle et al., 2003, for relevant discussion). Similarly, Chen et al. (2003) found that various factors at the character, word, and sentence levels can account for eye movement patterns in Chinese readers of different proficiencies.

Given the sensitivity of eye movement indices to the reading process, Inhoff et al. (1999) investigated how lexical factors such as encounter frequency affect readers' fixation times in reading Chinese sentences. Consistent with the reaction time data from lexical decision or naming tasks, they found that fixations were longer on low than high frequency words (28 ms and 37 ms differences for first fixations and gaze durations respectively). Their data also suggested a detrimental effect when the context-fit character was replaced with an inconsistent one. Moreover, the most interesting part of their finding is the differential harm induced by different types of replacement. Specifically, when being replaced with a homophone, reading slowed down by 90 ms in first fixations and 66 ms in gaze durations, compared with the original, unchanged target. The harm was much smaller for an orthographically similar replacement (29 ms for first fixations and 49 ms for gaze durations). Therefore, when the misfit character shares visual features with the actual target, it does not interfere too much with the retrieval of the correct meaning so that the difficulty produced in reading the text is smaller. However, homophonic replacements appear to produce a larger difficulty, producing much longer fixations. This finding, thus, is not consistent with a phonological mediation account of semantic access, because otherwise a homophonic replacement should create a smaller interference.

Comparing the overall eye movement patterns between orthographic and phonological replacements in Inhoff et al. (1999) reveals another important difference: Going from first fixations to gaze durations, the harm produced increases in the orthographic condition, but decreases in the homophonic case. Recall that the two indices are considered to be reflecting different time points during lexical access, with first fixation revealing the relatively early processes. Such a pattern appears to suggest that phonological information has a larger role to play at a somewhat later stage of lexical processing in Chinese. This suggestion has been confirmed by the results from other studies (e.g., Feng, Miller, Shu, & Zhang, 2001; Liu, Inhoff, Ye, & Wu, 2002; Wong & Chen, 1999). For instance, Wong and Chen (1999) employed the same replacement procedure as the one used in Inhoff et al. so that the first character in a two-character word (e.g., "栽" in "栽培") was replaced with an orthographically and phonologically similar character ("哉"), an orthographically similar character ("截"), a homophonic character ("災"), or an unrelated character ("紗"). With the four factorial conditions, Wong and Chen investigated the contributions of the orthographical and phonological factors independently. The results showed that while orthographic similarity revealed its effect in first fixations and gaze durations on the target words, the homophonic effect was delayed to total reading times or appeared as spillover effects on the characters following the targets.

Similarly, Feng et al. (1999) directly compared the roles of orthography and phonology across English and Chinese. Although in English, a robust early phonological effect could be observed with the more sensitive distributional analysis under specific circumstances, in Chinese the homophonic effect was again delayed to total reading times. These researchers attributed the late benefits induced by homophonic characters as evidence for its role in error recovery (i.e., readers may try to use the phonological information to recover the correct characters only after early lexical access and integration prove that the homophones are in a wrong place).

More recently, Liu et al. (2002) investigated the extraction of orthographic and phonological information in parafoveal vision using the boundary paradigm (Rayner, 1975) in which a specific target word changes when the gaze of a reader passes a pre-defined invisible boundary. They varied the orthographic and phonological relationship between the actual target and that in the parafoveal preview and found that homophonic preview benefits (compared with the unrelated control) emerged at a later time point relative to the condition with graphemically similar preview. More importantly, they demonstrated that even when the previewed characters shared the phonetic radicals with the targets (e.g., "味" and "妹"), benefits were indeed orthographic in nature. This is because the same pattern of results was found no matter if the phonetic radical provided a valid phonological cue to the pronunciation of the whole character or not. Therefore, the eye-movement studies reviewed seem to converge on the idea that Chinese lexical access relies more on visual features than on phonological information. This is in sharp contrast to the phonological mediation hypothesis proposed in English and thus provides an important piece of evidence against the view of universal phonological principle in semantic activation (Perfetti, Zhang, & Berent, 1992).

However, although it is very scanty, there are eye movement experiments that claim to have found early phonological effects in processing Chinese. For example, using the same boundary paradigm as in Liu et al. (2002), Tsai, Lee, Tzeng, Hung, and Yen (2004) reported a homophonic preview benefit for orthographically similar distractors in first fixation duration, and a similar effect for orthographic dissimilar distractors in gaze duration. However, there are a number of noteworthy points in this study. First, for instance, these researchers used only experimental stimuli without involving any additional error-free fillers, whereas Liu et al. included an equal number of experimental trials and error-free fillers to avoid inducing strategic processing. Thus, after being repeatedly exposed to the experimental stimuli, the participants in Tsai et al. might have developed task-specific strategies not appearing in conventional reading. Moreover, the results of Tsai et al. were only significant in one-tailed tests, indicating the results may not be very robust and should be interpreted with caution. Also, their target characters were embedded in low frequency two-character words. It remains to be seen whether the same results can be found using medium and high frequency words as stimuli. These points jeopardize the possibility of using the results of Tsai et al. to back up the assertion that phonological activation is vigorous and appears rapidly and early in conventional reading of Chinese.

A better-controlled study was reported by Pollatsek, Tan, and Rayner (2000), in which a parafoveally available homophonic cue was found to facilitate naming responses. However, the naming response required in their procedure might have biased their participants to the use of phonological information. Indeed, Shen and Forster (1999) demonstrated a robust orthographic effect in both lexical decision and naming, but a phonological effect was only found in naming, indicating that task demand can dramatically alter the use of phonological information in lexical processing. Moreover, it is not clear how "early" the homophonic effect in the study of Pollatsek et al. really was, because they presented the results of naming latencies, but not the corresponding eye-movement data.

In short, summarizing a number of independent studies, it appears that the visual route in lexical access is more robust in processing written Chinese (for related findings and discussions, see, e.g., Chen & Juola, 1982; Chen & Shu, 2001), and that whether or not a phonological effect can be obtained depends on a number of factors such as task demand, word frequency, and the time point at which measurements are made.

Semantic integration in Chinese text

Up to this point, we have reviewed a number of eye-monitoring studies which provide valuable information concerning visual encoding and lexical processing during Chinese reading. However, eye movement data are also useful in illuminating another important cognitive process necessary for reading, namely meaning integration across different portions of text. To illustrate this point, we will discuss two specific issues in this section: Factors involved in pronoun resolution (Bai, Zhang, & Yan, 2005; Wang, Yan, & Bai, 2006) and the immediacy of textual integration (Wang, Chen, Yang, Wu, & Wang, 2006; Wang, Chen, Yang, & Mo, 2008). Note that there are other issues in reading Chinese that have been investigated using the eye-monitoring technique, including, for example, lexical ambiguity resolution. However, they are topics of other chapters in this volume and thus are not discussed here.

In an attempt to test whether pronoun resolution requires a reactivation of the referent of the corresponding pronoun, Wang, Yan, et al. (2006) manipulated the word frequency of the antecedent that the pronoun referenced. They reasoned that if a full re-access is necessary for pronoun resolution (Garnham, Oakhill, Ehrlich, & Carreiras, 1995), then analyzing the pronoun is like accessing the antecedent again and will therefore be influenced by a frequency manipulation. On the other hand, if pronoun resolution only requires partial reactivation of the referent, antecedent frequency will not influence the fixation times of the pronoun. Wang et al. recorded Chinese readers' eye movements when they read sentences containing antecedents and their pronouns. The results showed that although the frequency manipulation strongly affected the fixation times when the antecedents were read, this effect did not penetrate into the analysis of the target pronouns. These results are more in line with the partial reactivation hypothesis.

While Wang, Yan, et al. (2006) were interested in the fundamental lexical activation during pronoun resolution, Bai et al. (2005) studied how the subtle causality within a sentence affected later pronoun interpretations. Following Garnham, Traxler, Oakhill, and Gernsbacher (1996), Bai et al. induced an implicit causality through the use of different verbs. For instance, in (1) "A approaches B because he...", readers usually interpret the pronoun "he" as referring to "A". In contrast, when reading (2) "A envies B because he...", people tend to believe that it is some properties of B which cause A to have the feeling of envy, and "he" is thus referring to "B". Bai et al. wanted to examine whether the implicit causality could immediately constrain the interpretation of the pronoun. They constructed sentences that started with clauses similar to the examples just presented and completed with other clauses that were either consistent or inconsistent with the implicit causality. If pronoun resolution is immediate, readers will have difficulty comprehending the incongruent continuations. If, however, resolution is delayed until sentence ends, fixation times will not be affected by causality congruence. However, their results did not provide clear-cut support to either position; whether an immediate effect was obtained depended on the type of causality: When those sentences similar to the first example were read, congruence had no early effect, whereas congruence exerted a significant impact on reading the second type of sentences.

Although it is unclear why different types of sentences could create distinctive results in Bai et al. (2005), their study at least suggests that some background information can be immediately retrieved and integrated with the currently fixated information. This immediacy hypothesis (Just & Carpenter, 1980; Thibadeau, Just, & Carpenter, 1982) is also consistent with the results obtained in Wang, Chen, et al. (2006; see also Wang et al., 2008), who investigated the role of prior semantic context in Chinese reading. In their study, narratives written in Chinese were presented to the participants. Half of the passages contained conflicting information prior to the target sentence (e.g., mentioning "warm climate" in the earlier part of the text would induce a conflict with "heavy snow" in the target sentence). Their results revealed a robust increase in first-pass reading times, and a decrease in skipping rates, when conflicts were noticed in the target sentence. Besides these immediate influences, second-pass reading times and regression rates also increased because of the conflicts. These results seem to suggest that Chinese reading is best described as an incremental process that adds each piece of new linguistic information to the existing internal text model. Whenever conflicting information is perceived, it seeks for immediate resolution and thus causes trouble right at the point of incongruence.

Thus, on the basis of the findings reviewed above, it seems reasonable to say that, unlike those lower processes such as visual encoding, higher mental processes in reading Chinese share relatively more similarities with those found in reading alphabetic scripts (for related findings, see, e.g., Chen, Cheung, Tang, & Wong, 2000).

Conclusions

There has been considerable progress over the past few years in understanding the importance of conducting reading research in non-alphabetic scripts such as Chinese. The eye movement research reviewed in this chapter suggests that script-specific properties can indeed affect the pattern of eye movements in reading Chinese, though there are also notable similarities in readers' eye movements across different scripts. However, much work remains to be done. Thus, identifying the processes that all scripts share and those that are script-specific and building a comprehensive theory of reading that can account for both should continue to be a challenge to reading researchers in the future.

Acknowledgments

This work was supported by a grant from the Research Grants Council of the Hong Kong Special Administrative Region, China (CUHK4142/04H) to Hsuan-Chih Chen.

References

Bai, X., Zhang, X., & Yan, G. (2005). The eye movement research on the time course of verb's implicit causality in pronoun resolution. *Psychological Exploration, 25,* 19-23.

Chen, H. C. (1992). Reading comprehension in Chinese: Implications from character reading times. In H. C. Chen, & O. J. L. Tzeng (Eds.), *Language processing in Chinese* (pp. 175-205). Amsterdam: North-Holland.

Chen, H. C. (1996). Chinese reading and comprehension: A cognitive psychology perspective. In M. H. Bond (Ed.), *The handbook of Chinese psychology* (pp. 43-62). Hong Kong: Oxford University Press.

Chen, H. C. (1999). How do readers of Chinese process words during reading for comprehension? In J. Wang, A. W. Inhoff, & H. C. Chen (Eds.), *Reading Chinese script: A cognitive analysis* (pp. 257-278). Mahwah, NJ: Lawrence Erlbaum Associate Inc.

Chen, H. C. (2006). Language processing: Implications from the study of Chinese. In Q. Jing, M. R., Rosenzweig, G. d'Ydewalle, H. Zhang, H. C. Chen, & K. Zhang (Eds.), *Progress in psychological science around the world (Vol. 1)* (pp. 367-381). New York: Psychology Press.

Chen, H. C., & Chen, M. J. (1988). Directional scanning in Chinese reading. In I. M. Liu, H. C. Chen, & M. J. Chen (Eds.), *Cognitive aspects of the Chinese language* (pp. 15-26). Hong Kong: Asian Research Service.

Chen, H. C., Cheung, H., Tang, S. L., & Wong, Y. T. (2000). Effects of antecedent order and semantic context on Chinese pronoun resolution. *Memory & Cognition, 28,* 427-438.

Chen, H. C., & Juola, J. F. (1982). Dimensions of lexical coding in Chinese and English. *Memory and Cognition, 10,* 216-224.

Chen, H. C., & Shu, H. (2001). Lexical activation during the recognition of Chinese characters: Evidence against early phonological activation. *Psychonomic Bulletin and Review, 8,* 511-518.

Chen, H. C., Song, H., Lau, W. Y., Wong, K. F. E., & Tang, S. L. (2003). Developmental characteristics of eye movements in reading Chinese. In C. McBride-Chang, & H. C. Chen (Eds.), *Reading development in Chinese children* (pp.157-169). Westport, CT: Praeger Publishers.

Chen, H. C., & Tang, C. K. (1998). The effective visual field in reading Chinese. *Reading and Writing, 10,* 245-254.

Daneman, M., Reingold, E. M., & Davidson, M. (1995). Time course of phonological activation during reading: Evidence from eye fixations. *Journal of Experimental Psychology: Learning, Memory, and Cognition, 21,* 245-254.

Feng, G., Miller, K., Shu, H., & Zhang, H. (2001). Rowed to recovery: The use of phonological and orthographic information in reading Chinese and English. *Journal of Experimental Psychology: Learning, Memory, and Cognition, 27,* 1079-1100.

Garnham, A., Oakhill, J., Ehrlich, M. F., & Carreiras, M. (1995). Representations and processes in the interpretation of pronouns: New evidence from Spanish and French. *Journal of Memory and Language, 34,* 41-62.

Garnham, A., Traxler, M., Oakhill, J., & Gernsbacher, M. A. (1996). The locus of implicit causality effects in comprehension. *Journal of Memory and Language, 35,* 517-543.

Hoosain, R. (1991). *Psycholinguistic implications for linguistic relativity: A case study of Chinese.* Hillsdale, NJ: Erlbaum.Associates.

Inhoff, A. W., & Liu, W. (1997). The range of effective vision during the reading of Chinese sentences. In H. C. Chen (Ed.), *The cognitive processing of Chinese and related Asian languages* (pp.243-265). Hong Kong: The Chinese University Press.

Inhoff, A. W., & Liu, W. (1998). The perceptual span and oculomotor activity during the reading of Chinese sentences. *Journal of Experimental Psychology: Human Perception and Performance, 24,* 20-34.

Inhoff, A. W., Liu, W., & Tang, Z. (1999). Use of preleixcal and lexical information during Chinese sentence reading: Evidence from eye-movement studies. In J. Wang, A. W. Inhoff, & H. C. Chen (Eds.), *Reading Chinese script: A cognitive analysis* (pp.223-238). Mahwah, NJ: Erlbaum Associates.

Just, M. A., & Carpenter, P. A. (1980). A theory of reading: From eye fixations to comprehension. *Psychological Review, 87,* 329-354.

Liu, W., Inhoff, A. W., Ye, Y., & Wu, C. (2002). Use of parafoveally visible characters during the reading of Chinese sentences. *Journal of Experimental Psychology: Human Perception and Performance, 28*, 1213-1227.

McConkie, G. W., & Rayner, K. (1975). The span of the effective stimulus during a fixation in reading. *Perception and Psychophysics, 17*, 578-586.

Perfetti, C. A., Zhang, S., & Berent, I. (1992). Reading in English and Chinese: Evidence for a "universal" phonological principle. In R. Frost, & L. Katz (Eds.), *Orthography, phonology, morphology, and meaning* (pp. 227-248). Amsterdam: North-Holland.

Pollatsek, A., Bolozky, S., Well, A. D., & Rayner, K. (1981). Asymmetries in the perceptual span for Israeli readers. *Brain and Language, 14*, 174-180.

Pollatsek, A., Tan, L. H., & Rayner, K. (2000). The role of phonological codes in integrating information across saccadic eye movements in Chinese character identification. *Journal of Experimental Psychology: Human Perception and Performance, 26*, 607-633.

Rayner, K. (1975). The perceptual span and eye movements in reading. *Cognitive Psychology, 7*, 65-81.

Rayner, K. (1979). Eye guidance in reading: Fixation locations within words. *Perception, 8*, 21-30.

Rayner, K. (1998). Eye movements in reading and information processing: 20 years of research. *Psychological Bulletin, 124*, 372-422.

Rayner, K. (2004). Eye movements, cognitive processes, and reading. *Studies of Psychology and Behavior, 2*, 482-488.

Rayner, K., Fischer, M. H., & Pollatsek, A. (1998). Unspaced text interferes with both word identification and eye movement control. *Vision Research, 38*, 1129-1144.

Rayner, K., Li, X., Juhasz, B. J., & Yan, G. (2005). The effect of word predictability on the eye movements of Chinese readers. *Psychonomic Bulletin and Review, 12*, 1089-1093.

Rayner, K., Li, X., & Pollatsek, A. (2007). Extending the E-Z model of eye movement control to Chinese readers. *Cognitive Science, 31*, 1021-1034.

Reichle, E. D., Rayner, K., & Pollatsek, A. (2003). The E-Z Reader model of eye-movement control in reading: Comparison to other models. *Behavioral and Brain Sciences, 26*, 445-526.

Schilling, H. E. H., Rayner, K., & Chumbley, J. I. (1998). Comparing naming, lexical decision, and eye fixation times: Word frequency effects and individual differences. *Memory & Cognition, 26,* 1270-1281.

Shen, D., Forster, K. I. (1999). Masked phonological priming in reading Chinese words depends on the task. *Language and Cognitive Processes, 14,* 429-459.

Sun, F., & Feng, D. (1999). Eye movements in reading Chinese and English text. In J. Wang, A. W. Inhoff, & H. C. Chen (Eds.), *Reading Chinese script: A cognitive analysis* (pp.189-205). Mahwah, NJ: Erlbaum Associates.

Sun, F., Morita, M., & Stark, L. W. (1985). Comparative patterns of reading eye movement in Chinese and English. *Perception and Psychophysics, 37,* 502-506.

Tang, C. K., Au Yeung, L. H., & Chen, H. C. (1997). The effective visual field in Chinese reading. In H. C. Chen (Ed.), *The cognitive processing of Chinese and related Asian languages* (pp.267-286). Hong Kong: The Chinese University Press.

Taylor, S. E. (1965). Eye movements in reading: Facts and fallacies. *American Educational Research Journal, 2,* 187-202.

Thibadeau, R., Just, M. A., & Carpenter, P. A. (1982). A model of the time course and content of reading. *Cognitive Science, 6,* 157-203.

Tsai, J., Lee, C., Tzeng, O. J. L., Hung, D. L., & Yen, N. (2004). Use of phonological codes for Chinese characters: Evidence from processing of parafoveal preview when reading sentences. *Brain and Language, 91,* 235-244.

Wang, S., Chen, H. C., Yang, J., & Mo, L. (2008). Immediacy of integration in discourse comprehension: Evidence from Chinese readers' eye movements. *Language and Cognitive Processes, 23,* 241-247.

Wang, S., Chen, H. C., Yang, J., Wu, Y., & Wang, R. (2006). Immediacy of integration in reading Chinese. *Acta Psychologica Sinica, 38,* 645-653.

Wang, W., Yan, G., & Bai, X. (2006). Antecedent frequency effects during processing of pronouns on eye movements in reading Chinese. *Psychological Exploration, 26,* 30-34.

Wong, K. F. E., & Chen, H. C. (1999). Orthographic and phonological processing in reading Chinese text: Evidence from eye fixations. *Language and Cognitive Processes, 14,* 461-480.

Yan, G., Tian, H., Bai, X., & Rayner, K. (2006). The effect of word and character frequency on the eye movements of Chinese readers. *British Journal of Psychology, 97,* 259-268.

Yang, H. M., & McConkie, G. W. (1999). Reading Chinese: Some basic eye-movement characteristics. In J. Wang, A. W. Inhoff, & H. C. Chen (Eds.), *Reading Chinese script: A cognitive analysis* (pp. 207-222). Mahwah, NJ: Erlbaum Associates.

Chapter 13

The perceptual span in Chinese reading

Deli Shen, Xuejun Bai, Guoli Yan, and Simon P. Liversedge

Basic issues associated with the perceptual span in reading

The perceptual span and the retina

The perceptual span is the area of effective vision from which useful information can be obtained during a fixation in reading (Rayner & Pollatsek, 1989). McConkie and Rayner (1975, 1976; see also Rayner & Bertera, 1979; Rayner, Well & Pollatsek, 1980) demonstrated for adults that the perceptual span for English readers is asymmetric about the point of fixation, extending approximately 3-4 characters to the left and 14-15 characters to the right. Our visual field in reading can be divided into three different regions with respect to our fixation point: the foveal region, the parafoveal region, and the peripheral region. The foveal region is the area from which high acuity information is obtained and includes 2 degrees of visual angle around the point of fixation. Where 1 degree of visual angle equates to three or four letters, then six to eight letters will fall on the foveal region. The parafoveal region extends beyond this to approximately 15 to 20 characters from the point of fixation, and finally, the peripheral region includes everything in the visual field beyond the parafoveal region (see Balota & Rayner, 1991). Reading efficiency is degraded when a smaller region of text than the perceptual span is made available to readers on any particular fixation. Readers are able to extract basic visual information from the entire region of the perceptual span. This information includes word spacing information and rough word shape information. They are able to identify letters from a smaller region of the span that extends less far from the point of fixation. Finally, the region of the perceptual span in which words can be successfully identified is reduced still more with respect to its extension from the point of fixation (Rayner, Well, Pollatsek, & Bertera, 1982; McConkie & Zola, 1987; Underwood & McConkie, 1985).

Techniques used to assess the perceptual span

The fixed-eye technique involves tachistoscopic presentation of words and letters in eccentric vision (Fisher & Lefton, 1976). Generally, in these experiments the participants were asked to fixate some point and then to identify stimuli presented at various distances from fixation. On the basis of the results from such experiments, estimates of word and letter identification in the perceptual span have been in the range of 2 or 3 words, or about 10 to 20 characters (Rayner & Pollatsek, 1989). While these early results are interesting, there are inherent problems associated with the technique (Rayner, 1978). First, what participants report from a brief presentation cannot necessarily be taken as a complete and veridical specification of what they actually perceived. Secondly, it is very likely that normal reading and tachistoscopic report are sufficiently different that they might induce different processing strategies in participants (Rayner, 1975). The tachistoscopic studies generally involved the isolated presentation of simple stimulus materials (words or letters). Thus, the estimate of the perceptual span obtained via such a technique could be quite different from that found in reading where the reader is faced with full sentences or even paragraphs of text. The data obtained from tachistoscopic studies are, however, valuable for determining acuity limitations and setting the upper bounds of the perceptual span.

A second method, the primitive "window" technique, involves the experimental control of what is seen on any given fixation, and the method is used to manipulate the amount of text that is visible to a reader at a given moment. Poulton (1962) had participants read aloud text over which a mask containing a "window" was passed. Only the text in the window could be seen and since the text was immobile as the window passed over it, only a certain amount could be seen at once. A different, yet clearly related procedure was adopted by Newman (1966) and Bouma and DeVoogd (1974). They reversed the procedure by having the participants' eyes fixed and having the text moving on a screen from right to left. The size of the "window" was manipulated by varying the number of letters on the screen at any moment. The results of these experiments showed that smaller windows created greater disruption to reading than larger windows.

The techniques mentioned above can be questioned on grounds of ecological validity since they may disrupt normal reading in that aspects of a reader's natural eye movement behavior (e.g. regressions) are inhibited (Rayner, 1978). In response to these shortcomings, the classic eye-contingent display change techniques were developed to estimate the perceptual span from natural reading. Specifically, three techniques were developed: the moving-window technique (McConkie & Rayner, 1975), the moving-mask technique (Rayner & Bertera, 1979), and the boundary technique (Rayner, 1975). Note, however, that the general principle underlying contingent change methodology, namely that the display is changed in some way contingent on where the eye is fixating, lends itself very well to a wide variety of experimental presentation paradigms.

In the moving-window technique, the text outside a pre-defined window region around the point of fixation is replaced by Xs or scrambled letters. Thus, wherever the reader looks, the text is visible within the window, but outside the window the text is disrupted in some way. When the reader moves their eyes, a new region of text is exposed while the region previously fixated reverts to a perturbed state. The rationale underlying this method is that when the window matches the maximum area from which the reader can extract useful visual and linguistic information, then eye movement behavior will not be disrupted relative to that observed for normally presented text. By varying the size and location of the window with respect to the point of fixation, the researcher can determine from what area of the text the reader is extracting useful information. Also, by varying the type of information outside the window, the researcher can determine how disruptive different types of non-text stimuli are. Figure 13.1 illustrates the moving-window technique for a Chinese sentence. Note also that the moving-window technique permits the reader to undertake normal reading behavior (McConkie & Rayner, 1975), so results obtained with this method yield a better estimation of the perceptual span than do the alternative methods described earlier.

The moving-mask technique, or the foveal masking technique (Rayner & Bertera, 1979), is similar to the moving-window technique in that saccade contingent changes are made to the text, except that a mask moves with the eyes rather than a window of clear text (see Figure 13.2). That is, the normal text is displayed outside the center of vision and a visual mask, moving in synchrony with the point of fixation, makes it impossible for the reader to obtain useful foveal information.

正常句子	陈教授的精彩讲评赢得了与会代表的阵阵掌声
A	陈教授X X X X X X X X X X X X X X X X X
	*
B	X 教授的X X X X X X X X X X X X X X X X
	*
C	X X 授的精X X X X X X X X X X X X X X X
	*

Figure 13.1 An example of the moving-window technique

Note: The asterisk represents the location of fixation on three successive fixations. The size of the window is three Chinese characters. The meaning of the sentence is "Professor Chen's excellent comments won the participants' warm applause."

正常句子	陈教授的精彩讲评赢得了与会代表的阵阵掌声
A	X X X 的精彩讲评赢得了与会代表的阵阵掌声
	*
B	陈X X X 精彩讲评赢得了与会代表的阵阵掌声
	*
C	陈教X X X彩讲评赢得了与会代表的阵阵掌声
	*

Figure 13.2 An example of a moving-mask technique

Note: The asterisk represents the location of fixation on three successive fixations. The masked areas were three Chinese characters.

Rayner and Bertera (1979) used the moving-mask technique and found that when foveal vision was masked, reading was still possible from parafoveal vision but the reading rate fell to only 12 words per minute. However, when foveal vision and part of parafoveal vision (i.e. the central 11 to 17 character spaces around the fixation point) were masked, reading was almost impossible.

The third contingent change technique that we will discuss in detail is the boundary paradigm first introduced by Rayner (1975). Rayner first used this technique to investigate the kinds of information that can be extracted from the parafovea prior to direct fixation. In this paradigm, a target location is identified, and an invisible boundary is set just left of it. Prior to the reader making an eye movement to cross the boundary, an initial display stimulus (the preview) is presented, and when the reader's saccade crosses the boundary, the preview is replaced with the target word. Thus, in parafoveal vision the reader always sees the preview, but in foveal vision they only ever see the target word. Readers are unaware of the display change because it occurs during the saccade when extraction of clear visual information is not possible (the occasional trials on which the participant is aware of the change are discarded from the analysis). One benefit of this paradigm is that there is very minimal disruption of normal reading. Figure 13.3 illustrates the boundary technique.

正常句子	陈教授的精彩讲评赢得了与会代表的阵阵掌声
A	陈教授的精彩讲评赢得了与会代表的阵阵掌声
B	陈教授的精彩讲评赢得了与会代表的阵阵掌声
C	陈教授的精彩讲评赢得了与会代表的阵阵掌声

Figure 13.3 An example of the boundary technique

Note: The fixation point is denoted by an asterisk. The invisible boundary that triggers the display change is marked with a vertical bar. The box shows the target location.

The logic underlying this paradigm is that certain characteristics of the preview stimulus are processed parafoveally prior to fixation. Thus, by manipulating the characteristics of the preview in relation to those of the target word, and observing differences in oculomotor behavior that result, we can infer which characteristics of a parafoveal word are processed before it is fixated. An advantage of the boundary paradigm over the moving-window technique is that more precise control over parafoveal information is possible since only one word is selected for manipulation. In addition, since the region of abnormal text is small, normal reading is even more closely approximated (Rayner & Pollatsek, 1989).

The size of perceptual span

How much information can be obtained in a given eye fixation? McConkie and Rayner (1975) examined how many letters around the fixation point are needed in order that reading might proceed normally. They had participants read text when the window was 13, 17, 21, 25, 31, 37, 45, and 100 characters wide (with a window size of 100, the entire line was almost always present). They found when the window was up to 31 characters, or 15 character positions to each side of fixation, participants were able to read at normal speed with good comprehension. When the window size was smaller, they reduced their normal reading speed by about 60 percent, but normal comprehension was still attained. Rayner and Bertera (1979) also found no effect on comprehension unless the window was reduced to only 1 character (in which case, readers are literally reading letter by letter).

Rayner (1986) also employed the moving-window technique to examine the size of the perceptual span in second-, fourth-, and sixth-grade children, as well as adult skilled readers. In Experiment 1, reading level was manipulated (2nd, 4th, 6th grade, and adult readers were tested) and six window sizes were used (5, 11, 17, 23, 29 characters, and a full-line condition). Experiments 2 and 3 were conducted to determine whether or not beginning readers' perceptual spans were asymmetric. In Experiment 2, all words to the left of fixation were visible, and the number of words to the right of fixation was varied. The conditions in Experiment 3 were similar to those of Experiment 2, however, the position of the left boundary was manipulated. Rayner's results indicated that the perceptual span in beginning readers was slightly smaller than the perceptual span of skilled readers. It was also found that the perceptual span of beginning readers extended about 11 character spaces to the right of fixation (recall that for skilled readers, the span extends 14-15 spaces to the right of fixation). The size of the perceptual span increased with age, and again, the perceptual span was asymmetric to the right of fixation.

The perceptual span and word spacing information

As mentioned earlier, English readers can extract useful information from about 15 characters to the right of fixation but little beyond that. However, another important question concerns what kind of information is extracted from this region. Several studies have been carried out to investigate this question.

McConkie and Rayner (1975) investigated the perceptual span for word-boundary information by perturbing text in two ways outside the window. In one condition, all letters in words were replaced by X's but the spaces between words were preserved; in the other, the spaces were replaced by X's as well. They found when the window size was 25 character spaces or fewer (symmetric about the point of fixation), reading times were shorter when spaces were present among the X's outside the window than when they were not. By contrast, when the window size was 31 character spaces or greater, there was no difference between the background conditions. Thus, it appears that out to about 15 character spaces from fixation, participants use the spacing information to help guide their eye movements into that region. Also, Pollatsek and Rayner (1982) used the moving-window paradigm to compare reading when the word spaces were present with when they were replaced with an X. They found that saccade lengths were shorter when word space information was not available than when it was.

McConkie and Rayner (1975) also attempted to determine how far from fixation the information about the shapes of letters and words was extracted. They compared backgrounds in which the letters were visually similar to the letters in the text with backgrounds in which the letters were visually dissimilar. They found that letter shape information was not extracted as far out as word boundary information. There were differences between these two background conditions only for windows up to 21 character positions.

The asymmetry of perceptual span

In the original McConkie and Rayner (1975) experiment, the distance that the window of normal text extended was the same on both sides of fixation; hence, it was impossible to test whether readers extract more information from one side of fixation than the other. To test the symmetry of the perceptual span, McConkie and Rayner (1976) independently varied the left and right boundaries of the window of normal text and found that when the window extended 4 character positions to the left of fixation and 14 to the right, reading was virtually as fast as when the window extended 14 character spaces in both directions. In contrast, when the window extended 14 character spaces to the left of fixation and 4 to the right, reading was greatly impaired. Thus, for readers of English, the perceptual span is asymmetric, with processing extending to a greater degree beyond fixation to the right of fixation than to the left (see also Rayner et al., 1980).

Rayner, McConkie, and Ehrlich (1978) used a variation of the boundary paradigm to examine the asymmetry of the perceptual span. They found that an extrafoveal preview of a word in a location opposite to that in which the eyes were about to move, provided no facilitation in naming latency over having an incorrect preview, whereas a preview in the direction to which the eyes were about to move facilitated naming latency. The results suggest that little information is acquired from an extrafoveal location which is in the opposite direction to that in which the eyes are about to move, and that useful information is acquired prior to the eye movement from the position to which the eyes are about to move. These results are consistent with the findings of the moving window studies investigating the perceptual span previously described.

Several studies extend the work on the size of the perceptual span, and further demonstrate the asymmetry of the perceptual span (Rayner et al., 1980; Pollatsek, Bolozky, Well, & Rayner, 1981; Rayner, 1986). For example, Pollatsek et al., (1981) found for bilingual Israelis reading their native language, Hebrew, the perceptual span was asymmetric to the left of fixation, and when the same participants read English, their perceptual span was asymmetric to the right of fixation. So the perceptual span extended in the opposite direction during reading of Hebrew and flipped around, as appropriate, during reading of English. Thus, the asymmetry of the window is not fixed, but varies from language to language depending on the direction in which the language is read. The asymmetry of the perceptual span, and the flexibility of the direction in which it may project are interesting and important in that they suggest that attentional factors, rather than biological constraints associated with the retina play a central role in the acquisition of information from parafoveal words during a fixation in reading.

Age, reading skill, and the perceptual span

Several researchers have suggested that children have smaller perceptual spans than skilled readers. Taylor (1965) used a simple method to assess the amount of information readers were processing on any particular fixation. Taylor divided the number of words on a line by the number of fixations on the line. Using this measure, Taylor found that second-grade children were processing 0.57 words per fixation, fourth-grade children 0.72 words, and sixth-grade children 0.83 words. College students had a perceptual span of 1.11 words.

Fisher and Montanary (1977) had participants read text in which the spaces between words were filled with various types of letters or characters. They found the absence of word boundary cues interfered markedly with reading fluency in older children (fifth and sixth graders), but had much less influence on beginning readers (first and second graders). Thus, it was assumed that the more skilled readers were at a disadvantage with the text without spaces because they had developed more fluent and efficient skills through the use of non-foveal vision, and the mutilated word boundary cues interfered with their saccadic targeting strategy. In contrast, younger children were assumed to be far more dependent on foveal processing and therefore the missing boundary information in the parafovea was less disruptive.

By varying the availability of graphic information in the periphery of vision, Patberg and Yonas (1978) also investigated the development of the perceptual span in reading. The participants were low-ability eighth-grade readers, high-ability eighth-grade readers, and skilled adult readers. They read texts presented in a normal prose format, with a single space between words, and texts typed with 13 letter spaces between words. They found that removing peripheral information by wide spacing improved comprehension for low-ability eighth graders but did not affect their overall reading efficiency. By contrast, wide spacing decreased the reading efficiency of high-ability eighth-grade readers and skilled adult readers. The data from this experiment suggest that the perceptual span may increase as reading skill develops. Finally, consistent with these claims, Rayner (1986) also found the perceptual span was influenced by age: The perceptual span in beginning readers was slightly smaller than the perceptual span of skilled readers. Beginning readers devoted more of their processing to the foveally fixated word than more proficient readers.

Difficulty of foveal processing

In the Patberg and Yonas (1978) experiment, the normally spaced and widely spaced texts that were used were of two levels of reading difficulty. Patberg and Yonas hypothesized that participants might have a larger perceptual span with the easy text than with the difficult text. Their results showed that the difficulty of the text did not modulate the efficiency with which text was processed (both with respect to normally and widely spaced text). They took their results to show that processing demands associated with the text under fixation do not necessarily change the extent of the perceptual span during reading. Note, however, that the wide spacing manipulation employed in this experiment was very extreme and it is therefore not entirely clear whether reading could progress normally under such conditions.

In contrast to the findings of Patberg and Yonas, Rayner (1986) showed that the difficulty of the text being read did influence the extent of the perceptual span. Rayner argued that if difficulties associated with processing the foveal word can influence the size of the perceptual span, then it should be possible to reduce the area of effective vision by making the text more difficult. Thus, in his experiment, the difficulty of the sentence was manipulated in relation to the readers. The fourth grade participants were asked to read sentences that were appropriate for their reading level, and also to read sentences that were appropriate for college students. Rayner's results showed that difficulty processing the foveal word led to a reduction in the size of the effective visual field. When the sentences were difficult and participants had to devote more of their attention to processing the foveal word, the perceptual span was reduced. Consequently, Rayner concluded that size of the perceptual span became reduced as the text became more difficult to read.

Finally, Henderson and Ferreira (1990) employed the boundary paradigm to examine the effects of foveal processing difficulty on the perceptual span in reading. By changing the text contingent on the reader's current point of fixation, foveal processing difficulty and the availability of parafoveal word information were independently manipulated. In Experiment 1, foveal processing difficulty was manipulated through the use of either a high, or a low frequency word, and in Experiment 2 foveal difficulty was manipulated by using more or less syntactically complex structures immediately prior to a target word. In both experiments they found that less parafoveal information was acquired when foveal processing was difficult than when it was easy. They concluded that the extent of the perceptual span was variable and attentionally constrained such that increased foveal processing caused a reduction in the size of the span. More recently these results were replicated by White, Rayner, and Liversedge (2005).

Working memory

Working memory is often assumed to play a critical role in reading comprehension and sentence processing (e.g., Just & Carpenter, 1992). It is argued that a reader with sufficient working memory capacity is able to process texts efficiently, whereas a reader with insufficient capacity is less efficient in reading texts. Kennison and Clifton (1995) examined whether working memory capacity influenced parafoveal preview benefit. In their experiment, the Reading Span Test was used to assess working memory capacity. Also, they employed the boundary technique to examine whether working memory capacity influenced preview benefit. They found readers generally fixated closer to the beginning of the target word when the prior word was low frequency than when it was high frequency. Critically, however, the working memory capacity of the reader did not significantly influence parafoveal preview benefit. However, Kennison and Clifton did find differences in overall reading performance between high- and low- working memory capacity groups: Low-span participants experienced more difficulty during reading than high-span participants, as evidenced by longer total reading times and longer gaze durations on both the preview and target words.

Osaka and Osaka (2002) used the moving-window paradigm to examine individual differences in working memory in terms of the effective visual field size while reading Japanese text. Working memory capacity was measured by a Japanese reading span test, and the participants were divided into high-span and low-span groups. Reading performance was measured by reading time, sentence comprehension, and eye movement recordings. Their results indicated that as the window size in the moving-window paradigm decreased, the reading time increased significantly. Also, high-span participants had shorter reading times, better comprehension, and shorter fixation durations than low-span participants even with restricted visual fields. Interestingly, with reduced parafoveal vision, high-span participants showed better information integration than low-span participants during reading, indicating that reading performance was better for participants with larger working memory capacity under parafoveally restricted conditions.

Different writing systems

Since the invention of moving-window paradigm, cognitive psychologists have used it to study perceptual span in a number of different languages (e.g., Dutch, Japanese, and Hebrew). From these studies, and others, it is clear that writing systems affect not only eye-movement characteristics but also the size of the perceptual span. Similar to McConkie and Rayner's (1975) experiment, Den Buurman, Boersema, and Gerrissen (1981) used the moving-window technique to study Dutch readers. The window size was varied (13, 19, 25, 31, and 43 character positions, as well as a full text window). In the vertical direction this window always covered three lines. The results yielded a perceptual span of 25 to 31 character positions, or 12 to 15 positions to the right and left of the fixation point, approximately 4 to 5 degrees of visual angle (approximating the findings of McConkie & Rayner).

The Japanese writing system is a mixture of Kanji and Kana characters. Kanji characters are morphemic characters, and Kana characters are syllabic. Osaka (1987, 1992) used the moving-window technique to study Japanese readers. Osaka found that the perceptual span was larger for text consisting of a combination of Kanji and Kana than for text consisting only of Kana characters. For the combined Kana-Kanji script, the span extended 7 character spaces to the right of fixation. For the Kana script it extended 5 character spaces to the right of fixation. Osaka (1993) found that the perceptual span was asymmetric when reading vertically and horizontally. Thus, for the Japanese writing system, the perceptual span is considerably smaller than for English if one equates a Japanese character with a letter.

In contrast to English, Hebrew is printed, and therefore read, from right to left. Consequently, the asymmetry of the perceptual span in Hebrew has been an area of interest. As mentioned, Pollatsek et al. (1981) reported an experiment dealing with the characteristics of the perceptual span for native Israeli readers of Hebrew. The experiment also included bilingual English-Hebrew readers who read sentences in both English and Hebrew. The window area around a fixation point was either symmetric, extending 14 characters both left and right of fixation, or asymmetric so that it extended either 14 characters to the left and 4 to the right of fixation or 4 characters to the left and 14 to the right of fixation. As mentioned earlier, the results indicated that the perceptual span was asymmetric to the left when Hebrew was read, and asymmetric to the right when English was read. Also, for the bilinguals, the perceptual span switched its asymmetry contingent on whether English or Hebrew was being read. Thus, the asymmetry of the perceptual span varies across different languages. Rayner (1998) argues that readers allocate their attention to the material that is in the direction in which they are about to move their eyes in order to obtain new information from this portion of the text.

Studies of the perceptual span in Chinese reading

The Chinese writing system has one of the longest histories of any writing system in the world. Chinese writing is fundamentally logographic. Each character fits into a rectangle of the same size. Each character represents a syllable of spoken Chinese. Characters can be used on their own, in combination with other characters, or as part of other characters. Modern Chinese dictionaries contain up to about 8,500 characters and the language is used by one fifth of the world's population. Given its widespread use and its unique properties, it is an extremely interesting language to study experimentally.

Studies using the moving-window technique

Tsai and McConkie (1995) used the moving-window paradigm to study the perceptual span in Chinese reading. The participants read two passages, which were presented a single line at a time. They found that total reading time, mean fixation duration, mean forward saccade length, and mean number of regressions were affected by window size. On the basis of these data they estimated that the perceptual span in Chinese reading was one character to the left and two characters to the right of the fixated word.

Inhoff and Liu (1998) conducted two experiments to investigate Chinese readers' perceptual span. In their study, they also employed the moving-window paradigm to control the visibility of characters. Characters outside a window of legible text were masked by dissimilar characters. Eleven viewing conditions were created. In a no-preview condition, only the directly fixated character was visible during each fixation, creating a one-character window of visible text. There were right-side window conditions in which one to seven characters to the right of the fixated character were available. Additionally, there were conditions in which, the fixated character, seven characters to its right, and either one or two characters to its left were visible during each fixation. These conditions allowed Inhoff and Liu to explore both boundaries of the perceptual span in Chinese. A whole-line control condition in which the whole sentence was visible was also used. Once again, the results showed that the perceptual span was asymmetric. It extended further to the right of fixation than to the left, and the effective range of vision extended one character space to the left of the fixated character and three character spaces to its right when saccade size, landing locations, and gaze durations were analyzed.

While the majority of studies have used adults as participants, in a recent study Yan, Xiong, Bai, and Shen (2006), used the moving-window paradigm to study the size of perceptual span of Chinese fifth graders . Sixteen fifth graders with normal or corrected-to-normal vision participated in the experiment. Their mean age was 10.6 years old. 64 sentences were used. All sentences contained 17 to 21 characters. Care was taken to ensure that each sentence did not contain internal clausal boundaries or punctuation marks. Most of the words in each sentence contained 1 or 2 characters. The difficulty of the sentence and familiarity of the words were controlled. An SR Eyelink II eye tracker was used to record eye movements. Masking characters that appeared outside of the experimentally defined window had no meaningful interpretation. The stroke number of the masking characters was matched with corresponding characters that they had replaced. In the experiment, only one sentence was displayed on each trial and comprehension questions were included to ensure that the participants read the sentences conscientiously. There were 8 viewing conditions (see Figure 13.4). In the whole-line control condition the full line of text was visible during each fixation. In the no-preview condition, only the directly fixated character was visible during each fixation. Four right-side, window conditions were designed by revealing 1 to 4 characters to the right of the fixated character. These four conditions were referred to as R1, R2, R3, and R4 respectively. Two left-side window conditions were also created. Either one or two characters to the left of the fixated word were revealed while four characters to its right were visible. These conditions were referred to as L1R4 and L2R4 respectively.

该测验的目的是考查学生对生字的掌握情况	Whole line condition
抖欣括泥字层酒朴查矣汐收末田度渣膜栖迫	No-proview condition
抖欣括泥字层酒朴查学汐收末田度渣膜栖迫	R1 condition
抖欣括泥字层酒朴查学生收末田度渣膜栖迫	R2 condition
抖欣括泥字层酒朴查学生对末田度渣膜栖迫	R3 condition
抖欣括泥字层酒朴查学生对生田度渣膜栖迫	R4 condition
抖欣括泥字层酒考查学生对生田度渣膜栖迫	L1R4 condition
抖欣括泥字层是考查学生对生田度渣膜栖迫	R2R4 condition

Figure 13.4 An example of the eight viewing conditions used by Yan et al.

Note: The asterisk indicates the fixation location at which the different windows of text were displayed. The box represents the characters in the visible window.

Three eye-movement measures were considered: Mean first-pass reading time per character, mean fixation duration, and mean saccade size. The results revealed that window constraints did influence readers' rightward eye movements. As window size increased, both mean first pass time per character and mean fixation duration decreased, while mean saccade size increased. When only one character to the left of fixated point was visible all measures reached asymptotic values. Furthermore, the perceptual span appeared to extend about two or three characters to the right. Clearly, the perceptual span in fifth grade Chinese readers is reduced relative to that of English readers, but it is asymmetric like English, extending further in the direction that the reader is progressing.

Studies using the boundary technique

Hoosain (1991) assumed that Chinese readers obtained more useful linguistic information from the area near fixation than did readers of English text, due to the increased density of information in Chinese characters.

Several researchers have used the boundary paradigm to directly investigate what information is acquired from the parafovea during Chinese reading (Pollatsek, Tan, & Rayner, 2000; Liu, Inhoff, & Wu, 2002; Tsai, Lee, Tzeng, Hung, & Yen, 2004; Bai, Zang, Yan, & Shen, 2006). Pollatsek et al. (2000) used a variation of the boundary paradigm to examine parafoveal processing of Chinese characters. In the first experiment there were five preview types: (a) identical previews, (b) orthographically similar homophonic previews, (c) orthographically dissimilar homophonic previews, (d) synonyms (without orthographic overlap with targets), and (e) unrelated controls. The results showed that character-level phonological codes and orthographic information, but not semantic information, were extracted from the preview and affected identification of the target. In the second experiment phonetic regularity was manipulated in order to specifically investigate whether the phonological representations of phonetic radicals were available form the parafovea. Moreover, to systematically scrutinize the possible influence of orthographic similarity, semantic radicals were varied according to whether they were semantically related to whole characters. The data from Experiment 2 indicated that subcharacter-level phonological codes were accessed early during the recognition of high-frequency Chinese characters. Pollatsek et al. concluded that both lexical and sublexical phonological codes of Chinese characters were extracted from the parafovea. Also, orthographic information from the preview was used in character identification, with no reliable evidence for the extraction of semantic information from the parafovea.

Liu et al. (2002) also used the boundary paradigm to examine parafoveal processing of Chinese character previews during reading. In Experiment 1, previews consisted of target words (identity previews), graphemically similar previews, homophonic previews, or dissimilar characters. Preview benefits were greatest for target-word previews, less so for previews that were graphemically similar characters, and least for previews that were homophonic or dissimilar characters. Experiment 2 showed that parafoveal preview of graphemically similar characters yielded benefits primarily when they shared the phonetic radical with their targets. They concluded that Chinese-character processing initially involves the use of orthographic information from the phonetic radical, and thereby, activation of the character's phonological form.

Tsai et al. (2004) re-examined preview benefits using the boundary paradigm. In Experiment 1, the phonological and orthographic similarity of the preview and target characters were manipulated orthogonally according to whether they were homophones and whether they shared the same phonetic radical. The results revealed benefits from both phonological and orthographic previews in the parafovea. A second experiment directly manipulated the consistency of target characters to clarify whether the extent of character consistency modulated phonological preview benefit. The results showed that the phonological preview benefits were reliable only when the target and preview were consistent. Tsai et al.'s experiments suggested that rapid parafoveal effects and that phonological computation was influenced both at the level of the character and the radical during Chinese-character identification.

Similar to the experiments reported by Pollatsek et al. (2000), Bai et al. (2006) used the boundary paradigm to further examine the influence of phonological, graphemic, and semantic information in parafoveal processing during Chinese reading. In their study, the target-character frequency was manipulated to determine whether this modulated parafoveal preview benefit. Also, the graphemic and homophonic characteristics of the preview characters in relation to the targets were manipulated. The results indicated that the homophonic and graphemic information from the preview had an early facilitatory influence on the identification of the target character both at character and subcharacter level. In addition, there were no reliable modulatory effects of target frequency on parafoveal preview benefit.

Other related studies

Besides the experiments using the eye-contingent display change techniques mentioned above, there are some other experiments that are related to the issue of perceptual span in Chinese reading. Miles and Shen (1925) conducted the earliest eye movement study on Chinese reading. In their study, they examined some basic eye-movement characteristics of Chinese reading of text presented vertically and horizontally. In the experiment, a photographic recording technique was used to record eye movements. The participants were 11 Chinese students at Stanford University. Participants read four texts that were selected from magazine articles. Each text comprised a complete paragraph containing 10 to 12 lines of text. Selections A and B were vertical while C and D were horizontal. The data were analyzed in terms of the number of words "covered" by a fixation. Interestingly, they found that the average number of words per fixation was 2.3 for the text presented vertically, but only 1.9 for the text presented horizontally.

Gray (1956) reported a study that compared basic reading processes of mature readers in 14 languages (including Chinese). Eye movements were measured photographically. Records were obtained for both oral and silent reading. Gray estimated that during each fixation, the participants could recognize two or three words.

More recently, Sun and Feng (1999) used saccade size to assess the word identification span, and performed a comparative study of eye movements in reading Chinese and English. Participants consisted of one group of native Chinese graduate students and one group of native English-speaking graduate students. The results indicated that the recognition span of Chinese was 2.57±0.5 character spaces per fixation, equivalent to 1.7±0.3 words per fixation. And the recognition span of English was 1.75±0.6 words per fixation. Although, the visual forms of the two languages were strikingly different, their recognition spans in reading were very similar.

However, some of the above studies (Miles et al., 1925; Gray, 1956; Sun et al., 1999) refer to the word identification span, which measures the number of words that can be identified (on average) per fixation. It provides no information about the extent to which information beyond the span of word identification is obtained and used during a fixation. The method is based on the assumption that on successive fixations the perceptual spans do not overlap. A great deal of research with skilled readers has demonstrated that this assumption is false and that there is an overlap of information from fixation to fixation (Rayner, 1978).

Chen and Tang (1998) used a self-paced moving-window technique to study the perceptual span of Chinese readers. In their study, a mechanical mouse was connected to the computer to control stimulus display. The position of the mouse was represented on the screen by a pointer, which would move underneath horizontally arranged random masks. A character corresponding to a certain position was immediately displayed when the pointer moved under that position. By moving the mouse from left to right, a participant viewed successive characters of a sentence displayed in spatially appropriate locations on the screen. There were 10 different display conditions. There was one single-character condition, four preview-without-review conditions, four preview-with-review conditions, and one whole line condition.

In the single-character condition only the fixated character was visible in each successive display. In the four preview-without-review conditions, the fixated character with one, two, three, or four characters to its right were visible in each display. In the four preview-with-review conditions, the fixated character, the character(s) to its right, and the character to its left were visible in each successive display. The viewing time was taken to indicate reading effectiveness under various display conditions. It was concluded that the effective visual field in reading Chinese was asymmetric and skewed in the direction of scanning. Also, it was of limited extent, being comprised of the fixated character and two characters to its right.

Conclusions

Since McConkie and Rayner (1975) invented the moving-window paradigm there have been many studies to investigate the perceptual span across different languages. As we have described above, there have been a number of experiments that have specifically investigated this question, as well as more generally, examining parafoveal processing in Chinese. It is our view that issues related to reading in Chinese are of particular interest due to intrinsic characteristics of the language that are often quite different to those of other languages. A critical question in this area concerns the granularity of processing in Chinese, that is to say, it is vital to understand whether the character, or the word is the primary unit of information in Chinese reading. Note that this question is pervasive, in that foveal and parafoveal processing, and oculomotor control more generally, must (at least at some level) be characterized with respect to the Chinese characters or words that comprise the text. Clearly, substantially more research is required before we have developed a comprehensive understanding of issues related to this aspect of reading in Chinese.

References

Bai, X. J., Zang, C. L., Yan, G. L., & Shen, D. L. (2006). *The role of different linguistic codes in parafoveal processing*. Paper presented at the Second China International Conference on Eye Movement, Tianjin, China.

Balota, D. A., & Rayner, K. (1991). Word recognition processes in foveal and parafoveal vision: The range of influence of lexical variables. In D. Besner, & G. Humphreys (Eds.), *Basic processes in reading: Visual word recognition* (pp. 198-232). Hillsdale NJ: Lawrence Erlbaum Associates.

Bouma, H., & De Voogd, A. H. (1974). On the control of eye saccades in reading. *Vision Research, 14,* 273-284.

Chen, H. C., & Tang, C. K. (1998). The effective visual field in reading Chinese. *Reading and Writing, 10,* 3-5.

Den Buurman, R., Boersma, T., & Gerrissen, J. F. (1981). Eye movements and the perceptual span in reading. *Reading Research Quarterly, 16,* 227-235.

Fisher, D. F., & Lefton, L.A. (1976). Peripheral information extraction: A developmental examination of reading processes. *Journal of Experimental Child Psychology, 21,* 77-93.

Fisher, D. F., & Montanary, S. P. (1977). Spatial and contextual factors in beginning reading: Evidence for PSG-CSG complements to developing automacity? *Memory & Cognition,5,* 247-251.

Gray, W. S. (1956). *The teaching of reading and writing: An international survey.* Chicago: Scott Foresman.

Henderson, J. M., & Ferreira, F. (1990). Effects of foveal processing difficulty on the perceptual span in reading: Implications for attention and eye movement control. *Journal of Experimental Psychology: Learning, Memory, and Cognition, 16,* 417-429.

Hoosain, R. (1991).*Psycholinguistic implications for linguistic relativity: A case study of Chinese.* Hillsdale, NJ: Erlbaum.

Inhoff, A. W., & Liu, W. (1998). The perceptual span and oculomotor activity during the reading of Chinese sentences. *Journal of Experimental Psychology: Human Perception and Performance, 24,* 20-34.

Just, M.A., & Carpenter, P.A. (1992). A capacity theory of comprehension: Individual differences in working memory. *Psychological Review, 98,* 122-149.

Kennison, S. M., & Clifton, C. (1995). Determinants of parafoveal preview benefit in high and low working memory capacity readers: Implications for eye movement control. *Journal of Experimental Psychology: Learning, Memory, and Cognition, 2,* 68-81.

Liu, W., Inhoff, A. W., Ye, Y., & Wu, C. (2002). Use of parafoveally visible characters during the reading of Chinese sentences. *Journal of Experimental Psychology: Human Perception and Performance, 28,*1213-1227.

McConkie, G. W., & Rayner, K. (1975). The span of the effective stimulus during a fixation in reading. *Perception & Psychophysics, 17,* 578-586.

McConkie, G. W., & Rayner, K. (1976). Asymmetry of the perceptual span in reading. *Bulletin of the Psychonomic Society, 8,* 365-368.

McConkie, G. W., & Zola, D. (1987). Visual attention during eye fixations while reading. In M. Coltheart, *Attention and performance,* vol. 12 (pp. 385-401). London: Erlbaum.

Miles, R.S., & Shen, E. (1925). Photographic recording of eye movements in the reading of Chinese in vertical and horizontal axes: Method and preliminary results. *Journal of Experimental Psychology, 8,* 344-362.

Newman, E. B. (1966). Speed of reading when the span of letters is restricted. *American Journal of Psychology, 79,* 272-278.

Osaka, N. (1987). Effect of peripheral visual field size upon eye movements during Japanese text processing. In J. K. O'Regan, & A. Levy-Schoen (Eds.), *Eye movements: From physiology to cognition* (pp. 363-383). Hillsdale. NJ: Eribaum.

Osaka, N. (1992). Size of saccade and fixation duration of eye movement during reading: Psychophysics of Japanese text processing. *Journal of the Optical Society of America, 9,* 5-13.

Osaka, N. (1993). Asymmetry of the effective visual field in vertical reading as measured with a moving-window. In G. d'Ydewalle, & J. Van Rensbergen (Eds.), *Perception and cognition: Advanced in eye movement research* (pp. 275-283). Amsterdam: North Holland.

Osaka, N., & Osaka, M. (2002). Individual differences in working memory during reading with and without parafoveal information: A moving-window study. *American Journal of Psychology, 115,* 501-513.

Patberg, J. P., & Yonas, A. (1978). The effects of the reader's skill and the difficulty of the text on the perceptual span in reading. *Journal of Experimental Psychology: Human Perception and Performance, 4,* 545-552.

Pollatsek, A., & Rayner, K. (1982). Eye movement control in reading: the role of word boundaries. *Journal of Experimental Psychology: Human Perception and Performance, 8,* 817-833.

Pollatsek, A., Bolozky, S., Well, A. D., & Rayner, K. (1981). Asymmetries in the perceptual span for Israeli readers. *Brain and Language, 14,* 174-180.

Pollatsek, A., Tan, L. H., & Rayner, K. (2000). The role of phonological codes in integrating information across saccadic eye movements in Chinese character identification. *Journal of Experimental Psychology: Human Perception and Performance, 26,* 607-633.

Poulton, E. C. (1962). Peripheral vision, refractoriness and eye movements in fast oral reading. *British Journal of Psychology, 53,*409-419.

Rayner, K. (1975). The perceptual span and peripheral cues in reading. *Cognitive Psychology, 7*,65-81.

Rayner, K. (1978). Eye movements in reading and information processing. *Psychological Bulletin, 85*, 618-660.

Rayner, K. (1986). Eye movements and the perceptual span in beginning and skilled readers. *Journal of Experimental Child Psychology, 41*, 211-236.

Rayner, K. (1998). Eye movements in reading and information processing: 20 years of research. *Psychological Bulletin, 124*, 372-422.

Rayner, K., & Bertera, J. H. (1979). Reading without foveal. *Science, 206*, 468-469.

Rayner, K., McConkie, G. W., & Ehrlich, S. F. (1978). Eye movements and integrating information across fixations. *Journal of Experimental Psychology: Human Perception and Performance, 4*, 529-544.

Rayner, K., & Pollatsek, A. (1987). Eye movements in reading: A tutorial review. In M.Coltheart (Ed.), *Attention and performance* 12, London: Erlbaum.

Rayner, K., & Pollatsek, A. (1989). *The psychology of reading*. Englewood Cliffs, NJ: Prentice Hall.

Rayner, K., Well, A. D., & Pollatsek, A. (1980). Asymmetry of the effective visual field in reading. *Perception & Psychophysics, 27*, 537 544.

Rayner, K., Well, A. D., Pollatsek, A., & Bertera, J. H. (1982). The availability of useful information to the right of fixation in reading. *Perception & Psychophysics, 31*, 537-550.

Sun, F., & Feng, D. (1999). Eye movements in reading Chinese and English text. In Jian Wang et al. (Eds.), *Reading Chinese script: A cognitive analysis*(pp.189-203). New Jersey: Lawrence Erlbaum Associates Publishers.

Taylor, S. E. (1965). Eye movements while reading: Facts and fallacies. *American Educational Research Journal, 2*, 187-202.

Tsai, J., Lee, C., Tzeng, O. J. L., Hung, D. L., & Yen, N. (2004). Use of phonological codes for Chinese characters: Evidence from processing of parafoveal preview when reading sentences. *Brain and Language, 91*, 235-244.

Tsai, C. H., & McConkie, G. W. (1995). *The perceptual span in reading Chinese text: A moving-window study*. Paper presented at the Seventh International Conference on the Cognitive Processing of Chinese and Other Asian Languages, Hong Kong.

Underwood, N. R., & McConkie, A. (1985). Perceptual span for letter distinctions during reading. *Reading Research Quarterly, 20*,153-162.

White, S. J., Rayner, K., & Liversedge, S. P. (2005). Eye Movements and the modulation of parafoveal processing by foveal processing difficulty: A re-examination. *Psychonomic Bulletin & Review, 12*, 891-896.

Yan, G. L., Xiong, J. P., Bai, X. J., & Shen, D. L. (2006). *The perceptual span and oculomotor activity in fifth grade Chinese readers.* Paper presented at the Second China International Conference on Eye Movement, Tianjin, China.

Chapter 14

Lexical processing and eye movements in Chinese readers

Dingguo Gao, Ruijian Zhang, and Ju Chen

In the past three decades, there has been a tremendous amount of research on the characteristics of eye movements in reading (see review by Rayner, 1998). However, most of these studies have been dedicated to studying alphabetic writing systems (see Rayner, 1998), and few have been done with the Chinese language even though it is the main language of more than one billion people all over the world.

Written Chinese is considered to be a logographic script that differs in many aspects from alphabetic writing systems. First, each character is composed of strokes that are arranged vertically and horizontally, and all the characters typically occupy the same space as each other. An alphabetic word usually consists of horizontally distributed alphabetic letters. Second, all Chinese characters are monosyllabic and each carries a meaning except for bisyllabic words and a few other exceptions. More importantly, given the fact that many picto-phonetic characters (phonograms) exist in the Chinese language, it is almost impossible for a reader to orthographically spell out a character, regardless of the reader's experience in orthography and correctness of pronunciation. Third, a Chinese character is usually comprised of a phonetic determinative (or phonetic component) and a semantic determinative. This is called a picto-phonetic character. The semantic component in a Chinese character strongly implies the meaning and classification. For instance, if a character contains a component [yu(2)-fish], it is almost certain that it represents a kind of fish or has something to do with fish. Although there are word-stems in alphabetic words, it is more common that a Chinese character carries such a component. Fourth, Chinese words consist of characters. However, the distinction between words and characters is vague. Most of the characters can function both as independent words and as parts of other words. Most words in Chinese contain two characters, but some contain a single character or four characters (which are mostly Chinese idioms). There are also three-character words (particularly for Chinese names) and five-or-more-character words (particularly for proper nouns; see Hoosain, 1991). Finally, although there are small spaces between any two characters, no space is used to distinguish Chinese words in a sentence. In English, it's easy to know the number of words in a sentence, but in Chinese the concept of a word count is often controversial. Chinese readers know clearly the number of characters in a sentence but often feel confused about the number of words. Fortunately, no evidence shows that this confusion damages reading comprehension.

Most researchers have focused more on the differences between processing Chinese and processing other languages, particularly alphabetic languages such as English and German. However, processing Chinese is also similar to processing other languages. It has also been demonstrated that word frequency, complexity, predictability, and ambiguity influence the reading of Chinese as they do in other languages (see Rayner, 1998). Previous studies have been done for lexical processing of Chinese through priming (Tan, Hoosain, & Peng, 1995; Tan, Hoosain, & Siok, 1996; Zhou & Marslen-Wilson, 1999a, 1999b; Zhou, Shu, Bi, & Shi, 1999), semantic categorization (Chen, Flores d'Arcais, & Cheung, 1995; Leck, Weekes, & Chen, 1995), character identification (Ju & Jackson, 1995; Perfetti & Zhang, 1991), lexical decision (Cheng, 1992; Cheng, & Shih, 1988; Zhou, Marslen-Wilson, Taft, & Shu, 1999), and naming paradigms (Flores d'Arcais, 1992; Hung, Tzeng, & Tzeng, 1992). There are also increasing eye-movement studies of lexical processing for Chinese (Feng, Miller, Shu, & Zhang, 2001; Pollatsek, Tan, & Rayner, 2000). In this chapter, we will mainly review the studies on lexical processing of Chinese through the eye-movement recording technique and explore the future directions of these issues, because investigating lexical processing can contribute to an understanding of the nature of reading and cognitive processes.

Lexical features affecting Chinese reading

Yang and McConkie (1999) summarized the features of Chinese characters and words which will affect reading. One feature is the frequency of words used in the language. Just as frequency of use affects eye behavior in reading English, it also has effects on the eye movements of reading Chinese (e.g., Inhoff & Rayner, 1986; Pollatsek et al., 2000). However, in Chinese, a complication is that characters and character components also have their own frequencies of use respectively. So, we should also examine the effects of character frequency and character components. Another is the variation and configuration of a character in visual complexity. Words or characters vary greatly in stroke number. Moreover, compound words can show different complexities at different character positions within a word. Other lexical features include predictability and ambiguity of a word in a sentence (see Rayner, 1999).

Frequency

Previous studies using lexical decision or naming tasks have demonstrated a frequency effect such that high-frequency words are processed more efficiently than those with low frequency both in alphabetic languages and Chinese (see Gao, Zhong, & Zeng, 1995 for Chinese). In English, word frequency has a strong effect on fixation time on a word in reading (see Rayner, 1998). However, the concept of word is more complicated in written Chinese than it is in alphabetic languages. A word in Chinese can consist of a single character, or two characters, or three or four (or more) characters. Chinese characters are more like morphemes. Moreover, the distinction between character and word is not clear in Chinese. As we noted above, characters are spaced evenly in Chinese text and no extra spaces are used to segment words. It's reasonable to argue that reading Chinese will be less efficient than reading English because all character boundaries could be possible locations for word boundaries and accordingly it will be more difficult to distinguish words in Chinese than to do that in English. However, Chinese and English readers read equally fast and have comparable eye-movement patterns (Feng et al., 2001; Wong & Chen, 1999).

In Chinese, since a character is part of a word or independently functions as a word, we should consider the effects of both characters and words when investigating Chinese reading. Here we consider two-character words as an example. There are eight possible combinations for two-character words: A high frequency word can consist of (a) high-frequency initial and second characters, (b) a high-frequency initial character and low-frequency second character, or (c) a low-frequency initial character and high-frequency second character, or (d) low-frequency initial and second characters. Accordingly, a low-frequency word is also composed of one of those four possible combinations.

Yan, Tian, Bai, and Rayner (2006) used this classification to investigate the effect of word frequency on eye movements of Chinese readers. They found first-pass word frequency effects on fixation time on a target word. That is, Chinese readers look longer for low-frequency words than high-frequency words. The results are consistent with the findings by Yang and McConkie (1999) and Chen, Song, Lau, Wong, and Tang (2003), and are comparable in effect size to that typically shown with English readers (see Rayner, 1998). In addition, they also found that character frequency affects fixation time on the target word and the effect of the initial character in two-character words is more significant than that of the second character. Specifically, fixations are longer on words with a low-frequency initial character than on words with a high-frequency initial character. They also found that word frequency modulates the character frequency effect. The character frequency effect was weakened with high-frequency target words whereas it was quite apparent with low-frequency target words. Yan et al. (2006) argued that a two-character word with high frequency is accessed as a single entity in the mental lexicon of Chinese readers, whereas a word with low frequency needs to be accessed via the characters (and hence an effect of character frequency appears). The findings that character frequency primarily influenced first-pass reading times but not rereading times, whereas word frequency affected both first-pass and rereading times suggest that character frequency effects are more short-lived than those of word frequency.

Yang and McConkie (1999) examined frequency effects on target words, specifically two-character words. They adopted five types of material through varying the frequency of the word and the complexity (stroke number) of the initial and second characters. They found that low-frequency words have longer gaze durations and are refixated more often than high-frequency words, whereas high-frequency words are skipped more often than low-frequency words. Zhang and Yan (2005) obtained similar results showing that frequency and familiarity affect fixation time in Chinese reading. That is, the more frequent and more familiar a word was, the less time it was fixated on. Chen et al. (2003) through regression analyses argued that character complexity and frequency were more important than word frequency.

However, no eye-movement studies have been done to explore situations complicated by idioms and three-character words. Also, there are no studies adopting eye-movement techniques to investigate the frequency of components, and the relationship between lexical and sublexical processing.

Complexity

Chinese characters are made up of strokes, varying from 1 to more than 30 strokes, whereas words in alphabetic languages vary in length or number of constituent letters. Therefore, the more strokes a character has the more complex it should be. There are eight types of strokes. Chinese characters are not random arrays of strokes but are constructed in a systematic way and are related to perceptual principles (Gao & Kao, 2002). In fact, the number of strokes in a character is inversely proportional to frequency. The fewer strokes a character contains, the more frequently it is used (Gao & Kao, 2002; Loo, 1989). Most characters are composed of components, which are the basic units for most characters. There are two types of components, one is called the radical or signific (which often carries semantic information), and the other is called the phonetic (which often carries pronunciation information). Signific components are often located in the left or the top of a character, and phonetics in the right or the bottom. A character with two or more components is called a compound character. However, there are characters called independent characters (du-ti-zi) which consists of only one component or is only constructed with some strokes (but the stroke combination is not a component). Two components can be aligned either horizontally or vertically to form a character or a part of a more complex character.

Each character is placed in a standard and almost equal space. Therefore, the density or visual complexity among characters is quite different. Behavioral studies have shown that complex characters are usually more difficult to recognize than simple characters (Huang, Wang, & Liou, 1991), particularly in peripheral vision (Yang, 1994).

Few studies have been conducted to investigate the complexity effect when reading Chinese. Because both have central roles in lexical processing, complexity and frequency are always manipulated simultaneously. In most previous studies, researchers recorded the reaction time or eye movements to investigate this question.

Zhang and Feng (1992) manipulated both the frequency and the stroke and component numbers of a character and examined the reaction time and error rate through a naming task. For high-frequency characters, they found an interaction effect between frequency and complexity in which the more strokes or components a character contained, the more time was used, but such an effect appeared only when the number of strokes and the number of components were distinct.

Chen, Zhao, and Sun (1999) recorded eye movements in a similar naming task to investigate the effects of complexity and frequency on word identification. They failed to reveal a significant correlation between recognition time and number of strokes, but they did find a frequency effect that recognition time and number of fixations increase as character frequency decreases. Goonetilleke, Lau, and Shih (2002) also found that word complexity did not show any significant effect on search time in an eye-movement study.

These studies have explored the issue of complexity effects. Strictly speaking, however, word recognition (particularly naming and lexical decision) can't be considered reading. At least, they are somewhat different from real reading in task requirements and cognitive processes. Therefore, the recording of eye movements in reading is crucial to exploring complexity effects.

Yang and McConkie (1999) manipulated the frequency of a word and the complexity of characters in a two-character word and recorded eye movements during Chinese reading. The results showed that both the complexity of characters and words influenced the likelihood of skipping characters and of refixating words, as well as the gaze duration on a fixated word. That is, there was an increase in gaze duration, a decrease in skipping rate, and an increase in refixation rate for more complex words.

Surprisingly, no preferred viewing position phenomenon appeared in reading Chinese, which indicated that Chinese readers didn't parse the character string into words in their parafoveal/peripheral vision. This is not consistent with those English studies in which the eyes fixated more near the center of a word than its beginning or ending (McConkie, Kerr, Reddix & Zola, 1988; Rayner, 1979). Yang and McConkie (1999) argued that the no preferred-viewing-position phenomenon suggests that words or words-like units are not functioning as saccade targets in Chinese as they do in English.

The results raise questions on reading Chinese. How do Chinese readers read and understand texts? More specifically, when and where are characters combined into a word during reading? These important questions need more study. Unfortunately, few studies have been done to address these questions.

Adopting regression analysis techniques with eye-movement data of Chinese adults and children, Chen et al. (2003) claimed that character complexity and frequency are more important than word frequency in Chinese reading. However, Yan et al. (2006) argued that regression analysis may obscure certain aspects of data. Frequency effects will decrease due to more exposures to target words, so such effects may not as salient in regression analyses across the whole passage as they are in experiments. Also, multicollinearity may obscure the effects of predictor variables in regression analyses when those variables themselves are correlated (Yan et al, 2006).

Predictability

Word predictability refers to the extent to which a reader can predict the upcoming words from the preceding text. Predictability has been demonstrated to have a robust effect on the eye movements of English readers (Ehrlich & Rayner, 1981; Rayner & Well, 1996). However, only one eye-movement study on Chinese investigated this question. Rayner, Li, Juhasz, and Yan (2005) used sentences that contained target words that varied in terms of high, medium or low predictability from the prior context and recorded the eye movements of Chinese readers while reading these sentences. They found that Chinese readers fixate less time on high-predictable and medium-predictable target words than on low-predictable target words, and are also more likely to fixate on low-predictable target words than on high-predictable or medium-predictable target words. The results were highly consistent with those obtained from English readers by Rayner and Well (1996), indicating that Chinese readers, like English readers, exploit target-word predictability during reading. Rayner et al. (2005) argued that, in spite of some clear differences between Chinese and English readers in terms of initial encoding of print (due to the nature of the logographic vs. alphabetic writing systems), once the material is encoded, reading processes appear to be more similar than dissimilar for the two groups of readers. According to Rayner et al. (2005), the difference in skipping words between Chinese and English and the lack of a preferred viewing position effect in Chinese may be due to the fact that the next Chinese character to be fixated is closer to the current eye position in Chinese than in English.

The study by Rayner et al. (2005) clearly showed that Chinese readers exploit contextual constraint/predictability factors in much the same way as English readers do, with the control of word frequency, character frequency and character complexity. However, how these four factors interact with each other or work together is still not known. Further studies may choose these factors as variables.

Ambiguity

Ambiguous words are frequently encountered in daily life. When we read texts, talk to, or listen to people, there are occasions when we can not fully understand a word in a sentence because the word has more than one meaning or more than one orthographic form. In these situations, we need additional information to help us to get over the ambiguity. There are two types of ambiguous words. If an orthographical representation corresponds to more than one semantic representation, this ambiguous word is named a homograph. Under the same logic, if more than one orthographic form that shares the same pronunciation (of course with different meaning) will be activated when we listen to the ambiguous words, these ambiguous words are named homophones.

Homophone. The percentage of characters that are picto-phonetic compounds, having a pronunciation identical to or similar to (allowing change in tone) the phonetic component, increases from 48% of those taught in first grade to 87% of those taught in sixth grade in China (Shu & Anderson, 1999). Moreover, picto-phonetic characters also concomitantly increase from 29% to 43%. Low-frequency characters are much more likely to be regular in their pronunciation, with more than 96% of very low frequency (less than 1 per million) characters pronounced the same as their phonetic component (Perfetti, Zhang, & Berent, 1992; Shu & Anderson, 1999). From these data, it seems that most Chinese characters can be read regularly with reference to the phonetic components. However, Chinese is often characterized as having a very "deep" orthography, because, unlike languages such as German and Italian, there is not a transparent correspondence between characters and their pronunciations. Although there are many picto-phonetic compounds exhibited in the Chinese writing system, the validity of the phonological cues from phonetic components is often not ideal, indicating that orthographic cues to phonology are less useful in Chinese than they are in a more regular orthographies. Fan, Gao, and Ao (1984) estimated that 73% of the Chinese compound characters are pronounced differently in contrast to their phonetic components pronounced in isolation. To some extent, a majority of Chinese characters have irregular pronunciations. Thus, the relationship of phonetic components to the pronunciation of the character is in some way analogical to the relationship of the pronunciation of the "body" of a monosyllabic English word to the pronunciation of the whole word (Pollatsek et al., 2000). Chinese readers face problems in pronouncing or spelling a character correctly, even among the prototypical picto-phonetic characters.

Chinese characters correspond to syllables. There are 1,277 syllables in modern Mandarin, the official dialect of both Mainland China and Taiwan (Chao, 1976), in contrast to more than 8,000 syllables in English (DeFrancis, 1984). Although almost 100,000 Chinese characters have existed at one point or another in Chinese history (see Wan & Hsia, 1957; Zhou, 1999), there are only around 5,000 characters, which are in active use in the modern Chinese language (Ann, 1986; Suen, 1986; Wang & Chang, 1986). Wang and Chang (1986) reported that 3,500 commonly used characters have occupied 99.87% of usage and show a skewed distribution on frequency of usage. Generally, readers could on the average be able to read 99.87% of all the characters contained in a 1,000-character article if they had learned those 3,500 characters. On the basis of these data, each syllable contributes to about four different characters on average. Thus, it's reasonable to argue that Chinese is replete with homophonic characters, many of which have low visual similarity, so almost no unique mapping exists from a particular syllable to a single character.

In the past decade, researchers have fallen into a debate regarding how phonology affects lexical access in Chinese. Researchers often use homophones to probe whether phonological processing plays a crucial role in lexical access. The paradigms include naming, lexical decision, backward masking, semantic judgment, and eye movements (Feng et al., 2001; Pollatsek et al., 2000).

Pollatsek et al. (2000) adopted an eye-movement-contingent display-change paradigm to investigate the role of the phonological code in Chinese character identification. They manipulated preview information in the parafovea to explore a preview benefit effect in which substantial facilitation in naming when preview is orthographically, phonologically or semantically relative to the target. This paradigm has been extensively used in reading, particularly in phonological activation of reading. In this study, Pollatsek et al. asked subjects to move their eyes from a central fixation location to a to-be-named parafoveal target character to see if phonological information can facilitate naming. In Experiment 1, the preview of the target was either (a) the target, (b) an orthographically similar homophonic character, (c) an orthographically dissimilar homophonic character, (d) a synonymous character, or (e) a dissimilar (control) character. Eye-movement-contingent display changes presented the target when the eyes moved toward its location. Under these conditions, parafoveal preview of the target and of the two types of homophones produced a preview benefit effect. In Experiment 2 and 3, they further revealed that high-frequency phonetically regular characters are named faster than high-frequency phonetically irregular characters. Therefore, both lexical and sublexical phonological codes of Chinese characters play roles early in the process of character identification. However, orthographic information was also involved in character identification, because orthographically similar previews facilitated target identification as well.

However, the role of phonological information from a parafoveally visible Chinese character could be subject to task demands. For instance, naming a character may differ from reading a sentence silently. Naming is often thought of as requiring the use of phonological knowledge. Using a boundary paradigm (Rayner, 1975), in which subjects were reading sentences, Tsai, Lee, Tzeng, Hung, and Yen (2004) examined the role of phonological information in Chinese character identification in sentence reading. In Experiment 1, they manipulated the phonological and orthographical similarity of homophones. Consistent with Pollatsek et al. (2000), they found early phonological activation for a character (i.e., when the character was in the parafovea). In Experiment 2, they manipulated the consistency value of characters and found that phonological preview benefits are significant only when the targets are of high consistency. Tsai et al. argued that phonological processing in Chinese is rapid and early at both character and radical levels for Chinese character identification.

The view of early activation of phonological information in Chinese reading has been challenged by some researchers. Liu, Inhoff, Ye, and Wu (2002) also used an eye-movement-contingent display-change paradigm in normal sentence reading. In their Experiment 1, a preview consisted of the target character or of graphemically similar, homophonic, or dissimilar characters. Each preview was replaced with the corresponding target when the eyes reached the target region. They also found preview benefits for targets, for graphemically similar characters and for homophonic characters. In Experiment 2, they found that parafoveal preview of graphemically similar characters yielded preview-benefit effects primarily when they shared the phonetic component with their targets. Parafoveal visibility of a character with considerable stroke overlap or with the same semantic component as the target character produced relatively small preview-benefit effects that were not significant during first-pass reading. These results imply that the phonological relationship between previewed components and subsequently viewed targets is not an effective cue. They argued that benefits obtained from the structural overlap in the phonetic component condition thus cannot be due to readers' misperception of the preview for the target. Chinese character processing thus involves the initial use of orthographic information from the phonetic component and the activation of phonology of a character.

Feng et al. (2001) used a basic error disruption paradigm developed by Daneman and Reingold (1993) to investigate the time course of phonological activation in reading Chinese and English. Again, they selected homophones as stimuli, and manipulated simultaneously and independently the orthographic similarity between homophones and targets, word (character) frequency, and context predictability. Participants were asked to read passages in their native language that contained occasional spelling errors (graphemically or phonologically similar to the target word). The results showed that under some circumstances (i.e., when the word was orthographically similar to the target word and highly predictable from context), very early phonological activation could be identified but played only a limited role in the early stage of reading in English, and no such evidence of early phonological activation was found in Chinese. However, homophone errors revealed a benefit effect in late-stage of processing of both Chinese and English.

Wong and Chen (1999) conducted a similar study using a violation paradigm (Daneman, Reingold, & Davidson, 1995; Rayner, Pollatsek, & Binder, 1998) to examine orthographic and phonological processing in reading Chinese text. They also found that orthographic information has a reliable and early disruption in first fixation duration, whereas phonological information affects only the relatively late stage of processing (i.e., total reading time) at the target position and not early stages of processing.

These results (Feng et al., 2001; Wong & Chen, 1999) showed that, in contrast to an early activation of phonological code (as per Pollatsek et al., 2000, and Tsai et al., 2004), later processing of phonology helps readers recover from the disruptive effects of spelling errors. Wong and Chen (1999) even argue that orthography rather than phonology plays an early and dominant role in reading Chinese. The discrepancies between Feng et al., Wong and Chen, and Pollatsek et al. may be due to different task demands in the studies. In Feng et al. and Wong and Chen, participants just read normally, therefore it seems there was no need for early phonological activation, whereas in Pollatsek et al., naming obviously needed more involvement of phonology. On the other hand, Tsai et al. used a reading task and obtained evidence for early activation of phonological codes. Although many studies have been done to show the role of phonology in reading Chinese, the issue is still far from settled.

Homograph. As mentioned earlier, there is another type of ambiguous word, the homograph—which is an orthographical representation that corresponds to more than one meaning, often to two meanings. Homographs can be classified as either balanced or biased, depending on the relative frequency of alternative meanings (Rayner & Duffy, 1986). Balanced ambiguous words have two salient meanings (and possibly, other subordinate meanings), whereas biased ambiguous words have one dominant meaning and one or more subordinate meanings. For example, 分别 (*/fen/bie/*) is a balanced ambiguous word, which means either farewell or difference; whereas 弟妹 (*/di/mei/*) is a biased ambiguous word which means either brothers and sisters or sister-in-law.

From the syntactic role of the word, ambiguous words can be classified as syntactic category ambiguous words and lexical ambiguous words. The meaning of a syntactic category ambiguous word depends on the syntactic role it plays in a sentence. The most typical category is the noun-verb syntactic category. For example, *fire* means *light up* when it is a verb and means *blaze* when it is a noun in a sentence. This type of ambiguous words is common in Chinese. About 40% of one-character words have two meanings that play different syntactic roles in sentences (e.g., 花 */hua/* means *spend* when it is a verb in a sentence, and means *flower* when it is a noun). The two meanings of a lexically ambiguous word, usually a noun, play the same syntactic role in a sentence. For example, 仪表 (*/yi/biao/*) means either *appearance* or *instrument* in Chinese.

Research on lexical ambiguity has been focused on two general questions. One question is: When reading sentences that contain ambiguous words, which meaning(s) are retrieved in the early stage of processing ambiguous words? Another question is: How does context influence lexical access processes?

Much exploration on ambiguity resolution in alphabetic languages has adopted a crossmodal priming paradigm (Swinney, 1979; Tanenhaus, Leiman, & Seidenberg, 1979). In this paradigm, participants first listen to a sentence containing a lexically ambiguous target word. At some point relative to the target word, a probe word is then presented on a screen, and participants must respond to the probe in a lexical decision or naming task. The probe word is either related to one of the two meanings of the ambiguous word or is irrelevant to the ambiguous word.

When the probe is presented immediately after offset of the ambiguous prime, priming to both contextually appropriate and inappropriate meanings occurs relative to an unrelated control word, but when the probe is delayed by 200 ms or more, priming only to the appropriate meaning appears. Such results have generally been interpreted as supporting *exhaustive access* and the modularity of lexical processing, in which context only operates after a later, postlexical stage of processing after all meanings have been initially accessed (e.g., Fodor, 1983; Forster, 1979). However, some results are more consistent with *selective access* and interactivity, in which context directs the early, lexical selection of the appropriate meaning (McClelland, 1987; Morton, 1969).

But there are critiques about results from the *cross-modal priming paradigm*. It has been suggested that the technique is compromised by *reciprocal* or *backward priming* effects in which priming to the contextually inappropriate meaning of an ambiguous word may be more an artifact of secondary priming than a result of autonomous access (Glucksberg, Kreuz, & Rho, 1986).

Another critique is that, due to a cross-modal task, additional attention demands are placed on the participants by the requirements to switch modes and to respond to a visual target. It is possible that only the last one or two words of the auditory context are preserved in articulatory rehearsal when the target is visually presented. In this circumstance, participants can respond to the visual target on the basis of very little contextual information. Thus, multiple accesses may actually reflect context-free priming.

Rayner and Duffy (1986) designed an initial eye-movement study to examine the processing of lexical ambiguity. Since then, several eye movement studies on this issue have been reported (Binder & Morris, 1995; Folk & Morris, 2003; Rayner & Frazier, 1989; Rayner, Pacht, & Duffy, 1994; Sereno, 1995; Sereno, O'Donnell, & Rayner, 2006; Sereno, Pacht, & Rayner, 1992). In these eye-movement studies, three factors of ambiguous words have been manipulated. First, disambiguating information can precede the ambiguous word (biasing context) or follow it (neutral context). Second, the ambiguous word can be either the balanced or biased type. The last factor is the meaning instantiated by the context. Context can lead either to the dominant meaning or to the subordinate meaning (even in the case of balanced ambiguous words, the two meanings are rarely precisely equal in frequency).On the basis of the pattern of eye-movement data, two different models have been proposed: the *reordered access* model (Duffy, Morris, & Rayner, 1988) and the *integration* model (Rayner & Frazier, 1989). These models can be viewed as modified versions of the *interactive* (McClelland, 1987; Morton, 1969) and *modular* (e.g., Fodor, 1983; Forster, 1979) models. In both of the eye-movement ambiguity models, alternative meanings become available in the order of their meaning frequencies. In the *reordered access* model, both context and meaning frequency can influence the speed of lexical access. Thus, context may reorder the sequence of meaning activation for integration into the text. In the *integration* model, meaning frequency affects the speed of lexical access alone; contextual processes interact with only the outputs of the lexical processor.

Most studies of Chinese ambiguous words have been done through a cross-modal priming paradigm, and few studies have been conducted using an eye-movement technique. Through the cross-modal priming paradigm, Shu, Tang, and Zhang (2000) explored lexical access of two-character biased homophones in no prior context. In this study, participants were asked to lexically judge visual probes. They found that reaction times to probes that were either semantically related to the dominant meaning or related to the subordinate meaning of an ambiguous word were shorter than reaction times to controls. Both meanings of ambiguous words were activated as early as between 0 ms and 150 ms after onset of auditory homophones. They concluded that when there is no prior context (i.e., words in isolation), all meanings of an ambiguous word are initially accessed.

Wu and Shu (2001) further investigated the effect of meaning dominance on resolution of one-character biased homographs in no prior context. They manipulated SOA as a between-subject variable (43, 84, 200, and 400 ms, respectively) to examine the early lexical access stage and later integration stage. They found both meanings were activated without context restriction, with the dominant meaning retrieved earlier than the subordinate meaning. Moreover, after the initial activation, the less frequent meaning became less active, while the dominant meaning maintained a high level of activation. The finding reveals that relative frequency modifies the multiple activation process of Chinese ambiguous words.

In real reading, however, ambiguous words are rarely presented alone. Thus, the question of how context information influences lexical access processes or how context interacts with meaning dominance to influence the processing of ambiguous words needs more attention. Is the effect of meaning dominance as large when there is no prior context as when the ambiguous word follows useful context? Or, as *selective access* indicates, can context direct the early activation stage of appropriate meaning?

Zhang, Shu, and Zhang (1999), through the cross-modal priming paradigm, examined the effect of context on biased homographs. They found that responses to probes that were semantically related to the dominant meanings of ambiguous words were facilitated, whereas responses to probes that were related to the subordinate meanings were suppressed at 84 ms SOA (stimulus onset asynchrony). As SOA increased to 400 ms, effect of context became salient, with contextually appropriate meanings facilitated and inappropriate meanings suppressed. Zhou and Chen (2003) used the same paradigm as Zhang et al. (1999) but different SOAs to investigate the effect of context on biased homographs. Probes were presented either 200 ms or 400 ms after onset of auditory targets, and the probe was either related to the dominant meaning or to the subordinate meaning of an ambiguous word. Responses to probes that were related to the contextually appropriate dominant meaning were facilitated compared with the controls at 200 ms SOA. However, when probes were presented at 400 ms SOA, contextually appropriate meanings (both dominant and subordinate) were facilitated. Zhou and Chen (2003) concluded that both disambiguating context and meaning dominance have effects on the early stages of lexical access, but the effect of meaning dominance was larger than that of context. At the later, postlexical stage, the context effect became larger and the contextually inappropriate meaning was suppressed. Similar results were found in a study on resolution of one-character syntactic category ambiguous words (Wu & Shu, 2002).

Zhou, Chen, Yang, and Chen (2004) recently used a unimodal priming paradigm to explore the effect of suppression mechanisms on the processing of homographs. In this paradigm, sentences were visually presented character by character, and the ambiguous word was the last word in each sentence. The probe appeared in different ISI after the whole sentence was presented, and the probe was semantically inconsistent with the context-appropriate meaning. The results showed that responses to probes either related to the dominant meaning or related to the subordinate meaning of ambiguous words were disrupted compared with the controls at 200 ms ISI, but when probes were delayed by 800 ms, only the contextually inappropriate dominant meanings were disrupted.

These results from Chinese, through the cross-modal priming paradigm, are largely similar to those findings from English (Rayner & Duffy, 1987; Duffy et al., 1988; Rayner & Duffy, 1986). Recent eye-movement studies on Chinese reading (Gao, Rayner, Chen, Li, & Zhang, 2006; Chen, 2007) also support the view that reading Chinese ambiguous words is largely similar to reading English ambiguous words. Gao et al. (2006) used a paradigm used by Duffy, Morris, and Rayner (1988) and collected preliminary data on the resolution of ambiguous words through recording eye movements. In this study, both balanced and biased ambiguous words were used, and contexts were either before or after the ambiguous words. The contexts instantiated either the more salient meaning of a balanced ambiguous word or the subordinate meaning of a biased ambiguous word. Results showed that Chinese readers fixated longer on ambiguous words than on controls, and fixated longer on biased ambiguous words than on balanced ambiguous words. When reading sentences containing biased ambiguous words, subjects fixated longer at the disambiguating information than they did for the sentences that contained balanced ambiguous words.

Adopting a paradigm by Sereno et al. (2006), we conducted two experiments to explore how context influences resolution of lexically ambiguous words in Chinese sentence reading (Chen, 2007). The question focuses on whether context influences early lexical access processes, or whether it only influences the post-lexical integration stage. Three dependent variables (i.e. first fixation duration, gaze duration, and total fixation time) were measured in our study to examine the relative time course of resolution of ambiguity. In Experiment 1, eye movements were recorded when subjects read sentences containing either a biased ambiguous word or a word-form control word. Results showed a subordinate-bias effect (SBE) in Chinese sentence reading, in which fixation times on ambiguous words were longer than those on word-form control words when the disambiguating context instantiated the subordinate meaning of an ambiguous word. For ambiguous words and controls, the means of first fixation duration (FFD) were 229 ms and 185 ms respectively; the means of gaze duration (GD) were 272 ms and 220 ms respectively; and the means of total fixation time (TT) were 444 ms and 350 ms respectively. Experiment 2 was dedicated to further examine what factors influence the SBE by adding a set of non-ambiguous words that were matched with the meaning frequency, instead of the word-form frequency, of the ambiguous words. The control words used in Experiment 2 included low-frequency words (LF). In contrast, the control words used in Experiment 1 were high-frequency words (HF). Thus, the 3 stimulus conditions in Experiment 2 were ambiguous words, HF controls, and LF controls. Results showed that, in the target region, fixation times on ambiguous words were longer than those on HF controls, which replicates the results in Experiment 1. Otherwise, a frequency effect was also observed in which the fixation times on HF targets were much shorter than those on LF targets. Most interestingly, the FFD and GD for ambiguous words were shorter than those for LF controls. The means of FFD for ambiguous words and LF controls were 219 ms and 252 ms respectively and the means of GD for ambiguous words and LF controls were 267 ms and 324 ms respectively. In the spillover regions, fixation times were not significantly different between any two conditions, suggesting that participants did not feel any additional processing difficulty among the three conditions. The results are comparable with those from Sereno et al. (2006) and seem to support the integration model.

It is clear that meaning dominance plays an important role in lexical access. At the early, lexical access stage, meanings of an ambiguous word are retrieved in the order of meaning dominance, with dominant meaning activated faster and more actively than subordinate meaning. Contextually appropriate dominant meaning is facilitated, but context support for subordinate meaning is not as large as that for dominant meaning.

Although the pattern of results is comparable with the *integration* model and the *reordered access* model, the Chinese language results do not clearly support either the *integration* model or the *reordered access* model. Context mainly has effects on the output of the lexical processor in the processing of homographs: Contextually appropriate meanings are facilitated and contextually inappropriate meanings are suppressed.

Summary

Obviously, lexical access is necessary and crucial to reading, including Chinese reading. The original goal of this chapter was to bring together all the studies on eye movements in Chinese reading. However, the eye-movement technique, which has proved to be a very effective method to understanding reading processes, is still a relatively new approach used in investigating reading Chinese. Most of the work was done by overseas groups in the last decade. So, in this chapter, for some issues, we have to introduce the findings through other paradigms. However, our expectation is that there will be increasing numbers of studies on Chinese reading done through this technique. In fact, there are many issues that can be further explored through eye-movement recording, but unfortunately many experiments have not been conducted, at least not systematically and thoroughly. For instance, the eye-movement patterns of Chinese people reading Chinese and alphabetic languages, the eye-movement patterns of non-Chinese speakers reading Chinese, and the underlying processes are worthy to study but have not been explored.

The Chinese language is different in many aspects from alphabetic languages. Some psychologists are more interested in comparing the differences between Chinese and English, particularly the role of phonology in processing Chinese. When we examine the uniqueness of Chinese, however, we should keep in mind that Chinese reading actually shares more similarities than differences with reading any other language. This point of view has been demonstrated by many studies (e.g., Rayner et al., 2005; Yan et al., 2006; see also Rayner, Li, & Pollatsek, this volume).

Acknowledgments

This paper was supported in part by grants from the National Natural Science Foundation of China (No.: 30200079), the National Social Science Foundation (No.: 01BYY003) and the 985-2 program of Sun Yat-Sen University (No.: 90015-3272210).

References

Ann, T. K. (1986). *Cracking the Chinese puzzles* (Vol. 5). Hong Kong: Stockflow.

Binder, K. S., & Morris, R. K. (1995). Eye movements and lexical ambiguity resolution: Effects of prior encounter and discourse topic. *Journal of Experimental Psychology: Learning, Memory, and Cognition, 21*, 1186-1196.

Chao, Y. R. (1976). *Aspects of Chinese sociolinguistic: Essays.* New York, NY: Stanford University Press.

Chen, H. C., Flores d'Arcais, G. B., & Cheung, S. L. (1995). Orthographic and phonological activation in recognizing Chinese characters. *Psychological Research, 58,* 144-153.

Chen, H. C., Song, H., Lau, W. Y., Wong, K. F. E., & Tang, S. L. (2003). Developmental characteristics of eye movements in reading Chinese. In C. McBride-Chang, & H. C. Chen (Eds.), *Reading development in Chinese children* (pp. 157-169). Westport, CT: Praeger.

Chen, J. (2007). *Effects of disambiguating context on resolution of biased ambiguous word in Chinese sentence reading.* Unpublished master thesis, Sun Yat-Sen University, Guangzhou, China.

Chen, L., Zhao, X., & Sun, F. (1999). Eye movements in recognition of Chinese character: The character-frequency effect and the channel capacity. (in Chinese). *Acta Biophysica Sinica, 15,* 91-97.

Cheng, C. M. (1992). Lexical access in Chinese: Evidence from automatic activation of phonological information. In H. C. Chen, & O. J. L. Tzeng (Eds.), *Language processing in Chinese* (pp. 67-91). Amsterdam: North-Holland.

Cheng, C. M., & Shih, S. I. (1988). The nature of lexical access in Chinese: Evidence from experiments on visual and phonological prim ing in lexical judgment. In I. M. Liu, H. C. Chen, & M. J. Chen (Eds.), *Cognitive aspects of the Chinese language* (pp.23-37). Hong Kong: Asian Research Service.

Daneman, M., & Reingold, E. (1993). What eye fixations tell us about phonological recoding during reading. *Canadian Journal of Experimental Psychology, 47,* 153-178.

Daneman, M., Reingold, E. M., & Davidson, M. (1995). Time course of phonological activation during reading: Evidence from eye fixations. *Journal of Experimental Psychology, 21,* 884-898.

DeFrancis, J. (1984). *The Chinese language: Fact and fantasy.* Honolulu: University of Hawaii Press.

Duffy, S. A., Morris, R. K., & Rayner, K. (1988). Lexical ambiguity and fixation times in reading. *Journal of Memory and Language, 27,* 429-446.

Ehrlich, S. F., & Rayner, K. (1981). Contextual effects on word recognition and eye movements during reading. *Journal of Verbal Learning and Verbal Behavior, 20,* 641-655.

Fan, K. Y., Gao, J. Y., & Ao, X. P. (1984). Pronunciation principles of the Chinese character and alphabetic writing scripts. (in Chinese). *Chinese Character Reform, 3,* 23-27.

Feng, G., Miller, K., Shu, H., & Zhang, H. (2001). Rowed to recovery: The use of phonological and orthographic information in reading Chinese and English. *Journal of Experimental Psychology: Learning, Memory, and Cognition, 27,* 1079-1100.

Flores d'Arcais, G. B. (1992). Graphemic, phonological, and semantic activation processes during the recognition of Chinese characters. In H. C. Chen, & O. J. L. Tzeng (Eds.), *Language processing in Chinese* (pp. 37-66). Amsterdam: North-Holland.

Fodor, J. A. (1983). *The modularity of mind.* Cambridge, MA: MIT Press.

Folk, J. R., & Morris, R. K. (2003). Effects of syntactic category assignment on lexical ambiguity resolution in reading: An eye movement analysis. *Memory & Cognition, 31,* 87-99.

Forster, K. I. (1979). Levels of processing and the structure of the language processor. In W. E. Cooper, & E. Walker (Eds.), *Sentence Processing: Psycholinguistic studies presented to Merrill Garrett* (pp. 27-85). Hillsdale, NJ: Erlbaum.

Gao, D. G., & Kao, H. S. R. (2002). Psycho-Geometric analysis of commonly used Chinese characters. In H. S. R. Kao, C. K. Leong, & D. G., Gao (Eds.), *Cognitive neuroscience studies of the Chinese language* (pp. 195-206). Hong Kong: Hong Kong University Press.

Gao, D. G., Rayner, K., Chen, J., Li, X. S., & Zhang, R. J. (2006, June). *Resolution of ambiguous words in reading Chinese: An eye movement study.* Paper presented at the Second China International Conference on Eye Movements, Tianjin, China.

Gao, D. G., Zhong, Y., & Zeng, L. (1995). Research on how frequency influenced the recognition speed of common Chinese characters. (in Chinese). *Psychological Science (China), 18,* 225-229.

Glucksberg, S., Kreuz, R. J., & Rho, S. H. (1986). Context can constrain lexical access: Implications for models of language comprehension. *Journal of Experimental Psychology: Learning, Memory, and Cognition, 12,* 323-335.

Goonetilleke, R. S., Lau, W. C., & Shih, H. M. (2002). Visual search strategies and eye movements when searching Chinese character screens. *International Journal of Human-Computer Studies, 57,* 447-468.

Hoosain, R. (1991). *Psycholinguistic implications for linguistic relativity: A case study of Chinese.* Hillsdale, NJ: Erlbaum.

Huang, J. T., Wang, M. Y., & Liou, S. N. (1991). *Component diagnosticity and pattern complexity in object recognition.* Unpublished manuscript.

Hung, D. L., Tzeng, O. J. L., & Tzeng, A. K. Y. (1992). Automatic activation of linguistic information in Chinese character recognition. In R.

Frost, & L. Katz (Eds.), *Orthography, phonology, morphology, and meaning* (pp. 119-130). Amsterdam: North-Holland.

Inhoff, A. W., & Rayner, K. (1986). Parafoveal word processing during eye fixations in reading: Effects of word frequency. *Perception & Psychophysics, 40,* 431-439.

Ju, D., & Jackson, N. E. (1995). Graphic and phonological processing in Chinese character identification. *Journal of Reading Behavior: A Journal of Literacy, 27,* 299-313.

Leck, K. J., Weekes, B. S., & Chen, M. J. (1995). Visual and phonological pathways to the lexicon: Evidence from Chinese readers. *Memory & Cognition, 23,* 468-476.

Liu, W., Inhoff, A. W., Ye, Y., & Wu, C. (2002). Use of parafoveally visible characters during the reading of Chinese sentences. *Journal of Experimental Psychology: Human Perception and Performance, 28,* 1213-1227.

Loo, S. C. (1989, September). *Some characteristics of commonly used Chinese characters and words: A statistical viewpoint.* Paper presented at the Inter-Faculty Seminar on Application of Statistics, National University of Singapore, Singapore.

McClelland, J. L. (1987). The case of interactionism in language processing. In M. Coltheart (Ed.), *Attention and performance XII: The psychology of reading* (pp. 3-36). Hillsdale, NJ: Erlbaum.

McConkie, G. W., Kerr, P. W., Reddix, M. D., & Zola, D. (1988). Eye movement control during reading: The locations of initial eye fixations in words. *Vision Research, 28,* 1107-1118.

Morton, J. (1969). Interaction of information in word recognition. *Psychological Review, 76,* 165-178.

Perfetti, C. A., & Zhang, S. (1991). Phonological processes in reading Chinese characters. *Journal of Experimental Psychology: Learning, Memory, and Cognition, 21,* 633-643.

Perfetti, C. A., Zhang, S., & Berent, I. (1992). Reading in English and Chinese: Evidence for a "universal" phonological principle. In R. Frost, & L. Katz (Eds.), *Orthography, phonology, morphology, and meaning* (pp. 227-248). Amsterdam: North-Holland.

Pollatsek, A., Tan, L. H., & Rayner, K. (2000). The role of phonological codes in integrating information across saccadic eye movements in Chinese character identification. *Journal of Experimental Psychology: Human Perception and Performance, 26,* 607-633.

Rayner, K. (1975). Eye movements and the perceptual span in reading. *Cognitive Psychology, 7,* 65-81.

Rayner, K. (1979). Eye guidance in reading: Fixation locations in words. *Perception, 8*, 21-30.

Rayner, K. (1998). Eye movements in reading and information processing: 20 years of research. *Psychological Bulletin, 124*, 372-422.

Rayner, K. (1999). What have we learned about eye movements during reading? In R. Klein, & P. McMullen (Eds.), *Converging methods for understanding reading and dyslexia* (pp. 23-56). Cambridge, MA: MIT Press.

Rayner, K., & Duffy, S. A. (1986). Lexical complexity and fixation times in reading: Effects of word frequency, verb complexity, and lexical ambiguity. *Memory & Cognition, 14*, 191-201.

Rayner, K., & Duffy, S. A. (1987). Eye movements and lexical ambiguity. In J. K. O' Regan, & A. Levy-Schoen (Eds.), *Eye movements: From physiology to cognition*. Amsterdam: Elsevier.

Rayner, K., & Frazier, L. (1989). Selection mechanisms in reading lexically ambiguous words. *Journal of Experimental Psychology: Learning, Memory, and Cognition, 15*, 779-790.

Rayner, K., Li, X. S., Juhasz, B. J., & Yan, G. (2005). The effect of predictability on the eye movements of Chinese readers. *Psychonomic Bulletin & Review, 12*, 1089-1093.

Rayner, K., Pacht, J. M., & Duffy, S. A. (1994). Effects of prior encounter and global discourse bias on the processing of lexically ambiguous words: Evidence from eye fixations. *Journal of Memory and Language, 33*, 527-544.

Rayner, K., Pollatsek, A., & Binder, K. S. (1998). Phonological codes and eye movements in reading. *Journal of Experimental Psychology: Learning, Memory, and Cognition, 24*, 476-497.

Rayner, K., & Well, A. D. (1996). Effects of contextual constraint on eye movements in reading: A further examination. *Psychonomic Bulletin & Review, 3*, 504-509.

Sereno, S. C. (1995). Resolution of lexical ambiguity: Evidence from an eye movement priming paradigm. *Journal of Experimental Psychology: Learning, Memory, and Cognition, 21*, 582-595.

Sereno, S. C., O'Donnell, P. J., & Rayner, K. (2006). Eye movements and lexical ambiguity resolution: Investigating the subordinate-bias effect. *Journal of Experimental Psychology: Human Perception and Performance, 32*, 335-350.

Sereno, S. C., Pacht, J. M., & Rayner, K. (1992). The effect of meaning frequency on processing lexically ambiguous words: Evidence from eye fixations. *Psychological Science, 3*, 296-300.

Shu, H., & Anderson, R. (1999). Learning to read Chinese: The development of metalinquistic awareness. In J. Wang, A. W. Inhoff, & H. C. Chen (Eds.), *Reading Chinese script: A cognitive analysis* (pp. 1-18). Mahwah, New Jersey: Erlbaum.

Shu, H., Tang, Y., & Zhang, Y. X. (2000). A study on the resolution of lexical ambiguity of two-syllable homophones in Chinese. (in Chinese). *Acta Psychologica Sinica, 32,* 247-252.

Suen, C. Y. (1986). *Computational studies of the most frequent Chinese words and sounds.* Philadelphia, PA: World Scientific.

Swinney, D. A. (1979). Lexical access during sentence comprehension: (Re)consideration of context effects. *Journal of Verbal Learning and Verbal Behavior, 18,* 645-659.

Tan, L. H., Hoosain, R., & Peng, D. L. (1995). Role of presemantic phonological code in Chinese character identification. *Journal of Experimental Psychology: Learning, Memory, and Cognition, 21,* 42-54.

Tan, L. H., Hoosain, R., & Siok, W. W. T. (1996). The activation of phonological codes before access to character meaning in written Chinese. *Journal of Experimental Psychology: Learning, Memory, and Cognition, 22,* 865-883.

Tanenhaus, M. K., Leiman, J. M., & Seidenberg, M. S. (1979). Evidence for multiple stages in the processing of ambiguous words in syntactic contexts. *Journal of Verbal Learning and Verbal Behavior, 18,* 427-440.

Tsai, J., Lee, C., Tzeng, O. J. L., Hung, D. L., & Yen, N. (2004). Use of phonological codes for Chinese characters: Evidence from processing of parafoveal preview when reading sentences. *Brain and Language, 91,* 235-244.

Wan, G., & Hsia, T. T. (1957). *Most commonly used Chinese characters and how to find them in dictionaries without using radicals.* New Haven, CT: Far Eastern Publications, Yale University.

Wang, H., & Chang, B. Y. (1986). *A frequency dictionary in modern Chinese.* (in Chinese). Beijing: Beijing Language Institute Press.

Wong, K. F. E., & Chen, H. (1999). Orthographic and phonological processing in reading Chinese text: Evidence from eye fixations. *Language and Cognitive Processes, 14,* 461-480.

Wu, N. N., & Shu, H. (2001). Meaning activation of Chinese syntactic category ambiguous words in isolation. (in Chinese). *Acta Psychologica Sinica, 33,* 305-311.

Wu, N. N., & Shu, H. (2002). Meaning activation of Chinese syntactic category ambiguous words in sentence context. (in Chinese). *Acta*

Psychologica Sinica, 34, 454-461.

Yan, G., Tian, H., Bai, X., & Rayner, K. (2006). The effect of word and character frequency on the eye movements of Chinese readers. *British Journal of Psychology, 97,* 259-268.

Yang, H. M. (1994). Word perception and eye movements in Chinese reading (Doctoral dissertation, The University of Illinois at Urbana-Champaign, 1994). *Dissertation Abstracts International.*

Yang, H. M., & McConkie, G. W. (1999). Reading Chinese: Some basic eye movement characteristics. In J. Wang, A. Inhoff, & H. C. Chen (Eds.), *Reading Chinese script: A cognitive analysis* (pp. 207-222). Mahwah, NJ: Erlbaum.

Zhang, W., & Feng, L. (1992). A study on the unit of processing in recognition of Chinese characters. (in Chinese). *Acta Psychologica Sinica, 24,* 379-385.

Zhang, X., & Yan, G. (2005). Age of acquisition, familiarity, concreteness and frequency effects of words on college students' eye movements in reading. (in Chinese). *Studies of Psychology and Behavior, 3,* 194-198.

Zhang, Y. X., Shu, H., & Zhang, H. C. (1999). The time course of meaning access of homographs in Chinese sentence reading. (in Chinese). In C. N. Huang, & Z. D. Dong (Eds.), *A corpus on computational linguistics* (pp. 81-88). Beijing, China: Tsinghua University Press.

Zhou, W. B. (1999, November 29). A new Chinese character database by "Guo'an Informatics". *The Guangming Daily.* (in Chinese).

Zhou, X., & Marslen-Wilson, W. (1999a). The nature of sublexical processing in reading Chinese characters. *Journal of Experimental Psychology: Learning, Memory, and Cognition, 25,* 819-837.

Zhou, X., & Marslen-Wilson, W. (1999b). Phonology, orthography, and semantic activation in reading Chinese. *Journal of Memory and Language, 41,* 579-606.

Zhou, X., Marslen-Wilson, W., Taft, M., & Shu, H. (1999). Morphology, orthography, and phonology in reading Chinese compound words. *Language and Cognitive Processes, 14,* 525-566.

Zhou, X., Shu, H., Bi, Y., & Shi, D. (1999). Is there phonological mediated access to lexical semantics in reading Chinese? In J. Wang, A. W. Inhoff, & H. C. Chen (Eds.), *Reading Chinese script: A cognitive analysis* (pp.135-143). Mahwah, NJ: Erlbaum.

Zhou, Z. J., & Chen, Y. M. (2003). The processing of Chinese homographs in different tasks. (in Chinese). *Journal of Huazhong University of Science and Technology (Social Science Edition), 17,* 89-93.

Zhou, Z. J., Chen, Y. M., Yang, L. X., & Chen, H. C. (2004). Inhibition for ambiguous word inappropriate meaning. (in Chinese). *Acta Psychologica Sinca, 36*, 637-643.

Chapter 15

Word segmentation in Chinese reading

Jun Wu, Timothy J. Slattery, Alexander Pollatsek, and Keith Rayner

A very important issue with respect to Chinese reading is how Chinese readers segment sequences of characters into words. In English, and other alphabetic writing systems, this is quite easy because spaces are inserted between words. But in Chinese, there are no spaces between words. Given that spacing cues are not available to Chinese readers, how do they segment a text into words?

Inhoff and Wu (2005) contrasted two models of word-boundary finding strategies: the Multiple Activation Model and the Unidirectional Parsing Model. According to the Multiple Activation Model, (a) all Chinese characters within the effective area of vision (the perceptual span) are activated, (b) all the possible words which are consistent with the adjacent characters are activated in parallel, and, only later, (c) those that can fit in with the context are selected. To give some sense of how this would work, let's consider the following example: There is a four-character string ABCD, and AB and CD are words that fit in with the context—BC is also a word but BC does not fit with the prior context. The Multiple Activation Model predicts that AB, BC, and CD will all be activated at the same time, but BC will then be subsequently inhibited in some fashion.

In contrast, the Unidirectional Parsing Model posits that all Chinese characters within the perceptual span (which extends 1 character to the left and 2-3 to the right of fixation, see Shen, Bai, Yan, & Liversedge, this volume) are activated and whether or not the characters combine into a word is computed in a serial fashion after the activation of the individual characters. Again consider a string of four Chinese characters, ABCD. After the activation of individual characters (which may be serial or parallel), the system decides whether AB is a word. If AB is a word, then a decision about whether ABC is a three-character word will be made. If ABC is a word, ABC will be selected. If not, AB will be selected. After the system makes a decision that a word has been selected (in this case, either ABC or AB), processing of the next word will begin, starting with the first character after the word that has been selected (e.g., starting with D if ABC is selected and starting with C if AB is selected). Thus, according to the Unidirectional Parsing Model, the identification of Chinese words is sequential.

Inhoff and Wu (2005) reported the results of some experiments that led them to favor the Multiple Activation Model. In one of their experiments, they used two types of ABCD strings. In the ambiguous condition, AB, BC, and CD were all two-character words, but only AB and CD were consistent with the context. In the unambiguous condition, only AB and CD were two-character words (i.e., BC was not a word), and both of them were consistent with the context. Inhoff and Wu found that Chinese readers spent more time viewing both the whole region ABCD and the smaller region BC in the ambiguous condition than in the unambiguous condition.

It is clear that the Multiple Activation Model can account for this data pattern, as the activation of BC in the ambiguous condition would need to be suppressed by later context, which should take processing time. It is also true that a non-recursive variant of the Unidirectional Parsing Model cannot account for these data; however, a Recursive Unidirectional Parsing Model is capable of explaining the Inhoff & Wu data (see Wu, Slattery, Pollatsek, & Rayner, 2008). This raises the question of whether it is possible to discriminate between the Multiple Activation Model and the Recursive Unidirectional Parsing Model. Recent work by Wu et al. (2008) suggests that it may be possible to discriminate between these models. In fact, the Wu et al. data appear more consistent with the Unidirectional Parsing Model.

One of our experiments was similar to Inhoff and Wu's (2005) study but used the boundary technique (Rayner, 1975). As with Inhoff and Wu, there was a critical four-character region, which we will again denote as ABCD. However, when a saccade crossed an (invisible) boundary between characters B and C, the C and D characters changed. (Participants are rarely aware of these changes as they occur during an eye movement.) We will designate the four characters that appeared after the display change as ABCD and the ones that appeared before the display change as ABC′D′. In all conditions, the sequence ABCD consisted of two words, AB and CD, which were consistent with the sentence context. Moreover, the ABCD sequence was unambiguous, as neither BC, ABC, nor BCD formed a word. However, the ambiguity of the sequence ABC′D′ that appeared before the display change was manipulated. In the critical ambiguous preview condition, ABC′D′, BC′ was also a two-character word, but in the control condition, BC′ was not a word. Using the boundary technique in this way allowed us to investigate the time course of the disruption in reading caused by this type of ambiguity. Additionally, the frequency of the word AB, either high frequency (HF) or low frequency (LF), was factorially varied with whether BC′ was a word. Note that C′D′ was not a word in either ambiguity condition so that the word frequency of C′D′ was matched (at zero frequency), and the frequencies of all the characters were matched across conditions.

As one might expect, the frequency of the AB word had a marked effect on processing. This effect appeared early (a 26 ms effect on the first fixation duration on the AB region) and had a marked effect on the processing time on the whole ABCD region (e.g., a 139 ms effect on gaze duration). These and other effects of the frequency of the AB word were highly significant. In contrast, however, there was no significant effect of ambiguity (i.e., whether BC′ was a word). The strongest evidence for an interference effect due to ambiguity was a 21 ms effect on total time for the entire ABCD region; however, this was far from significant ($p>0.10$). Moreover, for gaze duration on the ABCD region, there was only a 1 ms interference effect due to ambiguity. There were barely hints of facilitation due to ambiguity on early measures before the display change (3 ms on first fixation duration and 2 ms on gaze duration, $Fs<1$).

These data are thus more compatible with a Unidirectional Parsing Model than with the Multiple Activation Model. That is, the Unidirectional Parsing Model predicts that the ambiguity should have no effect because ABC′ is not a word. Hence, the reader takes AB as a word and then starts looking for the next word starting with character C. In contrast, the Multiple Activation Model predicts that there should be interference because of the conflict between AB being a word and BC′ being a word. Moreover, the Multiple Activation Model would seem to predict an interaction between this effect and the frequency of AB; presumably, if AB is lower frequency, the interference effect from BC′

should be quite a bit larger. However, there was no significant interaction between ambiguity and AB frequency observed in the experiment; moreover, the pattern of this interaction across measures was quite inconsistent.

The null result of ambiguity, of course, raises the question as to why Inhoff and Wu (2005) observed an inhibitory ambiguity effect and we did not. We will discuss this in detail later. However, the difference between the two experiments suggests that the inhibitory effect observed by Inhoff and Wu is a late effect, possibly related to noticing that BC is a word when fixating C or D and then double-checking to be sure that the original parse was correct. Given our display-change methodology, this effect would be eliminated because BC is not a word when readers fixate on either C or D.

The second experiment was not primarily designed as a test between the Multiple Activation and the Unidirectional Parsing Models. Instead, it was intended as a test of one of the key assumptions of the Recursive Unidirectional Parsing Model. The key question is how the system deals with the ambiguity in ABCD when AB and ABC are both words. If both are activated in parallel, one might expect there to be little effect of ABC being a word because three-character words are much less frequent in the language than two-character words. However, the Recursive Unidirectional Parsing Model posits that in these cases of ambiguity, (a) the system has to activate both AB and ABC and (b) ABC would ultimately generally prevail. If not, then a serial parsing mechanism would have very little chance of successfully recognizing three-character words when the first two characters also form a word.

This was not a boundary experiment. Instead, there was a temporary ambiguity in each sentence frame between whether the next word in the sentence was AB or ABC. In fact, the word that fit into the sentence was ABC. (There was a "structural character" (的) to the left of character A in each sentence that unambiguously marked that A was the beginning of a word.) The key manipulation was the frequency of ABC (either 16.3 or 0.7 per million): Unavoidably, the average word frequency of AB was considerably higher (348.4 per million) and was equated in the high- and low-frequency ABC conditions. (Character frequencies and stroke complexities were also equated in the two conditions.)

It is clear that one should obtain a difference in reading time between the two frequency conditions and indeed there were significant differences when examining the entire ABC region: a 13 ms difference on first fixation duration, a 57 ms effect on gaze duration, and a 106 ms effect on total time. The key question, however, was how early in the reading measures the frequency of ABC surfaced. The answer was 'quite early': There was a 12 ms effect of the frequency of ABC on the first fixation duration in region AB and a 29 ms effect on the gaze duration in the AB region. (Both effects were significant.) Thus, the frequency of ABC was having a substantial effect on processing in the AB region. This would be incompatible with a model in which readers first identified the word as AB and then, only later, considered the possibility that ABC was also a word. However, it seems compatible with both the Unidirectional Parsing and Multiple Activation Models.

The third experiment sought to probe the time course of this effect by again using the boundary technique. As in the first experiment above, the critical region of the sentence was ABCD, and in the sentence seen after the boundary change, it was always unambiguous: AB and CD were words, but BC, ABC, and BCD were not. However, in one preview condition, ABC′ formed a word and in the other, it did not. In addition, the frequency of ABC′ was varied. As in the first experiment, the boundary was between the B and C characters. Again, the character frequencies and other character measures, such as stroke complexity were equated across conditions.

As in the second experiment, frequency effects appeared quite early. Thus, in the AB region, there was a 17 ms difference in first fixation duration between the word and nonword ABC′ conditions and a 18 ms difference in gaze duration. (The latter effect was only marginally significant.) However, perhaps the most surprising result of the experiment was that there was no evidence of interference due to the (misleading) ABC′ preview on earlier measures in the CD region. In fact, there was (non-significant) evidence of facilitation: 10 ms for the first fixation duration on CD and 14 ms for the gaze duration on CD. The evidence for inhibitory effects due to misleading ABC′ word preview only occurred later in second pass times on the AB and CD regions; these were due to regressions back to those regions. (Only the latter effect was significant.)

These data are consistent with the Unidirectional Parsing hypothesis we have posited, in which the segmentation process performs a check of the three-character sequence ABC′ before deciding that the final segmentation is AB. The frequency effect of ABC′ indicated that ABC′ was activated; this was true even though the three-character word (a) sometimes didn't fit into the sentence very well and (b) was no longer there when character C is fixated. This reinforces the finding of Experiment

2 that this effect of the ABC word occurs very early in the processing sequence. Although that finding is also compatible with the Multiple Activation Model, the finding is that this ambiguity effect is not inhibitory —or if it is, it surfaces no earlier than on the total time on the CD region. That is, the Multiple Activation Model would posit that both words AB and ABC′ were activated and the system then has to sort out which is the right one. It is hard to see how such a model would not predict an inhibitory effect of ABC′ being a word. The segmentation process we are positing avoids this inhibition because it assumes that readers always check the lexicality of three character sequences and that this checking process takes longest when the sequence is not a word (in this case the system must search the lexicon completely).

As a Chinese word-boundary-finding strategy, the Unidirectional Parsing Model is consistent with the E-Z Reader Model (Pollatsek, Reichle, & Rayner, 2006; Rayner, Ashby, Pollatsek, & Reichle, 2004; Reichle, Pollatsek, Fisher, & Rayner, 1998; Reichle, Rayner, & Pollatsek, 2003) in that both models assume lexical access to be a serial process. (We will clarify below in what way the Unidirectional Parsing Model is a serial model.) There are three main assumptions in the E-Z Reader Model. First, the cognitive system and the oculomotor system are two independent systems, but the cognitive system communicates to the oculomotor system in two ways: (a) it sends commands to execute saccades, and (b) it provides information about what should be the target of a saccade. Second, words are lexically processed one by one, with two stages of word processing: L_1 and L_2. L_1 is the initial processing of a word and L_2 is a higher level of processing of that word. L_1 and L_2 are both influenced by the frequency of the current word and that word's predictability from the prior text. After the completion of the L_1 stage, a signal to make an eye movement to the next word is sent from the cognitive system to the oculomotor system. After the completion of the L_2 stage, attention shifts from the current word to the next word, and the L_1 stage of the next word begins at the same time, but the processing of the next word proceeds more slowly since it is farther from the fixation point and thus its featural information is more difficult to process. Third, there are also two stages associated with the oculomotor system: m and M. The early stage in the oculomotor system (m) is a labile state and can be cancelled by subsequent command to execute another saccade. The second stage (M) is a nonlabile stage and it cannot be cancelled by the subsequent command to execute another saccade. Neither m nor M is influenced by language attributes since the oculomotor system is independent from the cognitive system. Upon completion of the nonlabile stage, a saccade is executed that usually has the center of the next word as its target. However, during this time, the cognitive system will continue its language processing. Figure 15.1 illustrates how the E-Z Reader works. The top panel illustrates how information flows from the cognitive system to the oculomotor system and the second panel shows how the saccade cancellation mechanism works. That is, when word n+1 is easy to process, the duration of $L_1(n+1)$ will be short, and if $L_2(n) + L_1(n+1)$ is less than m(n+1), the eye movement program to word n+2 will cancel the eye movement program to word n+1, and word n+1 will be skipped.

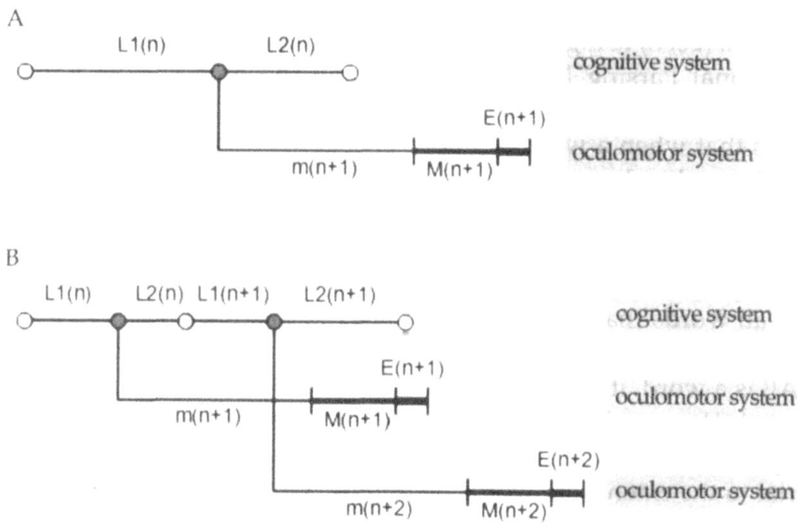

Figure 15.1 (A) This shows how E-Z Reader works by communication from the cognitive system to the oculomotor system. The top line stands for the cognitive system and the bottom line stands for the oculomotor system. The cognitive system has been divided into two stages: L_1 and L_2. After the completion of L_1 stage, the cognitive system will send a saccadic signal to the oculomotor system and continue to process word n in L_2 stage. After the completion of L_2 stage, attention will shift to the next word immediately. (B) This shows how the word will be skipped by the E-Z Reader model. When word n+1 is easy to process, the length of $L_1(n+1)$ will be short. If the length of $L_1(n+1) + L_2(n)$ is shorter than the length of m(n+1), the eye movement program to word n+2 will cancel the eye movement program to word n+1, and word n+1 will be skipped.

Eye movement control models like the E-Z Reader Model provide us with a clear mechanism for how the cognitive processing system could communicate to the eye movement system during reading. However, E-Z Reader, like most eye movement control models, is based on studies of English. This raises the question of whether an eye movement control model which can successfully simulate how Chinese is read will be different from a model for English even though Chinese readers must segment words during reading. Recent work by Rayner, Li, and Pollatsek (2007; see also this volume) suggests that that the answer is "no". That is, they demonstrated that with some relatively minor changes (related to the span of perception and saccade size) the E-Z Reader Model can reproduce Chinese eye movement data quite well. However, this claim must be qualified because Rayner et al. assumed that Chinese readers segmented characters into words without specifying how this happens.

In the remainder of this chapter, we present an overview of how the E-Z Reader Model may be extended to explain the results reported by Wu et al. (2008) using a model of word segmentation based on the Unidirectional Parsing Model. Although all the details have not been worked out, the basic idea of the model is as follows. First, the model posits that when a word has been encoded, attention shifts to the region immediately to the right of the last character of the word that has just been encoded. (In our experiments, this would be the region starting with character A.) Second, the model assumes that the characters in this region of text are processed in parallel (within acuity limits) and that all words that begin with character A that are present in the text are activated to some extent. That is, if A is a word, it will be activated, if AB is a word, it will be activated, and if ABC is a word, it will be activated. The speed of activation of these words is influenced both by the frequency of the word and by visual acuity factors. Thus, the model is serial to the extent that words beginning with B or C are not activated in the initial part of the word encoding process. The model then assumes that, if more than one word is activated within a certain time frame, the longest word will be selected as the word encoded. This will allow the model to encode three character words like ABC even when the first two characters AB also form a word. The model, however, also needs some "double checking" mechanisms to deal with ambiguities. For example, if both ABC and AB are words, an additional check of word CD will be performed such that if (a) CD is not a word, the meaning of ABC will be integrated into the sentence and the segmentation process will start over with characters DE, but if (b) CD is a word, context will be used to select the most appropriate meaning before moving on to segment the remaining text.

The basic outline for how these word encoding processes are connected to the eye movement system is as follows. First, when the excitation in the lexicon (related to the frequency of the candidate words being extracted) exceeds a threshold (i.e., the end of the L_1 stage), a signal is sent to the eye movement system to execute a saccade to the right. We are not sure exactly what the target of this saccade would be (e.g., whether it could be influenced by the length of words that are activated but not yet fully encoded), but assume that it would be something like 2-3 characters forward. However, attention would not move forward to the next word (i.e., the end of the L_2 stage) until a word is actually decided upon. Here, presumably, attention would shift to the region including the first character after the word that was just encoded and the following three characters.

Obviously, this model is incomplete, in that it doesn't account in detail for how all Chinese words are eventually encoded in reading. However, we think it represents a sensible initial step and can give a good account of the experiments above. First consider the second and third experiments described above. A key finding in both was that the frequency of the ABC word affected early measures such as the first fixation duration on the AB region. This is compatible with our model because the decision to move the eyes forward is driven by the sum of the activation of all words beginning with A. Thus, even though ABC is lower frequency than AB, it will contribute to the general excitation in the lexicon, and thus speed the decision to move forward. It will clearly take detailed modeling to determine whether this is consistent with a model in which the speed of activation is merely determined by the frequency of a word or something more complex, such as the frequency of a word relative to the frequencies of all words of the same length (and perhaps character frequency).

The second finding of some interest in the third experiment was that there was little, if any, indication that having a (misleading) three-letter word preview ABC′ produced any later interference. Although it will take detailed modeling to determine whether this result is consistent with our model, on the surface, it seems reasonable. That is, it is merely excitation from ABC′ that is causing the saccade off of the AB region—not the actual identification of it. (This is also consistent with the fact that the effect still occurred even though ABC′ often did not fit well into sentence context.) As a result, the L_2 stage is still likely ongoing after the eyes move across the boundary and C′ is replaced by C. Thus, further processing of ABC′ will cease. Moreover, as prior experiments in English and Spanish (Altarriba, Kambe, Pollatsek, & Rayner, 2001; Rayner, Balota, & Pollatsek, 1986) indicate that little, if any, of the meaning of parafoveal previews affect processing once a word is fixated, the lexicality of ABC′ is unlikely to have any further effect on processing.

The third finding was the one in our first experiment, in which we found no ambiguity effect from a preview. That is, if AB and C′D′ were words, it made no difference whether BC′ was a word. This result differed from that of Inhoff and Wu's (2005) study, which was not a display-change experiment. In their study, processing of the words AB and CD was slower when BC also a word. As we argued above, this difference indicates that the ambiguity effect is likely to occur in later, checking, stages of processing that would be part of the L_2 stage. According to our model, only words beginning with A would be activated in early stages of processing related to L_1, and hence to the eye movement off of the AB region. However, the lexicality of BC may be involved in a "double-checking" routine, and thus have slowed processing in the Inhoff and Wu study. However, in our first experiment, when the boundary was crossed, BC was no longer a word; hence, there was no longer any ambiguity and no double-checking routine needed to be employed.

In summary, in this chapter we have described some preliminary results from experiments we have completed dealing with word segmentation in Chinese (Wu et al., 2008). In addition, we have sketched out a preliminary model of word segmentation based on these results and also suggested how the model could fit within the context of the E-Z Reader Model. It should be clear at this point that our discussion of word segmentation is quite preliminary and that a concerted effort will be needed to spell out the details of the model and do the necessary computational modeling. Nevertheless, we think what we have presented represents a reasonable start.

Acknowledgments

Preparation of this chapter was supported by Grant HD26765 from the National Institute of Health. The work was completed when the first author was a Visiting Student at the University of Massachusetts.

References

Altarriba, J., Kambe, G., Pollatsek, A., & Rayner, K. (2001). Semantic codes are not used in integrating information across eye fixations in reading: Evidence from fluent Spanish-English bilinguals. *Perception & Psychophysics, 63*, 875-890.

Inhoff, A. W., & Wu, C. (2005). Eye movements and the identification of spatially ambiguous words during Chinese sentence reading. *Memory & Cognition, 33*, 1345-1356.

Pollatsek, A., Reichle, E. D., & Rayner, K. (2006). Tests of the E-Z Reader model: Exploring the interface between cognition and eye-movement control. *Cognitive Psychology, 52*, 1-56.

Rayner, K. (1975). The perceptual span and peripheral cues in reading. *Cognitive Psychology, 7*, 65-81.

Rayner, K., Ashby, J., Pollatsek, A., & Reichle, E. D. (2004). The effects of frequency and predictability on eye fixations in reading: Implications for the E-Z Reader model. *Journal of Experimental Psychology: Human Perception and Performance, 30*, 720-732.

Rayner, K., Balota, D. A., & Pollatsek, A. (1986). Against parafoveal semantic preprocessing during eye fixations in reading. *Canadian Journal of Psychology, 40*, 473-483.

Rayner, K., Li, X., & Pollatsek, A. (2007). Extending the E-Z Reader model of eye movement control to Chinese readers. *Cognitive Science, 31*, 1021-1034.

Reichle, E. D., Pollatsek, A., Fisher, D. L., & Rayner, K. (1998). Toward a model of eye movement control in reading. *Psychological Review, 105*, 125-157.

Reichle, E. D., Rayner, K., & Pollatsek, A. (2003). The E-Z Reader model of eye-movement control in reading: Comparisons to other models. *Behavioral and Brain Sciences, 26*, 445-476.

Wu, J., Slattery, T. J., Pollatsek, A., & Rayner, K. (2008). *Eye movement control and Chinese word segmentation*. Submitted for publication.

Chapter 16

Immediacy of processing intra-sentential and inter-sentential information in reading Chinese

Suiping Wang, Jinmian Yang, and Hsuan-Chih Chen

As a language used by nearly a quarter of the world's population, Chinese is a logographic writing system drastically different from alphabetic languages in how meaning and speech are represented. Such language-specific properties can serve as crucial test cases for theories or models of psycholinguistics, thus helping to explore both universal and language-specific processes associated with the processing of different languages.

Although nowadays people's understanding of the cognitive processes and mechanisms of Chinese comprehension is much better than before, it is far from comprehensive and systematic. Most of the recent studies on Chinese focus mainly on how separately presented Chinese characters or words are processed, while only a few studies have focused on how Chinese readers integrate those characters or words to form a coherent representation during text reading. However, the dramatic differences between Chinese and alphabetic languages (such as English) not only exist at the lexical level, the level of the character or word, but they also contribute to the various contrasts of morphological and syntactic rules, which may in turn result in different high-level comprehension processes during reading.

The purpose of this chapter is to explore how readers integrate the incoming word with both local and global context during the reading of Chinese sentences and texts. This chapter consists of four parts. The first part reviews the evidence for this issue from the studies of alphabetic languages. The second part describes the peculiar properties of Chinese that are related to the processing we focus on. The third part reports some recent studies on the time course of information integration during sentence and text reading in Chinese. The last part discusses universal and language-specific mechanisms associated with the processing of different writing systems.

The time course of reading comprehension — Evidence from alphabetic languages

A fundamental task of reading comprehension is to build up a coherent mental representation, in which readers integrate the incoming information with both the local context (i.e., intra-sentential information that is still active in working memory) and the distant information, or global context (i.e., backgrounded information that is no longer in working memory). This task can be accomplished naturally and quickly by a skilled reader, yet the construction of a coherent mental representation, in fact, involves a lot of processes. Take the processing of a word for example; to build up a coherent representation, word recognition must be initiated first, as well as the identification of the context-dependent syntactic and semantic properties of this word. Meanwhile, the related background information is activated, so that the reader can integrate the word with it and further build up a global-coherent representation of the meaning. Therefore, answers to when the above processes are initiated, how long they last, and when they come to an end are essential to the construction of language comprehension models.

So far, most evidence appears to be in line with the immediate processing position, which postulates that readers can start all levels of processes immediately (Just & Carpenter, 1980). For example, there is not too much delay concerning the recognition of words (e.g., Marslen-Wilson, 1987; Rayner & Duffy, 1986) even if the current word is ambiguous (e.g. Rayner & Duffy, 1986; Duffy, Morris, & Rayner, 1988; Rayner & Frazier, 1989; Sereno, O'Donnell, & Rayner, 2006). Moreover, based on the results from behavior and event-related potential studies, readers could immediately detect whether a word was semantically congruent with the preceding context or not (e.g., Braze, Shankweiler, Ni, & Palumbo, 2002; Boland, Tanenhaus, Garnsey, & Carlson, 1995; Federmeier & Kutas, 1999; Kutas & Hillyard,1980; Ni, Fodor, Crain & Shankweiler, 1998; Murray & Rowan, 1998; Rayner, Warren, Juhasz, & Liversedge, 2004; Rosler, Putz, Friederici,& Hahne, 1993; van Berkum, Hagoort, & Brown, 1999). Also, garden-path effects, which strongly support the notion that syntactic analysis begins very rapidly, were observed in many studies (e.g., Bader & Lasser, 1994; Crocker, 1994; Frazier, 1987; Frazier & Rayner, 1982; Sturt & Crocker, 1996). There is also some evidence showing that readers immediately try to interpret the incoming information during reading. (e.g., Altmann, Garnham, & Dennis, 1992; Britt, Perfetti, Garrod, & Rayner, 1992; Clifton, 1993; Cook & Myers, 2004; Ehrlich & Rayner, 1983; Garrod, Freudenthal, & Boyle, 1994; Kambe, Rayner, & Duffy, 2001; O'Brien, Shank, Myers, & Rayner, 1988; Rayner, Cook, Juhasz, & Frazier, 2006; Traxler, Foss, Seely, Kaup, & Morris, 2000; Traxler & Pickering, 1996; Trueswell, Tanenhaus, & Garnsey, 1994). It seems that immediacy is one of the important mechanisms of language processing.

However, it is worth noting that although most recent studies support the idea that even higher-level language processing can be initiated without delay, they were mostly conducted in alphabetic languages. Since languages differ in many important aspects, it is not self-evident that the same processes can be applied to comprehend information across different languages. Indeed, there is behavioral and neural evidence showing that language-specific processes are involved in processing alphabetic and non-alphabetic languages (e.g., Chen & Juola, 1982; Cheung, Chen, Lai, Wong, & Hills, 2001; Cutler & Otake, 1994; Feng, Miller, Shu, & Zhang, 2001; Gandour et al., 2002; Schirmer, Tang, Penney, Gunter, & Chen, 2005). Hence, it is not clear to what extent the immediate integration position can account for reading comprehension in a distinctively different orthography, namely logographic Chinese. In this chapter, we will report some recent studies which were designed to explore this question and to decide whether or not the immediate integration position is suitable only for reading alphabetic scripts.

In the following section, we first discuss some peculiar properties of Chinese that might account for the difference between Chinese and English reading comprehension. Particularly, we focus our attention on the properties of Chinese words, because words are generally considered the basic unit of semantic and syntactic analysis during alphabetic language processing (e.g. Rayner & Pollatsek, 1989).

Some properties of Chinese words

Unlike readers of alphabetic languages, Chinese readers have only vague ideas about what a word is (Chao, 1968; Chen, 1996, 1999). As a matter of fact, processes from identifying a word in the text to understanding its semantic and syntactic properties are all highly context dependent, which can be further elaborated in three ways.

First, word boundaries are extremely vague in written Chinese. Unlike English (and other alphabetic writing systems), Chinese is a logographic script, the written text of which is formed by strings of equally spaced box-like characters with identical spaces in between. Most Chinese words consist of one or two characters (though some are three or four characters or longer), and there are no explicit physical markers between words (the width of the space between words is identical to that between characters within a word); so the notion of words in Chinese is very vague and Chinese readers can disagree somewhat concerning where word boundaries are located. Characters, therefore, are the basic perceptual units in the reading of Chinese. To the contrary, texts written in alphabetic scripts are typically constructed by horizontal strings of words with spacing in between. Thus, words are the basic perceptual units of alphabetic languages and the identification of individual words in reading these languages is simpler and more straightforward than that in reading Chinese.

Second, the lack of explicit markers of word boundaries sometimes results in the ambiguous meaning of Chinese words. This is because a character can be a single-character word or a morpheme of a multiple-character word, and the meaning of this character can be totally different in these two situations. To indicate the influence of the lack of word length cues on the semantic processing of Chinese words, the typical sentence "花生长在屋后的田里" is frequently quoted (Hsu & Huang, 2000). In this sentence, the first character 花, can either form a word on its own (flower) or combine with the next character, 生, (birth), to form a different word, 花生 (peanut). The third character, 长, could also form a word on its own (growing) or combine with the second character 生, that is, 生长, to represent the same meaning. Thus, this sentence could be understood in two different ways: (1) Flowers (花) grow (生长) in the field behind the house; or (2) Peanuts (花生) grow (长) in the field behind the house. This does not mean that Chinese texts are full of ambiguity. While writing, people will always try to avoid ambiguous expressions. However, the high possibility that a character may be a word itself or a morpheme of a totally different word may still bear some impact on some on-line processes, for readers may have to spend more resources referring to the context now and then to acquire the precise meaning.

Third, the grammatical properties of Chinese words are also very vague and the identification of them is highly context-dependent. This is because words in Chinese do not generally have explicit markers or inflectional indicators, such as lexical categories, number, gender, tense, and other aspects, to specify different types of syntactic information, as is the case in English and other alphabetic languages; neither does Chinese have intra-sentence concordance rules such as subject-verb agreement. Indeed, a particular Chinese word can be used as a verb or as a noun in a sentence without any morphological change. For example, the same Chinese word "调查" is used as a noun in the sentence "调查是一个重要的环节" and as a verb in the sentence "他们调查苹果价格", whereas "investigation" and "investigated" need to be used in the corresponding English sentences (i.e., "Investigation is an important step" and "They investigated the price of apples"). Since there are no explicit markers indicating the syntactic role of a word, syntactic analysis must be based on the context. For example, in the former sentence, "调查" was located in the beginning and followed by a verb "是 (is)", the predicate of the sentence. Thus, "调查" can only be identified as a noun, serving as a subject of the sentence. Whereas in the second example, "调查" is sandwiched between a pronoun (他们, they) and a noun (苹果, apple), with no other words being a predicate in the sentence. Therefore, it can be judged as a verb and the predicate of the sentence. The manner of identifying the grammatical properties of words in Chinese contrasts dramatically with that applied in the alphabetic languages. Compared with written Chinese, the writing systems of alphabetic languages, like English, have explicit markers (e.g., inflectional or derivational morphology) to mark lexical categories and indicate various syntactic functions of the words. Hence, readers of English can easily determine whether a sentence is grammatically right or not without referring to the semantics of the sentence. In other words, syntax and semantics are relatively independent in English.

How do the above mentioned differences between Chinese and alphabetic languages affect the time course of high-level processes during reading in Chinese? As we mentioned in the first section, most studies of alphabetic languages support the idea that comprehension processing is generally quite immediate, which is reflected by readers' immediate activation and application of the semantic and syntactic information in constructing both local and global coherent representations (some studies indicated that the processing of grammatical information comes before that of the semantic information (see e.g. Braze et al, 2002; McElree & Griffith, 1995), but generally these results are in line with the view that both kinds of processing are initiated quite immediately). In Chinese comprehension, however, given that the meaning of a single Chinese character is context-dependent, semantic and syntactic attributes are usually carried out by the sentential context as a whole. Thus, more resources are presumably needed to resolve the ambiguities arising from local context, and fewer resources would therefore be available for more global processes, such as integrating the incoming information with the backgrounded information. In addition, to build intra-sentential coherence, a delayed rather than immediate comprehension strategy would seem more suitable for reading Chinese because it can maximize the amount of information available and minimize the ambiguities encountered. In fact, some researchers (e.g., Aaronson & Ferres, 1986) have actually argued that higher-level mental processes in Chinese comprehension would not be expected to function in an immediate manner. The Chinese language thus provides a vigorous test for the immediate integration position. If we can find evidence for the idea that higher-level text processing like intra-sentential and inter-sentential integration can still be conducted on-line in reading Chinese, then the immediacy position may be considered to be a universal principle in reading comprehension.

Thus, the following sections are devoted to two sets of studies that explore to what extent the processing of different levels, i.e., intra-sentential and inter-sentential integration, will occur immediately when readers fixate on separate words while reading Chinese.

Processing of intra-sentential and inter-sentential information in reading Chinese

Before moving to the studies, we would like to introduce the research paradigm, the violation paradigm, which was used in the following studies. The basic manipulation is to change a critical word (or character) in the reading material so as to introduce an anomaly into the text. By observing and comparing the normal patterns and the patterns of disruptions caused by different types of anomalies on character/word viewing times, researchers can infer how and when the information that caused the anomaly can be processed by readers (Chen, 1992, 1999; Danks, Bohn, & Fears, 1983; Rayner et al., 2004).

Different types of anomalies can be presented according to the issue addressed in an experiment. For example, to investigate how the coherence of intra-sentence information, such as semantic or syntactic coherence, influences the processing of current information, we replaced the critical word to make changes in semantic category (i.e., a semantic violation), or substituted a semantically anomalous and syntactically inappropriate word for the original word (i.e., a syntactic + semantic violation), so as to see whether different types of violations have different effects on word reading. The same procedure was used to study inter-sentential integration. The only difference is that the target word was made congruent or incongruent at the discourse level by changing the inter-sentential preceding information in the passage. In other words, the critical word was congruent with the currently read context but incongruent with the background information that had been processed and driven out of working memory. Still, the time course of global integration processing can be inferred by the reading time on critical words.

So far, the violation paradigm has been widely used to study different levels of comprehension processes in reading, including semantic and/or syntactic processing of sentence reading (e.g. Frisson & Frazier, 2005; Ni et al., 1998; Braze et al., 2002; Deutsch & Bentin, 2001; Murray & Rowan, 1998; Pearlmutter, Garnsey, & Bock, 1999; Rayner et.al., 2004), as well as higher level processing, such as maintaining global coherence in discourse comprehension (e.g., Albrecht & O'Brien, 1993; McKoon & Ratcliff, 1992; Myers, O'Brien, Albrecht, & Mason, 1994; O'Brien & Albrecht, 1992; O'Brien, Rizzella, Albrecht, & Halleran, 1998; Traxler et al., 2000). Moreover, it has proven to be an effective research paradigm in studies on reading Chinese (see e.g., Chen, 1992, 1999; Schirmer et al., 2005; Wang & Mo, 2001). Therefore, our studies address the time course of intra-sentential and inter-sentential processing during Chinese reading.

Intra-sentential processing

As mentioned, the syntactic properties of the currently read word must be identified so as to build an intra-sentential coherence. However, due to the generally opaque semantic and syntactic features of Chinese words, can readers immediately activate and use the linguistic information of individual words, or do they have to wait until reaching the end of a phrase or sentence boundary to start relevant semantic and syntactic analyses? Using the violation paradigm, Chen (1999) first tried to solve this problem. In his study, a critical word was modified to form three types of violations (i.e., lexical, semantic, and syntactic + semantic). With a word-by-word self-paced reading procedure, he recorded and analyzed the patterns of disruptions caused by different types of violations on character viewing times. The results showed that when reading the stimuli with nouns as critical words, various types of violations triggered distinctively different patterns of disruptions: Lexical disruption appeared at exactly the target word, while both semantic and syntactic + semantic violations showed patterns of delayed disruption at the word +1 position. Additionally, no difference in disruption effects were found between the semantic and syntactic + semantic violations.

However, the slightly delayed effect found in Chen's study (1999) may have resulted from the self-paced reading procedure. Since readers can't press the response button as fast as they can comprehend, they may employ a strategy to press the key rapidly and then wait until the end of a clause or a unit to process the material. Hence, the data collected through the self-paced reading paradigm should be interpreted with caution (Danks, 1986; Magliano, Graesser, Eymard, Haberlandt, & Gholson, 1993).

As a result, recently we (Yang, Wang, & Chen, 2005) used a more ecological and sensitive method (i.e., the eye tracking procedure) to conduct a study similar to Chen's (1999). In this experiment, all the target stimuli were single-character words[1] and they were modified to form three kinds of conditions: consistent (CON), semantic violation (SEM), and syntactic and semantic violation (SYN + SEM). More importantly, since a syntactic violation is always accompanied by a semantic violation in written Chinese, we strictly matched the degree of semantic plausibility of SEM and SYN + SEM conditions. In this way, any possible difference in eye-movement patterns between the two violated con-

1 While words are considered the basic unit of comprehension processes, characters are the basic unit in perception in Chinese written text. Thus the experiment reported here used single-character words as the target stimulus to make sure semantic and syntactic properties were manipulated with in a basic perception unit.

ditions can be attributed to the syntactic processing.

A sentence structure used in this experiment is presented in Table 16.1. The target word in sentence 1a was "饼 (cake)", which was appropriate for the sentence context; and the target word in sentence 1b was "绳 (rope)", a different semantic category from "饼 (cake)" and inappropriate for the sentence. Both the target words in the consistent (CON) and semantic violation (SEM) conditions were nouns. Furthermore, a semantically anomalous and syntactically inappropriate word was developed as the target in the syntactic plus semantic violation (SYN + SEM) condition, like "跌 (fall down)" in sentence 1c. In this condition, all of the target words were verbs in the sentences. Moreover, all target words were located in the middle of the sentences, at least three characters away from the beginning and the end.

Table 16.1 Examples of a stimulus sentence used in the experiment

Consistent (CON):
1a. 刘卓今天早餐吃了一个饼*和一碗粥。 Liu Zhuo had a cake* and a bowl of porridge for breakfast this morning.
Semantic violation (SEM)
1b. 刘卓今天早餐吃了一个绳*和一碗粥。 Liu Zhuo had a rope* and a bowl of porridge for breakfast this morning.
Syntactic + semantic violation (SYN + SEM)
1c. 刘卓今天早餐吃了一个跌*和一碗粥。 Liu Zhuo had a fall down* and a bowl of porridge for breakfast this morning.

* The critical word

In order to ensure that any experimental effect was triggered by the relation between the target word and the contextual information, lexical properties of the three kinds of target words were controlled. In the sentences, character frequency, number of strokes and structure (the way to combine radicals) of the target words were matched. More importantly, to make sure the SEM and SYN + SEM conditions were equally plausible, 52 students who had not participated in the main experiment were asked to rate the plausibility of the sentences. The results indicated that the semantic plausibility of the CON sentences was significantly higher than that of SEM and SYN + SEM sentences; while the latter two did not differ from each other.

Twenty-eight skilled Chinese readers participated in the main experiment, with each subject receiving 48 experimental sentences for comprehension. Each sentence was presented on a Dell 17-inch SVGA monitor, with the target word in the middle of the line. Participants' eye movements were recorded via an SR Eyelink II eye-tracking system that calculated the x- and y-coordinates of the readers' point of fixation every 2 ms.

Given the high skipping rate of single characters, the results presented here are all based on a regional analysis[2]. From the third character before the critical character/word (N) to the fourth after it (i.e., N-3 to N+4), every two characters were combined. In other words, character N-3 was combined with N-2, N-1 with N, N+1 with N+2, N+3 with N+4 as different regions, which were linked to target regions T-1, T, T+1, and T+2. In addition, the last two characters and the period were combined as the last region (LR)[3]. This analysis reduced the skipping rate to about 15 percent (no difference among the three conditions), although the skipping rate for the last region remained as high as 50 percent.

The average first-pass reading time of the three conditions is plotted in Figure 16.1. The results showed that consistency effect was significant in regions T and T+1, because readers fixated longer in the SEM and SYN + SEM conditions than in the CON, but a significant difference between the SEM and SYN + SEM conditions was only found in T+1 but not T. No other significant differences were found.

Furthermore, a reliable consistency effect was revealed by the second-pass reading time (see Figure 16.2) in all the reported regions except the LR; reading time in the two incongruent conditions was significantly longer than in the congruent one. Moreover, the SYN + SEM violation triggered significantly longer fixation time on region T than the SEM violation, suggesting that readers encountered more difficulty in SYN + SEM violation condition. This effect did not appear in other regions.

2 A similar analysis was also conducted on character basis and the results were basically the same.

3 There were some exceptions in combining regions for the 48 experimental sentences. For 3 of the sentences, we did not make region T+2 and LR as those sentences only have 3 characters following the target word; and for 8 of the sentences having 4 to 6 characters after the target word, we did not have region T+2 either but we still had the LR as other sentences.

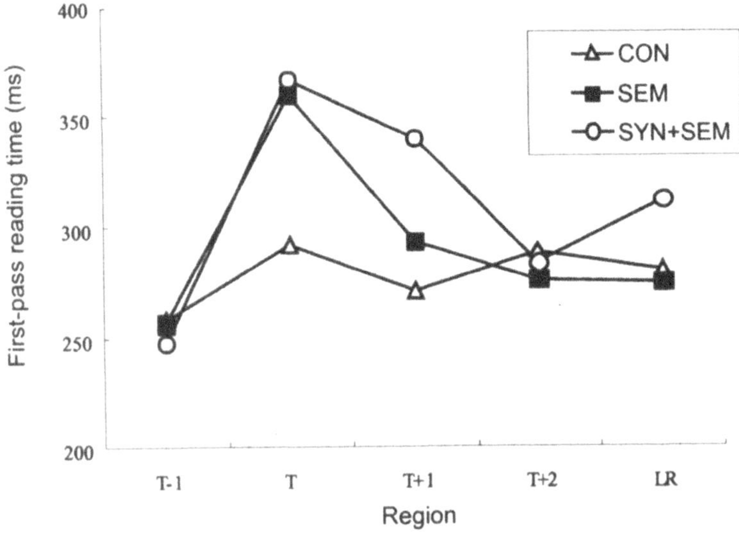

Figure 16.1 Mean first-pass reading times of the congruent, semantic (SEM) and syntactic+semantic (SYN+SEM) violation conditions. T refers to the target region. LR refers to the last two characters and the period in the sentence.

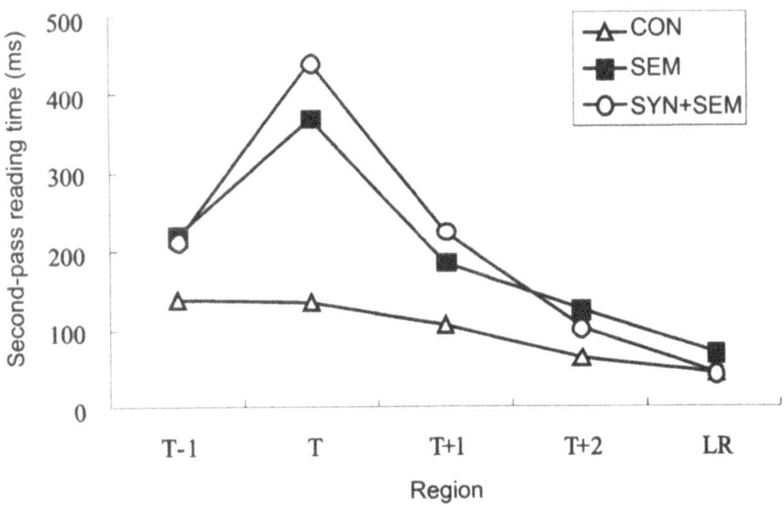

Figure 16.2 Mean second-pass reading times of the congruent, semantic (SEM) and syntactic+semantic (SYN+SEM) violation conditions. T refers to the target region. LR refers to the last two characters and the period in the sentence.

We also calculated the go-past reading time, which includes the amount of time that the readers looked at the target region as well as any time they spent in rereading earlier parts of the sentence. It is supposed to reflect both lexical processing and integration processes, because the reader was likely to realize that there were some problems with the target region and thus made a regression back to some earlier parts of the sentence (Rayner et al., 2004). The results suggested that readers had longer go-past reading time in the two violation conditions than in the CON condition in T and T+1 regions. Again, longer fixation time in the SYN + SEM condition than in the SEM condition was only found in region T+1.

In short, these results revealed that when local coherence was interrupted, no matter by a semantic or syntactic violation, readers showed processing difficulties right at the target region, as reflected by the longer fixation times in the SEM and SYN + SEM conditions than in the CON condition, although they could not discriminate the difference between the two incongruent conditions until they processed the post-target region and reprocessed the target region.

Before further discussing the implications of these results on understanding the properties of syntactic and semantic processing in Chinese reading, we would like to introduce another experiment, the aim of which was to further explore whether readers could still detect the incongruence immediately if the interruption occurred at a global (inter-sentential) coherence level.

Inter-sentential integration processing

The variation of the violation paradigm which we used in this study was originally developed by Albrecht and O'Brien (1993). The main manipulation of this paradigm is the degree of consistency between the backgrounded information and the target sentence that was coherent with the local context. For example, in one of the reading materials, the protagonist Mary was described either as a vegetarian (i.e., in the incongruent version) or as a health nut (i.e., in the neutral version). Such description was followed by several sentences that changed the topic of the discourse. Following that, participants read a sentence in which the protagonist engaged in a target action that was locally coherent but was either consistent or inconsistent with the target characteristic (e.g., Mary ordered a hamburger). Results from most studies (see e.g., Albrecht & O'Brien, 1993; McKoon & Ratcliff, 1992; Myers et al., 1994; O'Brien & Albrecht, 1992; O'Brien et al., 1998) showed that it took significantly longer to read the target sentence in the incongruent condition than in the congruent condition. Similar results were also found in some studies using Chinese passages as reading materials (see, e.g. Wang & Mo, 2001; Wang, Chen, Mo & Zou, 2004), indicating that the backgrounded traces were reactivated immediately to influence the understanding of the target sentence even though the sentence was coherent with the local context.

However, it should be noted that the evidence is still inadequate regarding whether global integration is initiated the very moment readers notice the critical word or after their analysis of the whole target sentence, for the critical information manipulated in the studies mentioned above was a whole sentence rather than a word. Based on this argument, we (Wang, Chen, Yang, & Mo, 2008) made an improvement on the aforementioned paradigm such that the violation effect was exactly triggered by one single character/word, which was always located in the middle of the target sentence. Thus, we could discriminate whether the integration with background information starts right on the critical character or not.

A stimulus passage used in our experiment (and the corresponding manipulations) is presented in Table 16.2. Each passage began with a brief introduction to the protagonist of the story, followed by an elaboration that was either congruent or incongruent with the information presented in the target sentence appearing in a later section. Next was a filler section (approximately six to seven sentences) which, being neutral with the information presented in the target sentence, mainly served to background the elaboration. Following the filler section was a target sentence (11 to 15 characters in length), which was identical in different versions. In the middle of every target sentence, there was a single-character target word that was either congruent or incongruent with the elaboration part of the passage. A concluding section of one or two sentences ended the story.

To make sure the consistency effect was triggered by the critical word, we conducted two rating experiments. First, 24 additional students were asked to rate the rationality of target sentences. The results showed that the target sentences were more rational in the congruent condition than in the incongruent one. Then, the critical words in incongruent passages were replaced by a word that was congruent with the information in the elaboration section. The idea was that if the critical words indeed triggered the incongruence, the resulting incongruence effect would disappear after changing the incongruent word to a congruent one. For example, in one passage, the elaboration was about a warm and sultry

Table 16.2 An example of a stimulus passage

Section 1: Introduction

上星期林伟酒后驾车，不幸被一辆迎面而来的货车撞昏。(Lin Wei's car crashed into a truck when he drove after drinking alcohol last week. Unfortunately, he was knocked into a coma.)

Section 2: Elaboration

2a. Neutral description

当他恢复知觉时，医生说他的大脑受到震荡，虽然现在看来他的行动跟受伤前一样自如，但需要住院观察一段时间。(When he became conscious, the doctor told him that he had suffered a cerebral concussion and that although he looked as normal as before, he should stay in the hospital for observation for several days.)

2b. Inconsistent description

当他恢复知觉时，医生同情地告诉他，他的双腿因为受到严重压迫已经做了截肢手术，后半生只能在轮椅上度过了。(When he became conscious, the doctor told him sympathetically that his legs had been amputated due to severe pressure. He had to spend the rest of his life in a wheelchair.)

Section 3: Filler

在住院这段时间，林伟常常想起刚工作时那段艰苦的日子。那时候身边总有很多朋友。如今朋友们和自己疏远了，这些天也没人来看他。他感到很失落。妻子知道他的心事，每天尽量陪着他。这天，他妻子又是一早就来到医院。(During the period of hospitalization, Li Wei often thought of the hard days when he first started working. At that time, he had many friends around him. But now his friends all alienated him and nobody came to see him. He felt depressed. His wife understood him and accompanied him every day. As usual, that day his wife was the first to arrive at the hospital.)

Section 4: Target sentence

①她 看见 李 伟/ ②正 站* 在/ ③窗 边 往 外 眺望。
①She saw Li Wei / ②standing / ③beside the window looking outside.

Section 5: Closing

怎么样才能让林伟的情绪好转起来呢，妻子觉得一定要想个办法才行。(His wife thought that she must find a way to help Li Wei to get emotionally better.)

* The critical word; ① the pre-target region; ② the target region; ③ the post-target region.

spring, but the target sentence contained information about heavy snow. If it were the target word "snow" that produced the inconsistency, changing it to "rain" would make the effect vanish. Thirty additional students rated the rationality of both the original target sentences in the incongruent passages and those in the revised ones. The results showed that the target sentences became more neutral after rewriting, suggesting that the incongruence between the target sentences and the elaboration in the incongruent passages was brought about by the critical words.

Forty skilled readers of Chinese participated in the main experiment, with each subject receiving 30 passages (including 2 practice and 14 filler ones) for comprehension. Each experimental passage was displayed across three pages, and the target sentence always appeared in the first line of the third page and the critical word was always located in the middle of this line. The eye movements of the participants were recorded.

As in our previous study, due to the high skipping rate of single characters, we extended the target region by combining the pre-target, target, and post-target characters[4]. The target sentences were divided into three regions: A target region, including the critical character (N) and the characters before and after the critical one (i.e., N-1 and N+1, respectively), a pre-target region (i.e., about 5-8 characters, including those characters from the beginning of sentence to N-2, the last character before the target region), and a post-target region (i.e., about 4-7 characters, including those characters starting from N+2 to the last character and the period at the end of the sentence).

Figure 16.3 and Figure 16.4 show the first-pass reading time and second-pass reading time, respectively, of different regions under the different conditions. The analysis of the first-pass reading time showed that there was an immediate disruption in the target region caused by the disruption of the global coherence, indicating that the first-pass reading time in the critical region was longer in the incongruent condition, which clearly shows that readers detected the inconsistency when they fixated on the region containing characters N-1, N, or N+1.

4 We first combined the pre-target and critical characters together. However, the initial skipping rate of the two-character region was still as high as 32%, indicating that nost data on fixation daration was still not available. So a 3-character rather than a 2-character region was used in the data analysis.

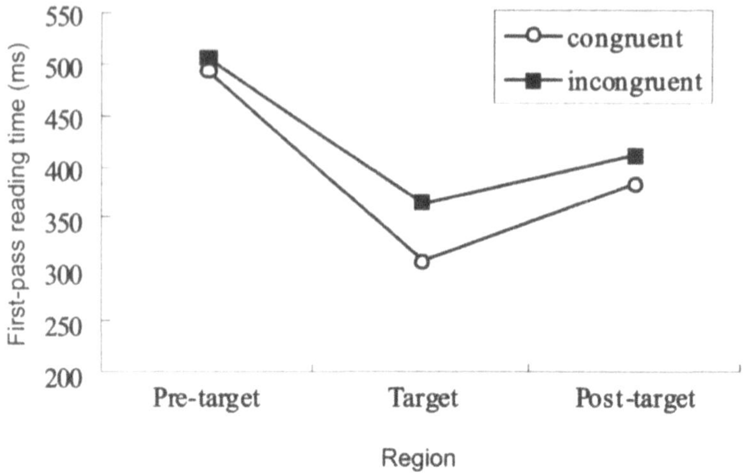

Figure 16.3 Mean first-pass reading time of the congruent and incongruent conditions

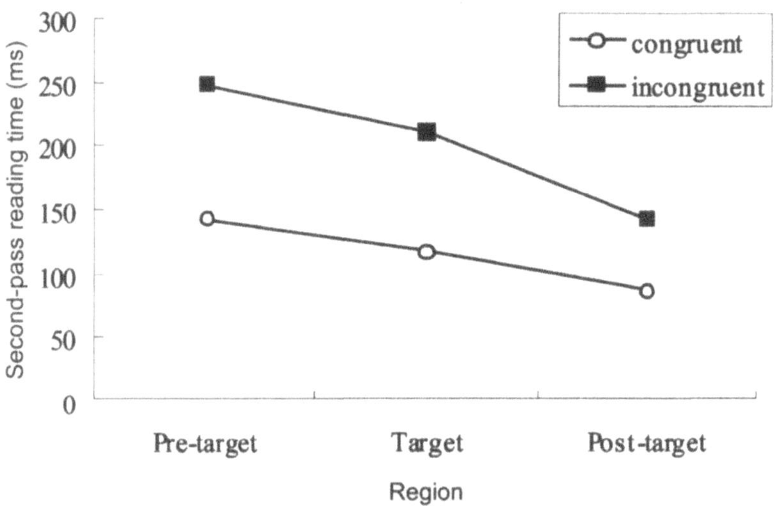

Figure 16.4 Mean second-pass reading time of the congruent and incongruent conditions

However, given that the target region includes a character after the target character, we also calculated the first fixation duration (FFD, which is mostly used in character/word based analyses) of the target region, trying to exclude the possibility that the information would not be integrated until the post-target character. It has been demonstrated that the perceptual span (effective visual field) for Chinese extends about 1 character to the left of fixation to 2-3 characters to the right when reading from left-to-right (Chen & Tang, 1998; Tang, Au Yeung & Chen, 1997; Inhoff & Liu, 1997, 1998); thus, no matter on which character the first fixation lies in the 3-character target region, readers could gain some information from the target character. FFD of the target region, therefore, can be a good index reflecting the initial processing of the critical word. Similar to the pattern of the first-pass reading time in the target region, analysis of FFD showed that the consistency effect was reliable in the target region: Readers fixated significantly longer in the incongruent condition (260 ms) than in the congruent condition (241 ms). No such effect was found in the pre-target and post-target regions. Such a pattern confirmed that readers did detect the violation right on the critical word.

Also, the manipulation of the global coherence produced obvious effects on the second-pass reading time in all three regions (Figure 16.4). Analysis of the index of regressions showed that readers regressed more often to the target region and the pre-target region in the inconsistent conditions.

Overall, these results suggest that Chinese readers are able to detect the inconsistency right at the target position. They slowed down and read more carefully as shown by the longer first fixation duration in this region. There were also reliable effects reflected by relatively late processes, suggesting that readers were trying to use contextual information to resolve the inconsistency.

Discussion

We have reviewed two studies on how readers process intra-sentential and inter-sentential information while reading Chinese. But what can be learned from these studies? We will first look at some properties of intra-sentential processing. Particularly, we are interested in the following questions: What's the time course of semantic and syntactic processing? And can they be separated from each other during on-line reading processing?

Clearly, based on the results of our study, syntactic + semantic violations and pure semantic violations can be detected immediately, and yield similar disruption effects right on the target region. However, since the two kinds of violations made no difference in the first-pass reading processing at the target region (the disruption effect neither appeared earlier, nor became more severe after introducing the syntactic violation to the semantic violation), it is difficult to identify the timing of syntactic anomaly detection. We are not sure whether or not it is as immediate as detection of semantic anomaly, because the immediate disruption effect in the syntactic + semantic violation might be caused by the pure semantic violation. But from our data, at least we can say that syntactic processing can't be conducted quicker than semantic processing during Chinese reading, which differs from the results of many studies using alphabetic languages.

Indeed, there are some studies (Boland, 1997; McElree & Griffith, 1995; Braze et al., 2002) suggesting that both syntactic violations and semantic violations were detected quite immediately during alphabetic language reading, with the syntactic violation detected a little faster than the semantic one. Such results are not difficult to understand because most alphabetic languages have some explicit markers to help readers specify the word categories and the syntactic role played by a word in a sentence; it's possible for readers to use these kinds of markers immediately, even without needing to understand the meaning of the word in the sentence. But since Chinese lacks such markers, syntactic processing can't be conducted so fast.

However, though the introduction of a syntactic violation didn't change the pattern of first-pass reading time on the target region, it does not mean that the syntactic + semantic and the semantic violations yield the same effect. With both types of violations being detected immediately, significant differences between them came up in the second-pass reading time, based on which we inferred that the syntactic violation did bring about more difficulty for understanding (although this effect was not revealed immediately). It seems that when coming across information that involves both syntactic and semantic violations (e.g., in one of the reported experiments, the object (a noun) of a verb was replaced by a verb), readers needed to reanalyze the sentence structure to find an appropriate explanation, which thus made it more difficult to integrate the target information, as shown by the longer second-pass reading time on the target region in the SYN+SEM than in the SEM condition. While compared with syntactic + semantic violations, the resolution of a semantic violation is not so difficult, though readers still needed to depend on the context to integrate the anomaly information, a fact reflected by the longer second-pass reading time at the target region and the region before and after it in the SEM condition compared to the CON one. The same effect was also revealed in the SYN+SEM condition for it also triggers a semantic violation.

Note that the different eye movement patterns for the syntactic + semantic violation can not be attributed to different degrees of semantic plausibility in the two violation conditions, for they were strictly controlled in the experiment. Therefore, the findings seem to support the hypothesis that there is a principled distinction between semantic and syntactic processing procedures within the Chinese language processing system. In this respect, the result is consistent with evidence from our recent functional neuroimaging study (Wang, Zhu, Xiao, Xiang, Zhang, & Chen, 2008), which suggested that there is a dissociation between semantic and syntactic processing in reading Chinese sentences. Compared with a SEM violation condition, the left inferior frontal area (BA44) was more strongly activated in the SYN + SEM condition, implying a prominent role of this area in Chinese syntactic processing.

What is also worth mentioning is, although both Chen (1992, 1999) and we found that a pure semantic violation and a syntactic + semantic violation were detected without too much delay, due to the more sensitive and elaborate technique we used (the eye-movement tracking technique), we found the detection of the violation occurred right at the critical character/region, and thus occurred earlier than Chen's studies indicated. Moreover, despite no difference found in terms of the time when detection occurs, we have discovered the difference between the two types of violations in the processing following the detection. No such effect was found in the previous Chen studies. Based on these results, we believe that eye movement data are highly informative with respect to understanding reading as they allow researchers to acquire a deeper and more precise understanding of the psychological integration processes during language comprehension.

The next issue of concern is immediate versus delayed integration of intra-sentential and inter-sentential semantic information. Although the identification of both meaning and grammatical properties of Chinese words is highly context-dependent, which may result in the greater possibility of ambiguity in Chinese than that in alphabetic languages (such as English), the presented experiment still indicates that different kinds of violations, from those caused by the preceding intra-sentential information to those caused by the more distant, backgrounded information, can all immediately result in the disruption of reading processing. Combined with the results from previous studies on other languages, immediate comprehension is likely to be a universal reading principle. Such immediate processing includes not only what Just and Carpenter (1987) stated, namely, "The immediacy of interpretation pervades all levels of comprehension, such as encoding a word, accessing its meaning, and determining its referent and semantic and syntactic status in the sentence", but also the immediate integration of an incoming word with relevant background information provided by previous discourse context (Pickering & Traxler, 2000). In other words, readers can update their "situation model" (Kintsch, 1988) continually as each word is processed.

One thing that we should keep in mind is that the critical characters in the studies reported in this chapter were all single-character words (instead of a morpheme of a multi-character word). Therefore, the conclusion drawn from these studies is only that integration processes may start immediately when a target character itself is a word; the question of whether the global integration could occur immediately or not when the critical character is only a morpheme still needs further study.

Moreover, even though we found that the violation was detected immediately, the change in reading patterns were not consistent with the most radical view of immediate processing (Just & Carpenter, 1980), which proposes that semantic interpretations are computed on a word-by-word basis as text is read. This is because the disruption effects arising from semantic, syntactic, or global context violations were also found in the second-pass processing in both pre-target and post-target regions, suggesting that readers were trying to use contextual information to resolve the inconsistency. Thus, as a whole, the results of the current study are in agreement with the intermediate view (i.e., the weak version of the immediacy hypothesis) that different levels of integration start immediately but the completion of it may last until the post-critical region.

Conclusions

Overall, the research reviewed in this chapter generally indicates that despite great differences between Chinese and alphabetic writing systems, there are still many similarities in comprehension processing between them. First, though the identification of the syntactic properties of words in Chinese sentences depends greatly on the semantic processing of the sentence context, evidence from eye-tracking data confirms that the parser's responses to the two anomalous types are distinct: Pure semantic violations perturbed the processor briefly, but the effect of anomaly (due to the addition of a syntactic violation) was prolonged and longer lasting, despite the degree of plausibility being matched in both conditions. Another similarity lies in the fact that both inter-sentential processing and intra-sentential processing can be initiated quite immediately, which is particularly striking, because Chinese is considered to be a highly context-dependent language. Such results support the claim that the tendency of immediate processing may be a universal reading principle , which may be suitable for all levels of processing (from intra-sentential to inter-sentential), and may be applied to both a structurally transparent language—such as English, and a structurally opaque language—such as Chinese.

However, some of the evidence from the experiments reported in this chapter also suggests that some language-specific characteristics did appear in Chinese reading. For example, compared with alphabetic languages, syntactic anomaly detection is no faster than semantic anomaly detection. This reminds us of the importance of conducting cognitive research across languages. Similar studies will help to explore both universal and language-specific processes associated with the processing of different systems, and further help to build a genuinely comprehensive theory of human language processing.

Acknowledgments

This work was supported by grants from the National Natural Science Foundation of China (30670700) , Guangdong Natural Science Foundation(06200524, 06025045), as well as a Grant 200208 from the Foundation for the Author of National Excellent Doctoral Dissertation, China.

References

Aaronson, D., & Ferres, S. (1986). Sentence processing in Chinese-American bilinguals. *Journal of Memory and Language, 25,* 136-162.

Albrecht, J. E., & O'Brien, E. J. (1993). Updating a mental model: Maintaining both local and global coherence. *Journal of Experimental Psychology: Learning, Memory, and Cognition, 19,* 1061-1070.

Altmann, G. T. M., Garnham, A., & Dennis, Y. (1992). Avoiding the garden path: Eye movements in context. *Journal of Memory and Language, 31,* 685-712.

Bader, M., & Lasser, I. (1994). German verb-final clauses and sentence processing: Evidence for immediate attachment. In C. Clifton, Jr., L. Frazier, & K. Rayner (Eds.), *Advances in sentence processing* (pp. 225-242). Hillsdale, NJ: Erlbaum.

Boland, J. E. (1997). The relationship between syntactic and semantic processes in sentence comprehension. *Language and Cognitive Processes, 12,* 423-484.

Boland, J. E., Tanenhaus, M. K., Garnsey, S. M., & Carlson, G. N. (1995). Verb argument structure in parsing and interpretation: Evidence from wh-questions. *Journal of Memory and Language, 34,* 774-806.

Braze, D., Shankweiler, D., Ni, W., & Palumbo, L. C. (2002). Readers' eye movements distinguish anomalies of form and content. *Journal of Psycholinguistic Research, 31,* 25-44.

Britt, M., Perfetti, C.A., Garrod, S., & Rayner, K. (1992). Parsing in discourse: Context effects and their limits. *Journal of Memory and Language, 31,* 293-314.

Chao, Y. R. (1968). *A grammar of spoken Chinese.* Berkeley: University of California Press.

Chen, H. C. (1992). Reading comprehension in Chinese: Some implications from character reading times. In H. C. Chen, & O. Tzeng (Eds.), *Language processing in Chinese* (pp.175-205). Amsterdam: North-Holland (Elsevier).

Chen, H. C. (1996). Chinese reading and comprehension: A cognitive psychology perspective. In M. H. Bond (Ed.), *Handbook of Chinese psychology* (pp. 43-62). Hong Kong: Asian Research Service.

Chen, H. C. (1999). How do readers of Chinese process words during reading for comprehension? In J. Wang, A. W. Inhoff, & H. C. Chen (Eds.), *Reading Chinese script: A cognitive analysis* (pp. 257-278). Mahwah, NJ: Erlbaum.

Chen, H. C., & Juola, J. F. (1982). Dimensions of lexical coding in Chinese and English. *Memory & Cognition, 10,* 216-224.

Chen, H. C., & Tang, C. K. (1998). The effective visual field in Chinese. *Reading and Writing, 10,* 245-254.

Cheung, H., Chen, H. C., Lai, C. Y., Wong, O. C., & Hills, M. (2001). The development of phonological awareness: Effects of speech experience, orthography, and literacy. *Cognition, 81,* 227-241.

Clifton, C. Jr. (1993). Thematic roles in sentence parsing. *Canadian Journal of Experimental Psychology, 47,* 222-246.

Cook, A., & Myers, J. L. (2004). Processing discourse roles in scripted narratives: The influences of context and world knowledge. *Journal of Memory and Language, 50,* 268-288.

Crocker, M. W. (1994). On the nature of the principle-based sentence processor. In C. Clifton, Jr., L. Frazier, & K. Rayner (Eds.), *Advances in sentence processing* (pp. 245-266). Hillsdale, NJ: Erlbaum.

Cutler, A., & Otake, T. (1994). Mora or phoneme? Further evidence for language-specific listening. *Journal of Memory and Language, 33,* 824-844.

Danks, J. H., Bohn, L., & Fears, R. (1983). Comprehension processes in oral reading. In G. B. Flores d'Arcais, & R. J. Jarrvella (Eds.), *The process of language understanding* (pp.193-223). Sussex, England: Wiley.

Danks, J. H. (1986). Identifying component processes in reading: Comment on Haberlandt and Graesser. *Journal of Experimental Psychology: General, 115,* 198-200.

Deutsch, A., & Bentin, S. (2001). Syntactic and semantic factors in processing gender agreement in Hebrew: Evidence from ERPs and eye movements. *Journal of Memory and Language, 45,* 200-224.

Duffy, S. A., Morris, R. K., & Rayner, K. (1988). Lexical ambiguity and fixation times in reading. *Journal of Memory and Language, 27,* 429-446.

Ehrlich, K., & Rayner, K. (1983). Pronoun assignment and semantic integration during reading: Eye movements and immediacy of processing. *Journal of Verbal Learning and Verbal Behavior, 22,* 75-87.

Federmeier, K. D., & Kutas, M. (1999). A rose by any other name: Long-term memory structure and sentence processing. *Journal of Memory and Language, 41,* 469-495.

Feng, G., Miller, K., Shu, H., & Zhang, H. (2001). Rowed to recovery: The use of phonological and orthographic information in reading Chinese and English. *Journal of Experimental Psychology: Learning, Memory, and Cognition, 27,* 1079-1100.

Frazier, L. (1987). Sentence processing: A tutorial review. In Coltheart, M. (Ed.), *Attention and performance XII* (pp. 559-286). Hillsdale, NJ: Erlbaum.

Frazier, L., & Rayner, K. (1982). Making and correcting errors during sentence comprehension: Eye movements in the analysis of structurally ambiguous sentences. *Cognitive Psychology, 14,* 178-210.

Frisson, S., & Frazier, L. (2005). Carving up word meaning: Portioning and grinding. *Journal of Memory and Language, 53,* 277-291.

Gandour, J., Wong, D., Lowe, M., Dzemidzic, M., Satthamnuwong, N., Tong, Y., & Li, X. (2002). A cross-linguistic fMRI study of spectral and temporal cues underlying phonological processing. *Journal of Cognitive Neuroscience, 14,* 1076-1087.

Garrod, S., Freudenthal, S., & Boyle, E. (1994). The role of different types of anaphor in the resolution of sentences in a discourse. *Journal of Memory and Language, 33,* 39-68.

Hsu, S. H., & Huang, K. C. (2000). Effects of word spacing on reading Chinese text from a video display terminal. *Perceptual and Motor Skills, 90,* 81-92.

Inhoff, A.W., & Liu, W. (1997). The perceptual span during the reading of Chinese text. In H. C. Chen (Ed), *The cognitive processing of Chinese and related Asian languages* (pp. 243-266). Hong Kong: The Chinese University Press.

Inhoff, A., W., & Liu, W. (1998). The perceptual span and oculomotor activity during the reading of Chinese sentences. *Journal of Experimental Psychology: Human Perception and Performance, 24,* 20-34.

Just, M. A., & Carpenter, P. A. (1980). A theory of reading: From eye fixations to comprehension. *Psychological Review, 87,* 329-354.

Just, M. A., & Carpenter, P. A. (1987). *The psychology of reading and language comprehension.* Boston: Allyn & Bacon, Inc.

Kambe, G., Rayner, K., & Duffy, S. A. (2001). Global context effects on processing lexically ambiguous words: Evidence from eye fixations. *Memory & Cognition, 29,* 363-372.

Kintsch, W. (1988). The role of knowledge in discourse comprehension: A construction- integration model. *Psychological Review, 95,* 163-182.

Kutas, M., & Hillyard, S. A. (1980). Reading senseless sentences: Brain potential reflect semantic incongruity. *Science, 207,* 203-205.

Magliano, J. P., Graesser, A. C., Eymard, L. A., Haberlandt, K., & Gholson, B. (1993). Locus of interpretive and inference processes during text comprehension: A comparison of gaze durations and word reading times. *Journal of Experimental Psychology: Learning, Memory, and Cognition, 3,* 704-709.

Marslen-Wilson, W. D. (1987). Functional parallelism in spoken word recognition. *Cognition, 25,* 71-102.

McElree, B., & Griffith, T. (1995). Syntactic and thematic processing in sentence comprehension: Evidence for a temporal dissociation. *Journal of Experimental Psychology: Learning, Memory, and Cognition, 21,* 134-157.

McKoon, G., & Ratcliff, R. (1992). Inference during reading. *Psychological Review, 99,* 440-466.

Murray, W. S., & Rowan, M. (1998). Early, mandatory, pragmatic processing. *Journal of Psycholinguistic Research, 27,* 1-22.

Myers, J. L., O'Brien, E. J., Albrecht, J. E., & Mason, R. A. (1994). Maintaining global coherence during reading. *Journal of Experimental Psychology: Learning, Memory, and Cognition, 20,* 876-886.

Ni, W., Fodor, J. D., Crain, S., & Shankweiler, D. P. (1998). Anomalous strings: Eye movement patterns. *Journal of Psycholinguistic Research, 27,* 515-539.

O'Brien, E. J., & Albrecht, J. E. (1992). Comprehension strategies in the development of a mental model. *Journal of Experimental Psychology: Learning, Memory, and Cognition, 18,* 777-784.

O'Brien, E. J., Rizzella, M. L., Albrecht, J. L., & Halleran, J. G. (1998). Updating a situation model: A memory-based text processing view? *Journal of Experimental Psychology: Learning, Memory, and Cognition, 24,* 1200-1210.

O'Brien, E. J., Shank, D. M., Myers, J. L., & Rayner, K. (1988). Elaborative inferences during reading: Do they occur on-line? *Journal of Experimental Psychology: Learning, Memory, and Cognition, 14,* 410-420.

Pearlmutter, N. J., Garnsey, S. M., & Bock, K. (1999). Agreement processes in sentence comprehension. *Journal of Memory and Language, 41,* 427-456.

Pickering, M. J., & Traxler, M. J. (2000). Parsing and incremental understanding during reading. In M. W. Crocker, & M. Pickering (Eds.), *Architectures and mechanisms for language processing* (pp. 238-258). New York: Cambridge University Press.

Rayner, K., Cook, A. E., Juhasz, B. J., & Frazier, L. (2006). Immediate disambiguation of lexically ambiguous words during reading: Evidence from eye movements. *British Journal of Psychology, 97,* 467-482.

Rayner, K., & Duffy, S. A. (1986). Links Lexical complexity and fixation times in reading: Effects of word frequency, verb complexity, and lexical ambiguity. *Memory & Cognition. 14,* 191-201.

Rayner, K., & Frazier, L. (1989). Selection mechanisms in reading lexically ambiguous words. *Journal of Experiment Psychology: Learning, Memory, and Cognition, 15,* 779-790.

Rayner, K., & Pollatsek, A. (1989). *The psychology of reading.* Englewood Cliffs, NJ: Prentice Hall.

Rayner, K., Warren, T., Juhasz, B. J., & Liversedge, S. P. (2004). The effect of plausibility on eye movements in reading. *Journal of Experimental Psychology: Learning, Memory, and Cognition, 30,* 1290-1301.

Rosler, F., Putz, P., Friederici, A. D., & Hahne, A. (1993). Event-related brain potentials while encountering semantic and syntactic constraint violations. *Journal of Cognitive Neuroscience, 5*, 345-362.

Schirmer, A., Tang, S. L., Penney, T. B., Gunter, T. C., & Chen, H. C. (2005). Brain responses to segmentally induced semantic violations in Cantonese. *Journal of Cognitive Neuroscience, 17*, 1-12.

Sereno, S. C., O'Donnell, P., & Rayner, K. (2006). Eye movements and lexical ambiguity resolution: Investigating the subordinate bias effect. *Journal of Experimental Psychology: Human Perception and Performance, 32*, 335-350.

Sturt, P., & Crocker, M. (1996). Monotonic syntactic processing: A cross-linguistic study of attachment and reanalysis. *Language and Cognitive Processes, 11*, 449-494.

Tang, C. K., Au Yeung, L. H., & Chen, H. C. (1997). The effective visual field in the reading of Chinese text. In H. C. Chen (Ed.), *The cognitive processing of Chinese and related Asian languages* (pp. 267-286). Hong Kong: Chinese University Press.

Traxler, M. J., Foss, D. J., Seely, R. E., Kaup, B., & Morris, R. (2000). Visual and lexical association effects on priming in natural language processing. *Journal of Psycholinguistic Research, 29*, 581-595.

Traxler, M. J., & Pickering, M. J. (1996). Plausibility and the processing of unbounded dependencies: An eye-tracking study. *Journal of Memory and Language, 35*, 454-475.

Trueswell, J., Tanenhaus, M., & Garnsey, S. (1994). Semantic influences on parsing: Use of thematic role information in syntactic ambiguity resolution. *Journal of Memory and Language, 33*, 285-318.

van Berkum, J., Hagoort, P., & Brown, C. M. (1999). Semantic integration in sentences and discourse: Evidence from the N400. *Journal of Cognitive Neuroscience, 11*, 657-671.

Wang, S., Chen, H. C., Mo, L., & Zou, Y. (2004). Accessing backgrounded information in text comprehension: A situation-constrained resonance process. (in Chinese). *Acta Psychologica Sinica, 36*, 644-653.

Wang, S., Chen, H. C., Yang, J., & Mo, L. (2008). Immediacy of integration in discourse comprehension: Evidence from Chinese readers' eye movements. *Language and Cognitive Processes, 23*, 241-247.

Wang, S., & Mo, L. (2001). Accessing of backgrounded information in discourse comprehension. (in Chinese). *Acta Psychologica Sinica, 33*, 312-319.

Wang, S., Zhu, Z., Xiao, Z., Xiang, H., Zhang, J. X., & Chen, H. C. (2008). Broca's area plays a role in syntactic processing during Chinese reading comprehension. *Neuropsychologia, 46,* 1371-1378.

Yang, J., Wang, S., & Chen, H. C. (2005). *Parafoveal preview effect of Chinese sentence reading.* Paper presented at the 11th International Conference on Processing Chinese and Other East Asian Languages, Hong Kong.

Chapter 17

What is the place for Pinyin in beginning Chinese reading? Evidence from eye movements

Ming Yan, Kevin F. Miller, Hong Li, and Hua Shu

The utility of sound-based cues in the acquisition of Chinese characters has long been controversial. To most Westerners, alphabetic writing seems both fundamental and obligatory, in the same way that reading alphabetic text is obligatory for skilled readers of such orthographies (Stroop, 1935). To most adult Westerners learning Chinese, phonetic representations of Chinese characters seem an essential aid to the acquisition of this orthography. The efforts of missionaries such as Matteo Ricci to learn Chinese before the advent of such aids have been documented by Spence (1984) and represent an extremely impressive accomplishment.

A variety of orthographic systems have been developed to represent the pronunciation of Chinese characters, beginning with character-based systems such as *fan*3 *qie*4 (反切), which uses one character that shares an onset with the target with another that shares a rime with the target character. For example, the pronunciation of 同 *tong*2 can be represented with 徒 (*tu*2) and 红 (*hong*2), taking the onset "t-" from the first character and the rime and tone ("-*ong*2") from the second. As Yin and Rohsenow (1994) note, the *fan*3 *qie*4 (反切) system has several shortcomings. It requires the user to know the pronunciation of the characters used to represent the sounds, and so may not provide a clear representation of the sounds of the characters. This is particularly true for characters whose pronunciation varies across dialects, as the relations among the triplet of characters (target, onset-representing, and rime-representing) may not be preserved across dialects. Finally, unless the learner knows the standard pronunciation for the different onset- and rime-representing characters, then *fan3 qie4* (反切) will not provide it for them.

In Mainland China, the official system for representing the sounds of Mandarin Chinese is *han4 yu3 pin1 yin1* (汉语拼音), which uses the Western alphabet plus tone markings to write the pronunciations of characters in Mandarin (although tone markings are often omitted in practice). Children in Mainland China are taught Pinyin on school entry and it is a standard (although not universal) method for entering Chinese on computer systems.

Western linguists such as DeFrancis (1984, 1989) have argued that Pinyin should and ultimately will replace Chinese characters due to its superior ability to represent spoken Chinese. Mair (1996) provides a typical example of this perspective:

...pinyin is now poised to take on the role of a full-fledged script. For political and practical reasons, the government cannot now advocate such a move. Yet the facts are inescapable: while not yet securely established as an auxiliary script, pinyin has long been widely accepted as a handy notational system, and China may be said already to have entered a policy of digraphia, with pinyin and the sinograms used in complementarity. Whether or not pinyin gradually displaces sonograms remains to be seen. (p. 205)

It may be that the advocates of alphabets are correct in their predictions of the eventual demise of character-based orthographies. As computer systems have incorporated larger word-based and phrase-based dictionaries, Pinyin text input has become more viable. It is now possible to type in an entire phrase, such as "*wen2 zi4 gai3 ge2*" 文字改革 (orthographic reform), and have the computer recognize the correct phrase. Early Pinyin systems that involved typing individual Pinyin syllables (e.g., "*wen2*") and then selecting among the (18) characters sharing that pronunciation were less appealing for obvious reasons. So it is possible that the demands of text input into computers and cell phones will lead to increasing familiarity with Pinyin. Alternatively, pen-based or speech-based input systems may lessen its use.

The failure of Pinyin to replace Chinese characters has clearly puzzled linguists such as DeFrancis (1996) who argued that this is simply a matter of time, particularly if the Chinese government drops what he terms a policy of repression. Others, such as Logan (2004) have argued that alphabetic reading and writing are the keys to skills such as classification and scientific reasoning.

It is notable, however, that this enthusiasm for Pinyin seems largely a Western phenomenon. The second author has been struck, for example, by the frequency with which well-educated Chinese adults refer to Pinyin as *ying*1 *wen*2 (英文) or "English," and argue that the presence of Pinyin scripts on signs in Chinese cities is designed to help foreigners who don't know Chinese (even though this would be of limited use to anyone who doesn't speak Chinese).

Arguing against the idea that Pinyin is destined to replace characters as the primary script for writing Chinese are features of the coevolution of spoken and written Chinese that make alphabetic writing problematic. Modern spoken Mandarin has approximately 1,300 syllables, including tone, although about 200 are rarely used (Duanmu, 2006); this is roughly an order of magnitude fewer than English has. In an analysis of text containing nearly 200 million characters, Da (2004) found slightly fewer than 10,000 unique characters. This implies that there should be 7-8 homophones for each character on average. Analyzing the most frequent 6,000 characters identified by Da (2000) and ignoring tone, Duanmu (2006) reported that most syllables represented fewer than 20 characters, although there were more than 100 characters pronounced [ji].

Although the question of whether Pinyin can provide a substitute for Chinese characters is deeply controversial, there is evidence that learning to read Pinyin has consequences for those who learn it, by helping mediate the development of some of the kinds of phonological awareness associated with learning to read an alphabetic script (Bradley & Bryant, 1991). Setting the pattern in this area of research, Read, Zhang, Nie, and Ding (1986) compared the ability of adults in Mainland China who had grown up in periods where Pinyin was or was not emphasized due to the vicissitudes of language reform and educational policy. Those who had been taught Pinyin as children substantially outperformed their peers who had been taught characters only, even though many of the Pinyin group could no longer in fact read Pinyin. Cheung and Chen (2004) compared Cantonese-speaking Chinese college students who had grown up in Guangzhou (learning Pinyin) and those who had grown up in Hong Kong (who learned Chinese without learning Pinyin or an alternative sound-based system). This is a particularly interesting comparison, because one of the main uses of Pinyin is as a guide to the pronunciation of the official Mandarin dialect for speakers of other dialects such as Cantonese. Because Cantonese and Mandarin differ substantially, this can be thought of as a combination of second-language learning plus the acquisition of an alphabetic script. Cheung and Chen reported that participants who had been taught Pinyin outperformed their peers who had not been taught Pinyin as young children in orally presented phonological awareness tasks requiring them to match syllables based on rime, onset, or coda. The latter group performed at chance on coda-matching.

McBride-Chang, Bialystok, Chong, and Li (2004) reported that kindergarteners and first graders in Mainland China (who were learning Pinyin) exceeded their Hong Kong counterparts (who were not learning Pinyin) in tasks requiring them to delete syllables and onsets, indicating that there is an early effect of Pinyin on phonological awareness.

Thus there is good evidence that learning Pinyin helps in the development of phonological awareness, particularly the ability to compare syllables based on their sounds and to separate syllables into onsets and rimes, and that this effect occurs as children learn to read Pinyin. The focus of this chapter is on the utility of Pinyin as a learning aid in the acquisition of character-based reading. Once mastered, Pinyin provides the learner with a means to pronounce new characters. The prevalence of Pinyin-based dictionaries means that learners can use alphabetical order to look up unknown characters (rather than identifying radicals and counting strokes). Thus it has the potential to speed the day when children become independent readers, able to read a broad range of materials and look up characters they don't already know.

Learning to read Pinyin is a major activity in first-grade reading instruction in Mainland China (Wu, Li, & Anderson, 1999), with approximately 38% of instructional time devoted to learning Pinyin, primarily during the first semester. Pinyin, which was invented to represent pronunciation, is a completely shallow orthography and is acquired quickly. Taking the Beijing reading series as an example, the first semester textbook is entirely devoted to Pinyin and only introduces characters, with Pinyin written above them, in the titles of three stories presented at the very end of the semester. In the second semester of first grade, all text includes both characters and Pinyin (written above each character) until nearly the end of the semester, when two stories are presented with characters alone. In second grade, nearly all text contains Pinyin above the characters. Starting in third grade, Pinyin is only used in presenting new characters.

One of the few psychological studies to look at the effect of Pinyin on incidental learning of characters was reported by Wu, Li, and Shu (2002), who compared the addition of Pinyin in the context of a shared book-reading approach to teaching young children to read Chinese. Somewhat surprisingly, Pinyin did not have any systematic effect on children's character learning. However, when Wu et al. analyzed their data separately by reading ability, they found an interesting interaction. For high-ability children, adding Pinyin promoted character learning, while for low-ability children, adding Pinyin actually decreased character learning.

Informal discussions with teachers raised both some questions about whether students really take advantage of Pinyin when reading, and concerns that some students might rely on Pinyin as a crutch to avoid learning to read characters. These are both possibilities, and the present study was designed to look at how the presence of Pinyin affects eye movements of beginning readers. Adding Pinyin complicates the perceptual environment confronting beginning readers since they see two parallel texts. In order to use it effectively, they may need to possess metacognitive abilities sufficient to permit them to monitor their own comprehension quickly enough to attend to Pinyin in cases where they fail to recognize a character. For Pinyin to be a useful tool for learning characters, readers must then use that information to learn a character's pronunciation in a way that permits them to recognize the character on future occasions. Pinyin surely has the potential to aid beginning Chinese readers in developing independent reading skills, but effective use of this tool may require levels of control over the reading process that young readers may not possess.

In addition to the information that Pinyin provides, its presentation accompanying new characters may also serve to identify these as difficult characters. Von Restorff (1933) demonstrated that marking items in any fashion leads to better recall; presenting Pinyin above unfamiliar characters may serve to call attention to them, which might be a useful strategy for young readers. To look at such signaling effects, we included a format in which new characters were marked with a set of asterisks, providing marking without any guide to pronunciation.

The practice of presenting Pinyin above Chinese characters provides potentially useful cues to support the independent learning of Chinese characters by young readers, yet its use in early reading in China remains controversial. Providing such additional information complicates the task of reading (by providing an additional, potentially distracting cue). It could, in some circumstances provide an alternative script: one that a number of Western linguists argue could replace Chinese characters. If children read Pinyin rather than attending to the characters, Pinyin could arguably be an obstacle to the development of fluent reading of characters. A final concern with the use of Pinyin is that the metacognitive control required to use it effectively may only benefit more skilled readers. Stanovich (1986) used the term Matthew effect (coined by Merton, 1968) to describe the phenomenon by which initial differences in skills and understanding related to early literacy lead to a cascading series of effects that grow larger over time. To the extent that Pinyin provides a cue that only more advanced readers can utilize, it has the potential to lead to Matthew effects in the development of Chinese reading, in which those children who profit from Pinyin have an advantage over their peers in learning characters and becoming independent readers.

The current study provides evidence for how children use Pinyin when they encounter it in conjunction with unfamiliar words. Key questions are the extent to which children are able to use Pinyin to help in this context, the extent to which Pinyin serves as a distraction in reading characters, and the extent to which the ability to use Pinyin effectively differs among readers of varying abilities.

Methods

Participants

A total of 80 second graders from a primary school in downtown Beijing participated in this project in some way, although issues due to headsize and weight of the helmet (with the eye tracker) or problems with maintaining calibration meant that usable eye-tracking data were collected from a total of 57 students, with a median age of 8 years and 1 month (range 7 years, 5 months to 9 years, 3 months). All participants had either normal vision or corrected-to-normal vision.

Apparatus

Eye movements were recorded using the EyeLink II system, a video-based system with a sampling rate of 500 Hz and a spatial resolution of 0.005°. Because the system compensates for head movements, no head restriction was used. Eye-movement recording was binocular, but data from only the left eye were analyzed. Reading materials were presented on a 19-inch monitor with refresh rate of 100 Hz and resolution of

1024x768, 60-70 cm away from the reader. The Chinese materials were displayed in 48-point Kai font, corresponding to about 56 pixels or 2.6 visual degrees per character.

Stimuli

Stimuli consisted of short (8-12 character) sentences containing a two-character key word that involved a concept familiar to students in their spoken language but not using characters they had learned in class. All other characters were already learned. Each sentence fit on one line of the computer screen and the target characters were never the first or last two characters of the sentence. A total of 32 experimental sentences and 8 practice sentences were developed and piloted.

Cloze tests administered to 10 other children from the same classrooms who did not participate in the experiment showed that guessing rate for the target characters was less than 5% in all cases, indicating that children should not be able to figure out the characters from context without reliance on the Pinyin.

Presentation conditions

As noted above, four presentation conditions were used, as shown in Figure 17.1: (a) full-Pinyin condition, in which Pinyin was written above each character; (b) mark condition, in which new characters were marked with asterisks that provided no phonetic information; (c) partial-Pinyin condition, in which only new characters had Pinyin; and (d) no-Pinyin condition, where no Pinyin was presented. All stimuli were shown to all subjects, and the order of those four conditions was counter-balanced using a Latin Square method to make four versions of the stimuli. Each participant was randomly assigned to one version.

Although the Eyelink II system compensates for head position, we were worried about loss of accuracy due to head movement as well as fatigue due to the weight of the helmet. Therefore, participants were asked to put their head on a height-adjustable chin rest and to move as little as possible. A preliminary practice session was included before the experiment began to allow participants to become familiar with the eye-tracking equipment and the experimental procedure.

Procedure

Both the practice session and the experimental session started with a calibration and validation procedure, and they were repeated when necessary during the experiment. Each trial started with a drift-correction check (with a single fixation point in the center of the screen) and was adjusted in case the check was negative.

(a)
jiě jiě de kā fēi hǎo xiāng ā
姐 姐 的 咖 啡 好 香 啊 。

(b)
xx xxx
姐 姐 的 咖 啡 好 香 啊 。

(c)
kā fēi
姐 姐 的 咖 啡 好 香 啊 。

(d)
姐 姐 的 咖 啡 好 香 啊 。

Figure 17.1 Example stimulus with the four presentation conditions used. (a) Full Pinyin, where Pinyin is presented above all characters, both familiar and unfamiliar, (b) Mark, where asterisks are presented above unfamiliar characters, (c) Partial, where Pinyin is presented only above unfamiliar characters, and (d) None, where no Pinyin is presented. The sentence can be translated as "The older sister's coffee smells good," with "coffee" the unfamiliar two-character word.

Participants were asked to read the sentences silently as they ordinarily would and push a button when they had finished. After reading each sentence, they were presented with a choice of two pictures and asked to select which one was consistent with the sentence they had just read by pressing one of two buttons. This served to focus their attention on comprehension.

Results

Excluded participants and ability grouping

Because the focus of this study is the utility of Pinyin in learning unfamiliar characters, we wanted to find a way to exclude cases where children already knew the characters. We could not do a pretest without priming the unfamiliar characters, so we decided to use eye-tracking data to identify students who were already familiar with the set of "unfamiliar characters." We identified a set of 20 participants who had a skipping rate of >50% for the putatively unfamiliar characters. Sixteen of these subjects showed >70% performance on the comprehension measure described previously, suggesting that they were indeed familiar with the "unfamiliar" characters. Four additional participants showed <70% comprehension, which may indicate inattentiveness to the task. This left us with a total of 37 participants, who gave some indication of not being familiar with the characters of interest. The analyses discussed below are based on these participants.

We asked the children's teachers to group them into high- (12: 8 boys, 4 girls), middle- (14: 7 boys, 7 girls), and low- (11: 7 boys, 4 girls) ability groups, following the procedure used by Wu et al. (2002) and others. These ability groups will be used in the following analyses, in order to assess whether the utility of Pinyin is dependent upon reading ability.

Reading comprehension

The rates of correct answers to the comprehension questions averaged 78.4%, 82.1%, and 91.4%, for the low-, middle-, and high-ability groups, respectively, which leads to a significant ability difference, $F(2, 34) = 4.292$, $p < 0.05$. Further multiple comparisons show that there is no difference between the low- and middle-ability groups, but a significant difference between the high-ability groups and the others. This serves as a rough indicator of the accuracy of the ability classifications made by the teachers.

Reading speed

Figure 17.2 shows total reading time per sentence by ability group and presentation condition. An ability group (3: high, middle, low) and presentation condition (4: full Pinyin, partial Pinyin, no Pinyin, and mark) MANOVA, with presentation condition as a within-subjects factor, found a consistent effect of presentation condition $F(3, 102) = 12.422$, $p < 0.001$. The two conditions that do not provide meaningful supplemental phonological information (the no-Pinyin condition and the mark condition) were the fastest to read. Multiple comparisons did not find significant differences between the two Pinyin conditions (full versus partial). There were no overall effects of ability on reading speed ($F(2, 34) = 0.343$, n.s) nor interactions between presentation condition and ability ($F(6, 102) = 0.565$, n.s.). Thus, one effect of providing Pinyin is to slow reading time, presumably because it provides additional information that can or even must be incorporated into the reading process. The lack of significant differences between the full-Pinyin and partial-Pinyin condition suggests that even young readers may already be somewhat selective in their ability to use Pinyin when and as needed (as in the case of unfamiliar characters).

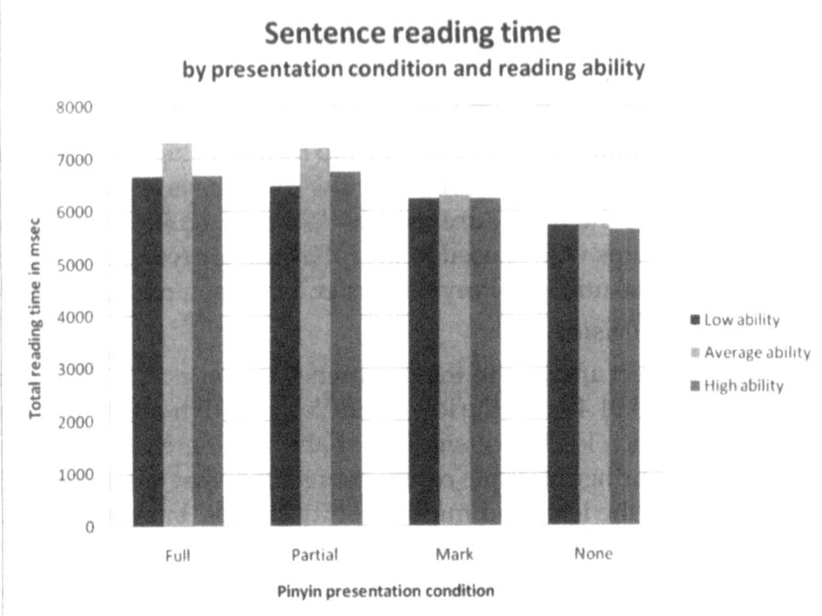

Figure 17.2 Effects of Pinyin presentation condition and reading ability on total sentence reading time.

Effects of Pinyin presentation condition on fixations on new characters

Number of fixations. The top panel of Figure 17.3 shows the total number of fixations on the unfamiliar two-character words as a function of Pinyin presentation condition. The only significant effect that emerged was a main effect of presentation condition ($F(3, 102) = 13.666, p < 0.001$), with no significant effect of ability group ($F(2, 34) = 0.832$, n.s.) nor a presentation by ability interaction ($F(6, 102) = 0.836$, n.s.). Further multiple comparisons of the four Pinyin presentation methods shows no difference between the full-Pinyin and partial-Pinyin conditions, a marginally significant difference between mark and no-Pinyin conditions, but a significant difference between other two conditions.

Looking time. The bottom panel of Figure 17.3 shows the total time spent looking at the unfamiliar characters as a function of Pinyin presentation condition. As with number of fixations, the only significant effect that emerged was a main effect of presentation condition ($F(3, 102) = 23.618, p < 0.001$), with no significant effect of ability group ($F(2, 34) = 0.406$, n.s.) nor a presentation by ability interaction ($F(6, 102) = 0.436$, n.s.). Multiple comparisons showed that there was no significant difference between the two Pinyin conditions (full and partial), but significant differences between these two and the mark and no-Pinyin conditions, which did not significantly differ from each other.

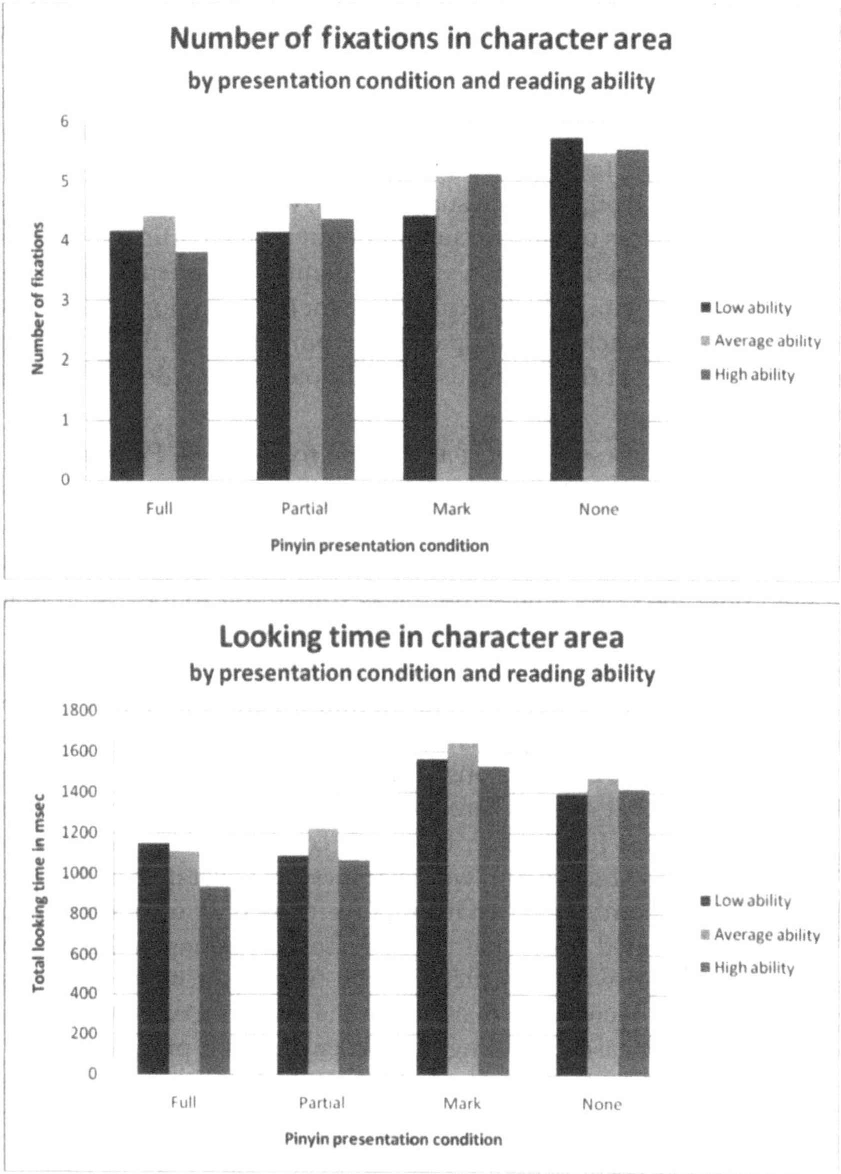

Figure 17.3 Effects of Pinyin presentation condition and reading ability on number of fixations (top panel) and total looking time (lower panel) for unfamiliar characters.

Simply put, when Pinyin is present, whether over all characters or only unfamiliar ones, it leads to fewer fixations on unfamiliar characters and lower total looking time. This is not simply due to the presence of something to look at above the characters, because the effect on number of fixations is smaller when unfamiliar characters are marked with an asterisk. There is some effect of having such marking, at least on number of fixations, though, because it does cause a reduction in number of fixations when compared to the no-Pinyin condition. The effects of Pinyin on reducing time spent looking at unfamiliar characters did not differ by reading groups, which suggests that, whether Pinyin was present for all characters or only for unfamiliar ones, the participants were able to redeploy their attention when unfamiliar characters were accompanied by Pinyin. A likely explanation for the reduction of fixations on unfamiliar characters accompanied by pinyin is that this is due to increased looking at the Pinyin as an additional cue to identifying the unfamiliar character.

Effects of Pinyin presentation condition on fixations on Pinyin area

Number of fixations. The top panel of Figure 17.4 shows the number of fixations in the Pinyin area above unfamiliar characters as a function of Pinyin presentation condition. In analyses of the Pinyin area, we considered only the cases where there was something to look at in that space: the full-Pinyin, partial-Pinyin, and mark conditions. The only significant effect that emerged was a main effect of presentation condition ($F(2, 68) = 46.041$, $p < 0.001$) with no significant effect of ability group ($F(2, 34) = 1.040$, n.s.) nor a presentation by ability interaction ($F(4, 68) = 1.177$, n.s.). Multiple comparisons of the three Pinyin presentation conditions showed that each differed significantly from the others, with significantly fewer fixations in the mark condition than in the full-Pinyin condition, which in turn were significantly fewer than in the condition where the unfamiliar characters were the only ones for which Pinyin was provided. Note that the increase in fixations in the Pinyin area when Pinyin was presented for the unfamiliar characters was greater than the decrease in fixations in the character area, which accounts for the increase in reading time when Pinyin is presented.

Looking time. The bottom panel of Figure 17.4 shows the total time spent looking in the Pinyin area as a function of Pinyin presentation condition. The same pattern was found as for number of fixations. The only significant effect that emerged was a main effect of presentation condition ($F(2, 68) = 41.638$, $p < 0.001$), with no significant effect of ability group ($F(2, 34) = 0.173$, n.s.) nor a presentation by ability interaction

($F(4, 68) = 0.210$, n.s.). Multiple comparisons of the three presentation conditions showed no difference between the full-Pinyin and partial-Pinyin conditions, and significant differences between the two Pinyin conditions and the other groups, which did not differ from each other.

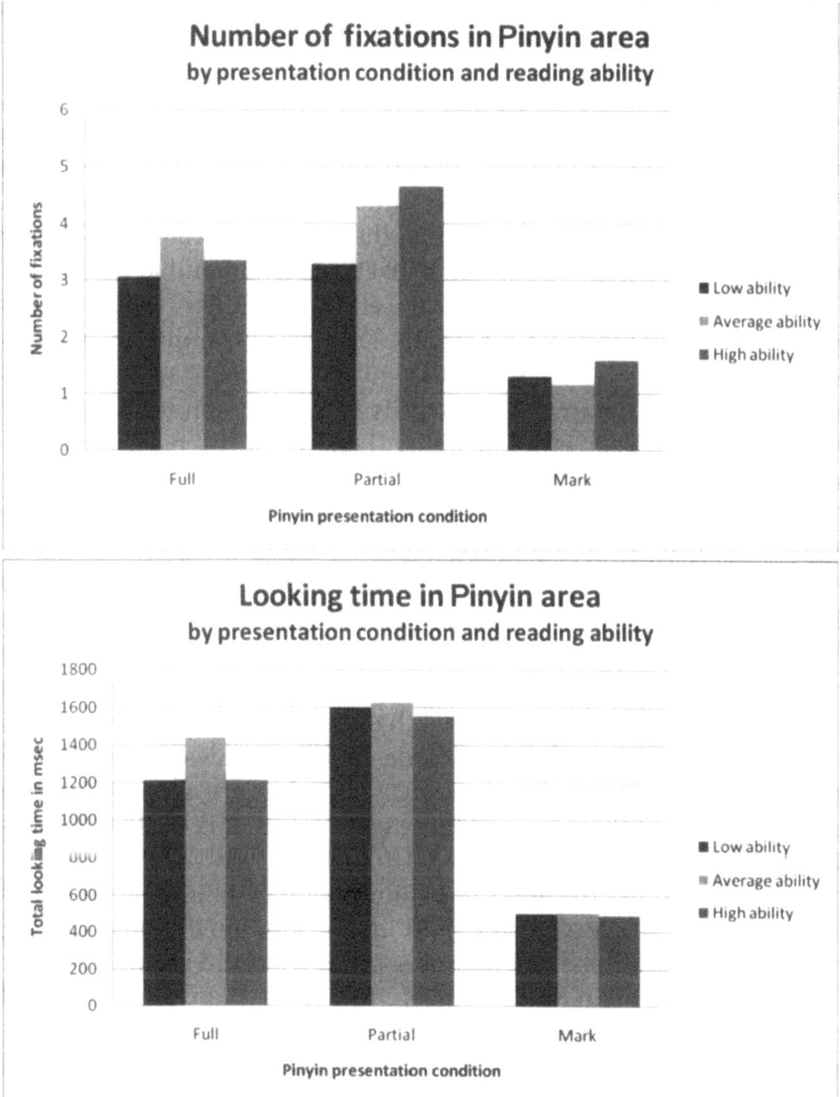

Figure 17.4 Effects of Pinyin presentation condition and reading ability on number of fixations in the Pinyin area (top panel) and total looking time (lower panel) in the three conditions where something was present in that area.

Results focusing on the Pinyin area, the area above a character where Pinyin is typically presented, show that second graders are responsive to its presence, in contrast to a low-information asterisk marking the unfamiliar character. There was some evidence that presenting Pinyin only for unfamiliar characters does serve as a signal to direct eye movements, with children more likely to look, and to look longer, when the presence of Pinyin also served to signal an unfamiliar character.

Comparing looking at familiar vs. unfamiliar words

The final analyses involved comparing looking at characters and Pinyin for unfamiliar versus familiar two-character words, after selecting a known two-character word in each stimulus sentence for this purpose. This comparison can only be done in the full-Pinyin condition, where pinyin was presented for familiar as well as for unfamiliar characters. The top panel of Figure 17.5 shows the effect of familiarity on the number of fixations in the character region. The effect of familiarity was significant ($F(1, 34) = 16.738$, $p < 0.001$); on average there was about one more fixation on the unfamiliar words in comparison to the familiar ones. But there was no effect of ability ($F(2, 34) = 0.761$, n.s.), and no interaction between ability and familiarity ($F(2, 34) = 0.294$, n.s.).

The bottom panel of Figure 17.5 shows the effect of familiarity on the number of fixations in the Pinyin region. The effect of familiarity was significant ($F(1, 34) = 191.096$, $p < 0.001$); on average there were almost three more fixations on the Pinyin above the unfamiliar words than on that above the familiar ones. But there was no effect of ability ($F(2, 34) = 0.600$, n.s.) and no interaction between ability and familiarity ($F(2, 34) = 0.829$, n.s.). Noteworthy is the fact that there were nearly no fixations on the Pinyin above the familiar words, which provides the clearest evidence that the eye-movements of second graders are already tuned to take advantage of Pinyin just in those cases where it is likely to be useful.

Figure 17.6 shows the effect of familiarity on looking time for familiar and unfamiliar words in the full-Pinyin condition (because looking at Pinyin above familiar words was so rare, we could not do a similar analysis for the Pinyin area). Looking time showed a pattern identical to that found for number of fixations. The effect of familiarity was significant ($F(1, 34) = 23.829$, $p < 0.001$); on average unfamiliar words were fixated for about 300 ms longer than familiar ones. But there was no effect of ability ($F(2, 34) = 1.222$, n.s.), and no interaction between ability and familiarity ($F(2, 34) = 0.461$, n.s.).

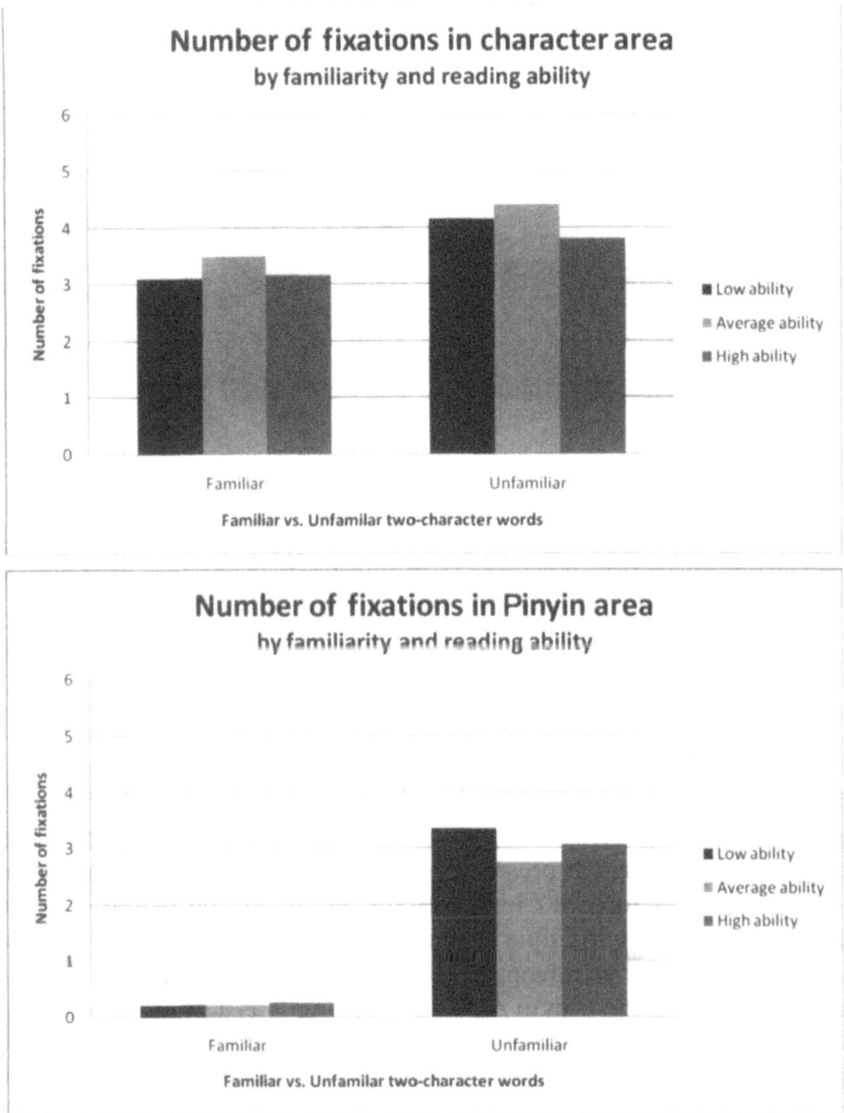

Figure 17.5 Contrast between familiar and unfamiliar two-character words in the full-Pinyin condition. Top panel shows mean number of fixations for the character area; bottom panel shows mean number of fixations for the Pinyin area.

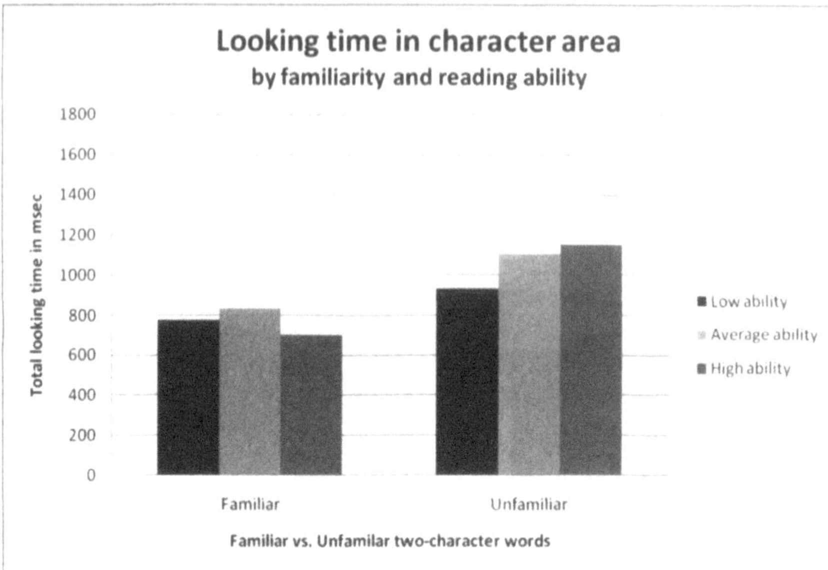

Figure 17.6 Contrast between familiar and unfamiliar two-character words in the full-Pinyin condition. Total looking time for the character area is shown. Results for Pinyin area are not show due to the extremely low incidence of fixations in this area for familiar characters (see Figure 17.5).

Discussion

Han4 yu3 pin1 yin1 (汉语拼音) is a shallow, alphabet-based orthography that provides a way to represent the sound of Chinese characters in the Mandarin dialect. It presents potentially useful cues to support the independent learning of Chinese characters by young readers, yet its use in early reading in China remains controversial. Pinyin could cause young readers to circumvent the hard task of learning to read in Chinese, by reading the Pinyin rather than using it as a guide to learning characters. Its use also may require a level of cognitive control over reading that is difficult for young readers, particularly those with fewer reading skills.

The results reported here suggest that even young children, and even those rated as low-ability readers by their teachers, are able to use Pinyin appropriately—looking at it when confronted by unfamiliar characters and finding it no distraction when presented with familiar characters. Eye-tracking evidence suggests that there is indeed a useful place for Pinyin in teaching young children to learn to read Chinese, and that by second grade, less than a year after children have learned to read Pinyin, they are already able to use it in the process of learning new characters from context.

Acknowledgments

The research reported here was supported in part by NSF grant BCS 00-79973 to the second author. We would also like to acknowledge the contributions of Di Wu, Lang Chen, and An Hong to this project.

References

Bradley, L., & Bryant, P. (1991). Phonological skills before and after learning to read. In S. A. Brady, & D. P. Shankweiler (Eds.), *Phonological processes in literacy: A tribute to Isabelle Y. Liberman* (pp. 37-53). Hillsdale, NJ: Lawrence Erlbaum Associates.

Chen, M. H., & Yuen, J. C. K. (1991). Effects of Pinyin and script type on verbal processing: Comparisons of China, Taiwan, and Hong Kong experience. *International Journal of Behavioral Development, 14,* 429-448.

Cheung, H., & Chen, H. C. (2004). Early orthographic experience modifies both phonological awareness and on-line speech processing. *Language and Cognitive Processes, 19,* 1-28.

Da, J. (1998). *Chinese text computing.* Retrieved from Middle Tennessee State University, Department of Foreign Languages. Web site: http://lingua.mtsu.edu/chinese-computing.

DeFrancis, J. (1984). *The Chinese language: Fact and fantasy.* Honolulu: University of Hawaii Press.

DeFrancis, J. (1989). *Visible speech: The diverse oneness of writing systems.* Honolulu: University of Hawaii Press.

DeFrancis, J. (1996). The prospects for Chinese writing reform. *Sino-Platonic Papers, 171,* 1-26.

Duanmu, S. (2006). Chinese (Mandarin): Phonology. In *The encyclopedia of language and linguistics, 2nd Edition* (Vol.2, pp. 351-355). Oxford, UK: Elsevier Publishing House.

Jenkins, J., & Cook, R. (2006). *Unicode Han database.* Retrieved May 17,

2007, from http://www.unicode.org/Public/5.0.0/ucd/Unihan.html.

Logan, R. K. (1986). *The alphabet effect: The impact of the phonetic alphabet on the development of western civilization.* New York: Morrow.

McBride-Chang, C., Bialystok, E., Chong, K. K. Y., & Li, Y. (2004). Levels of phonological awareness in three cultures. *Journal of Experimental Child Psychology, 89,* 93-111.

Merton, R. K. (1968). The Matthew effect in science. *Science, 159,* 56-63.

Read, C., Zhang, Y., Nie, H., & Ding, B. (1986). The ability to manipulate speech sounds depends on knowing alphabetic spelling. *Cognition, 24,* 31-44.

Spence, J. D. (1984). *The memory palace of Matteo Ricci.* New York: Viking.

Stanovich, K. E. (1986). Matthew effects in reading: Some consequences of individual differences in the acquisition of literacy. *Reading Research Quarterly, 21,* 360-407.

Stroop, J. R. (1935). Studies of interference in serial verbal reactions. *Journal of Experimental Psychology, 18,* 643-662.

von Restorff, H. (1933). Über die Wirkung von Bereichsbildungen im Spurenfeld (The effects of field formation in the trace field). *Psychologische Forschung, 18,* 299-334.

Wu, X., Li, H., & Shu, H. (2002). The role of Pinyin in Chinese children's shared book reading. (in Chinese). *Psychological Science, 25,* 548-551.

Yin, B., & Rohsenow, J. S. (1994). *Modern Chinese characters.* Beijing: Sinolingua.

Section 6
Cultural influences on eye movement

Chapter 18

How we see it: Culturally different eye movement patterns over visual scenes

Julie E. Boland, Hannah Faye Chua, and Richard E. Nisbett

It is blatantly obvious that culture is a powerful predictor of variance in overt human behavior. The foods we eat and the manner in which they are prepared, the holidays that we celebrate, and the languages that we speak are all strongly influenced by our cultural background. Culturally influenced behaviors like these seem to arise from a combination of conscious choices and environmental exposure. As such, cross-cultural differences in human behavior may be fairly superficial, overlaid onto underlyingly similar cognitive and perceptual processes. Alternatively, it is possible that our cultural backgrounds impact our cognition and perception at a more fundamental level. In this chapter, we explore the possibility that culture impacts basic aspects of visual perception.

Are cultural differences shallow or deep?

The superficiality of cultural differences is an assumption that is common in cognitive science. Within the Chomskian tradition of linguistics, this assumption is made explicit: we all share the same language organ, endowed with the same Universal Grammar (e.g., Baker, 2003; Chomsky, 1965). The syntactic differences among the world's languages arise from different settings for a small number of grammatical parameters (e.g., whether the verb starts or ends the verb phrase). Within psycholinguistics, the assumption that we comprehend, produce, and learn a language using the same cognitive mechanisms—regardless of the particular language involved—allows us to generalize experimental findings beyond the language in which the experiments were conducted. Yet, one can maintain the Chomskian assumptions about Universal Grammar and still ask whether habitually using English (or Chinese) influences how we think about the world. Whatever cross-linguistic differences do exist (e.g., in how temporal or spatial relations are expressed) could impact the way that we think within that domain. This is a version of the Sapir-Whorf hypothesis, which, in modified form, continues to capture the interest of cognitive scientists in domains such as color categorization (e.g., Kay & Regier, 2006; Roberson, Davies, & Davidoff, 2000), spatial reasoning (e.g., Majid, Bowerman, Kita, Haun, & Levinson, 2004), temporal comparisons (e.g., Boroditsky, 2001), and grammatical gender (e.g., Lucy, 1992; Sera, Elieff, Forbes, Burch, Rodriguez, & Dubois, 2002).

Of course, language is just one aspect of culture that might influence how we reason about the world, or even how we perceive it. There are numerous dimensions through which cultural differences might impact our thinking, including differences in social structure, educational practices, availability of resources, politeness norms, and so forth. Within the domains of cultural and social psychology, scholars have found that culture impacts a variety of high-level cognitive behaviors such as social judgments and verbal recall of visual scenes (e.g., Chua, Leu, & Nisbett, 2005; Kitayama, Duffy, Kawamura, & Larsen, 2003; Masuda & Nisbett, 2001; Morris & Peng, 1994). Most of this research has contrasted Americans with East Asians, leading to the conclusion that members of the two cultures view the world from quite different perspectives (Nisbett, Peng, Choi, & Norenzayan, 2001). For example, Chua, Leu, and Nisbett (2005) asked participants to recall everyday social events, including personal events and events concerning others. Regardless of the type of event, Americans recalled more events about the main character than East Asians did, and Americans were more likely than East Asians to mention the character's intentions.

Overall, this line of cross-cultural research has shown that Americans are inclined to focus their attention on central objects or entities, analyzing them in terms of their attributes, and categorizing objects in order to reason about them. The causal attributions of Americans tend to focus on the object in question, ignoring the broader context. In contrast, East Asians are likely to consider the broader context of the situation, noticing relationships and changes. East Asians are more likely to group objects based on family resemblance rather than category membership, and the causal attributions of East Asians tend to emphasize the context rather than unique properties of the central object. However, at just which representational levels culture influences cognitive processing has been unclear: Do East Asians and Americans really perceive the world differently? Or have we just been trained to interpret the task demands of each experiment differently?

Evidence from memory and change-detection paradigms

Most of the observed cultural effects rely upon off-line self-report, so it is possible that Americans and East Asians interpret the tasks differently, rather than actually experiencing the world differently. To illustrate, consider Masuda and Nisbett (2001), who asked Japanese and Americans to view 20-second underwater animations twice and then describe the animations from memory. In the animations, certain fish were considered focal on the basis of size, movement, etc. The animations also contained background fish, as well as other background objects, such as plants. During the recall phase, the Japanese participants mentioned background fish and objects 65% more than the American participants. Furthermore, after all ten videos were observed and tested, participants were given a recognition test in which they saw pictures of fish and were asked whether they had seen that fish in any of the ten videos. Although both Americans and Japanese participants correctly recognized focal fish against the original background, or against a white background, Americans were better at recognizing the fish if it was presented against a novel underwater background. Both the Japanese tendency to report more background fish and their difficulty recognizing a familiar fish on a novel background could be explained by differences in encoding the pictures: i.e., Japanese participants (more so than the Americans) encoded visual features from the background together with properties of the focal fish, such that properties of the fish could not be recalled without also recalling details about the context. Alternatively, Japanese and Americans might have encoded the same visual features from the scene in the same way, but had different response biases, based on cultural differences in what was deemed to be important and relevant. On this account, the Americans didn't mention the background fish because they didn't consider them important, while the Japanese failed to say that they recognized the familiar fish because the different background was considered relevant in their decision.

In another experiment, Masuda and Nisbett (2006) used a change blindness paradigm, in which two images alternated for up to one minute (or until the change was detected). The images were photographs of complex scenes, such as an airport. The difference between the two images was either a change to a focal object or a change to a background object. Each image appeared for 560 ms, with an 80 ms blank interval in between. East Asians detected changes to the focal object and background objects equally quickly, but Americans were faster to detect focal changes than background changes. In contrast to the memory study, this change blindness paradigm seems fairly on-line, but even here, it is not clear exactly how the East Asian and American participants differed. Did they represent the image differently, with the East Asians encoding more background details? Did they adopt different viewing strategies, with the Americans deciding to focus their attention on the focal object to a greater degree? Were the East Asians more adept at making mental comparisons between the current stimulus and their stored representation of the previous stimulus? Did the Americans have a response bias, such that they felt it was more important to report focal changes than background changes?

At the cognitively "shallow" end of the explanatory continuum, the cultural differences might reflect flexible strategies, capable of adapting to the perceived demands of the situation. In this case, the cultural differences reflect culturally different norms about what is deemed to be relevant and/or important in a given situation. At the cognitively "deep" end of the continuum, early enculturation experiences might lead to automatic and inflexible differences in the mechanisms supporting stimulus perception. For example, in the visual domain, East Asians and Americans might show stereotypically different fixation patterns when presented with the same visual scene. Because material close to the fixation point is known to be encoded in greater detail (e.g., Rayner & Bertera, 1979), this would lead to cultural differences in the amount of visual detail encoded for different regions of the scene. Another possible account, falling in between the "shallow" and "deep" endpoints, assumes that stimuli are perceived in the same manner cross-culturally, but that the representations of the information are structured differently, such that different details are most readily available for retrieval.

While it is not clear whether the observed cultural differences arise from differences in strategies, perception, memory, or something else entirely, the behavioral differences are quite stable. Across a range of tasks, Americans seem to emphasize central objects, representing background information only sparsely, while East Asians seem to bind their representations of focal objects together with rich representations of the background. In the current paper, we summarize recent evidence that the differences in overt behavior reflect cognitively deep differences in how information about the stimulus is perceived, rather than cognitively shallow differences in response patterns.

At this point, it is useful to review some well-accepted facts about scene perception. Within 100 ms of first viewing a scene, people can often encode the gist, e.g., "picnic" or "building" (Potter, 1976). Our mental representation of a scene, even after ample viewing time, is a woefully incomplete rendering of the original scene (e.g., Intraub, 1997; Potter, Staub, Rado, & O'Connor, 2002; Rensink, 2002; Simons & Rensink, 2005). Although the initial eye fixation on a scene is often not related to its contents (but rather where the eye happens to land), the following fixations are on the most informative regions of the scene for the task at hand (Henderson & Hollingworth, 1999). As noted above, fixation positions are important because foveated regions (i.e., the center of the fixated area) are encoded in greater detail than peripheral regions (e.g., Rayner & Bertera, 1979).

Can eye-tracking resolve the "shallow vs. deep" question?

In a recent experiment (Chua, Boland, & Nisbett, 2005), we asked graduate students at the University of Michigan to look at a series of pictures with a single focal animal or object and a richly detailed background. Two examples are in Figure 18.1. About half the students were raised in China, and about half were Americans of European descent. The Chinese and American students were drawn from a similar range of academic fields and all received the experimental instructions in English. We wanted a task that would be culturally neutral, so we asked the students to rate the pictures in terms of how much they liked each one. We tracked their eye movements for three seconds while they looked at the picture and verbally reported a rating. After the participants had seen

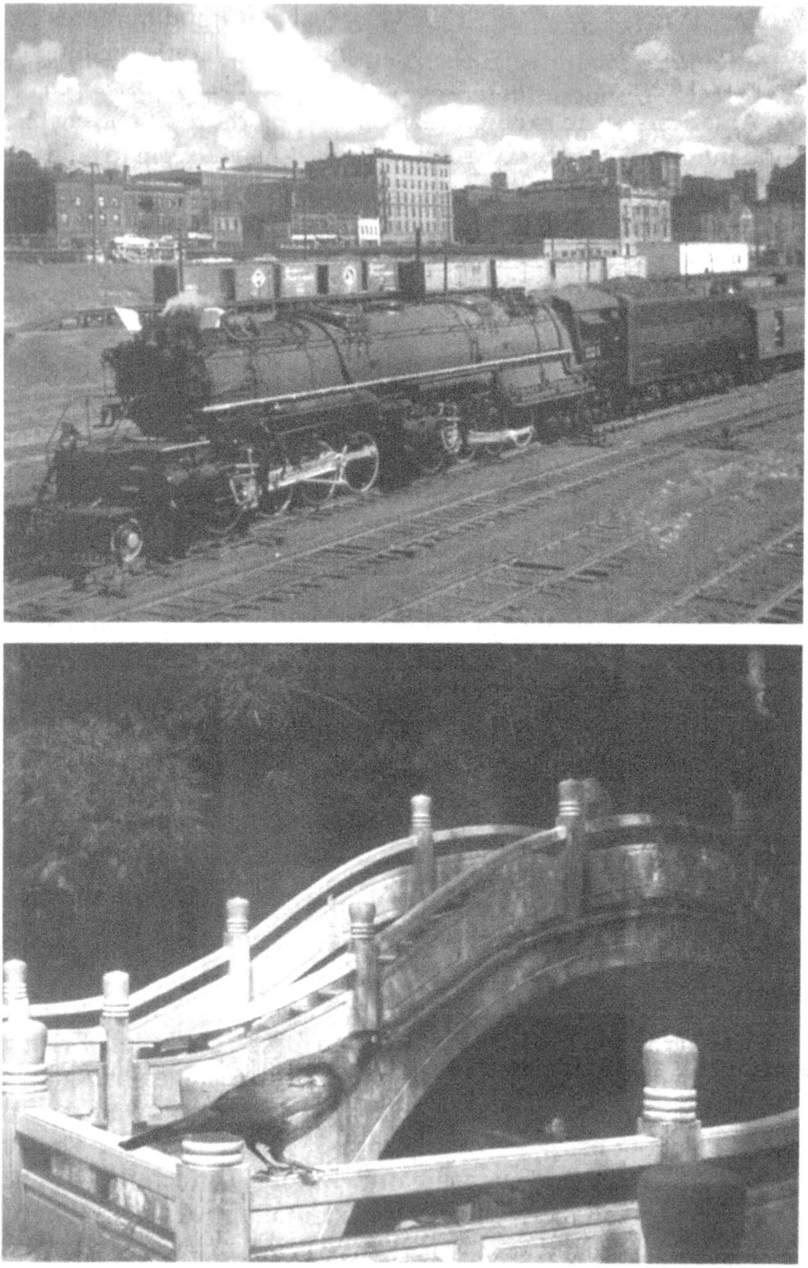

Figure 18.1 Two example scenes from Chua, Boland, and Nisbett (2005) illustrate the range in size and placement of our focal objects and the salience of the background objects. In the train yard picture, the train in the foreground was considered the focal object. In the bird/bridge picture, only the bird was considered the focal object. (*See Plate 12.*)

and rated each of the pictures, they were given an object recognition test, to confirm that we replicated the primary finding from Masuda and Nisbett (2001).

As reported in Masuda and Nisbett (2001), the Chinese participants were less likely than American participants to recognize one of the original focal objects if it was presented against a different background. We were happy to replicate the previous study, but were most interested in the pattern of eye movements during the initial exposure to the stimuli. We categorized each fixation as an object fixation or a background fixation, based on predefined segmentation of the images. Then, for each participant, we calculated several dependent variables: the target of the first saccade, the latency of the first look to the object, the number of saccades ending in a background fixation over a three-second interval, the mean fixation duration for both object fixations and background fixations over the three-second interval, and the probability of an object or background fixation across the three-second interval. Because people have quite limited awareness of their own fixation patterns, we assumed that these dependent measures capture largely unconscious, fairly automatic behavior. We also kept track of two overt judgments: how much participants reported liking the images (the Chinese participants reported liking them more), and how familiar participants rated the images to be in a post-test (Americans rated the pictures as more familiar, although we had taken pains to use primarily culturally neutral images, with a few specifically Chinese and specifically American scenes, in equal numbers).

Perhaps surprisingly, the eye movement patterns revealed cross-cultural differences in nearly every dependent measure we considered. Before the image came on the screen, we had participants look at a central fixation cross. So the first measurable fixation after the image appeared was usually in the center of the screen, where the fixation cross had been. Because our focal objects tended to be off center, this fixation was on the background portion of the scene more often than not. But on the very first saccade, Americans were more likely than Chinese participants to shift their gaze to the focal object. Because of this tendency to immediately orient visual attention toward the focal object, Americans had shorter latencies for the initial fixation on the object than the Chinese participants. The Chinese made more background fixations than the Americans, but because the Chinese fixations were generally shorter than the Americans, the Chinese did not spend significantly more time fixating the background than the Americans. Compared to the Chinese participants, the Americans had substantially longer fixations on objects than on backgrounds.

When we examined the pattern of object and background fixations across the three-second interval, we found that differences in the proportion of object and background fixations for American and Chinese participants began to emerge about 420 ms after stimulus onset. The period during which Americans were more likely to be looking at the focal object than the background spanned 420 to 1100 ms after stimulus onset. There was no temporal interval in which the Chinese participants were more likely to fixate the focal object than the background.

In sum, we did indeed observe cultural differences in the fixation patterns of Chinese and American participants, suggesting that we literally see the world differently. Our findings are consistent with a cognitively deep account of the much-reported cross-cultural differences in American and East Asian behavior. To be clear, we are not suggesting that there are cross-cultural differences in object recognition (i.e., recognizing the central object as a cow) or color perception, or the way in which visual information travels through the visual pathways in the brain. We assume that all of those basic vision processes are universal. The point is that the same stimulus is attended differently by people from different cultures. On one hand, this is not so surprising, because it is well-known that visual attention is influenced by high-level cognition, even if we are not consciously aware of how we are fixating a stimulus; in brief, we fixate regions of the stimulus which are deemed most relevant given the current task demands (Henderson & Hollingworth, 1999). On the other hand, differences in fixation patterns have deep implications for cognition, because only the foveated areas of a visual scene are represented in rich detail. We can't retrieve or reason about details that we don't encode in the first place.

Challenges to Chua, Boland & Nisbett (2005)

The finding that Chinese participants make more and shorter fixations than Americans has now been replicated by Rayner, Li, Williams, Cave, and Well (2007; see also Li, Williams, Cave, Well, & Rayner, this volume), who found that relative fixation durations are consistent across different visual tasks. Rayner et al. compared American and Chinese participants (similar to our participant groups) as well as English-dominant participants with some knowledge of Chinese. However, Rayner et al. reported mixed results with respect to cultural differences in looks to focal objects versus looks to the background. For the 18 scenes in which they were able to define (multiple) focal objects, they report no such cultural difference. For the six scenes[1] that they deemed most like those of Chua, Boland et al. (2005), they report a cross-cultural pattern that is similar to Chua, Boland et al. We will first outline our hypotheses about why they failed to replicate all of our effects in the 18-scene analysis.

Although the overt experimental task differed in the two studies Rayner et al. (2007) told participants that they would be given a memory test on the scenes, we doubt that the task difference was responsible for the diverging findings. While it is plausible that the memory instructions would have caused participants to view the pictures differently than they would have under our instructions, we assume that cultural differences in what is deemed relevant would remain, regardless of a main effect of task. Rather, we believe that differences in our findings are due to differences in the visual stimuli and in how the spatial regions of interest were defined.

In our study, the scenes always had exactly one focal object and its corresponding region of interest followed the contours of the object itself, to minimize the amount of background information that was included in the focal region of interest. In contrast, the 18 scenes that Rayner et al. (2007) analyzed had from one to more than 30 objects that they deemed to be foreground and treated as equivalent to our focal objects. The regions of interest (which never numbered more than six) could contain any number of objects and were always rectangular; thus their foreground regions sometimes contained considerable information that we would have defined as part of the background. For example, there is a kitchen scene in which a little boy is standing at a counter. We would have defined just the boy as the focal object, but Rayner et al. included (as separate foreground regions of interest) the overhead light, and various objects that were on the counter or stove. Another scene, set in an art museum, has just one region of interest, but it includes about 20 people and 15 statues or friezes. The only part of the image not included as foreground is the ceiling and the blank wall above the artwork.

1 For this analysis, Rayner et al. redefined some of their foreground regions as background, in order to make their definition of foreground more like our definition of focal object. Thus, the six-scene analysis is not simply a subset of the data from the 18 scene analysis.

In short, Rayner et al.'s (2007) images are simply not comparable with ours. The total area of their foreground regions tended to be larger than our focal object region, contain many more individual objects, and include portions of the region that we would have defined as background. Correspondingly, they report a dramatically higher proportion of focal-region fixations than Chua, Boland et al. (2005), for both Americans and Chinese. On the first fixation (Figure 4 of Rayner et al.), both the Chinese and American participants were fixated within a focal region about 80% of the time, while they fixated the background region only about 20% of the time. Looks to the focal objects increased on the next fixation for both groups, then fell and leveled off at around 70% looks to the foreground (and 30% looks to the background) for each group. In stark contrast, the first fixation in our study (Chua, Boland et al., Figure 4)[2] was on the focal object only about 30% of the time, for both Chinese and American participants, and our American participants spent roughly equal amounts of time on the focal object and background across the three-second interval, while our Chinese participants spent less time on the foreground than the background.

Clearly, differences in our images and how we defined the regions of interest caused this dramatic difference in the relative proportion of time spent looking at the background. We suspect that these differences are at the heart of Rayner et al.'s (2007) inability to replicate all of the cultural differences that we reported in Chua, Boland et al. (2005). When considering the 18 scenes used in their primary analysis, there seems to have been a difference in the information content of the backgrounds between the two experiments. In designing the Chua, Boland et al. stimuli, we took pains to ensure that the backgrounds were sufficiently interesting to attract a fair amount of attention. This was motivated by our theoretical assumption that Chinese, more so than Americans, gather details from the context that inform their interpretation of focal objects and actions. In other words, we would not predict a cultural difference in looks to the focal object versus looks to the background if the background was a blank wall, or a uniform texture. While the Rayner et al. backgrounds were not featureless, most of the visually interesting features of the images, including rocks, mountains, and distant build-

2 The percentages from the two figures are only roughly equivalent, because Chua, Boland, et al. (2005) graphed the data by time from picture onset, whereas Rayner et al. (2007) graphed the data in terms of fixation number. As a result, the Chua, Boland, et al. values sum to less than 1 (because at a given timepoint, some viewers were saccading rather than fixating), while Rayner et al.'s values sum to 1.

ings, were counted as foreground. Regardless of our intuitions about the images, the relatively few background fixations reported by Rayner et al. raises the concern that there was not sufficient content in the background to elicit a culturally different pattern of fixations. Support for this assertion comes from their analysis of six scenes similar to ours, which revealed similar gaze patterns to those reported in Chua, Boland et al. (2005).

We cannot dismiss the possibility that the Chua, Boland et al. (2005) eye movement results are limited to scenes with a single focal object. While this might seem to be an undesirable constraint, we designed our stimuli in this way because scenes with a single focal object allow for the clearest predictions for cultural differences, as motivated by the theoretical views outlined in Nisbett (2003). When there are multiple focal objects, each object plays a dual role; a given object may be considered focal to the scene, but it is also part of the context for another focal object. To illustrate, consider Li et al.'s (this volume) example of their scene with three bears near a mountaintop. In the 18-scene analysis, the foreground regions included all three bears and the mountaintop. In the six-scene analysis, only the bears were considered focal. Nonetheless, one of the most important aspects of the context for each bear is that it is in the company of two other bears. In a culture, such as Chinese, that stresses relationships over individuals, the perceived relationships (e.g., familial, aggressive, etc.) among the bears may be the most important aspect of the picture. On the other hand, Americans would tend to look at the three bears for the same reason that they looked at a single bear in our study—because the bears are the focal subject matter of the scene. In such cases, Nisbett's theory would not predict any cultural differences in the proportion of looks to the bears versus looks to the mountaintop, sky, and grass.

Some insight into the generalizability of our results can be gleaned from Rayner et al.'s (2007) six-scene analysis. The scenes had from one to three focal objects: a distant silo on the horizon, an elderly man and woman sitting across from each other at a table, a boy on a dock, the rear view of a car parked in front of a house, the three bears described above, and two rams on a snowy mountain. For five of the scenes, regions considered as foreground in the primary analysis were redefined as background for this analysis. Thus, these scenes all had richly detailed, interesting backgrounds and participants divided their gaze fairly evenly between foreground and background elements, as in Chua, Boland et al. (2005). Nonetheless, three of the six scenes had more than one focal animal/person, potentially diluting the cultural differences. We are not surprised therefore, that the predicted interaction was not significant (though they report that their Chinese participants spent significantly less time fixating on the focal objects and made significantly more fixations on the background, compared to the Americans).

In sum, the cross-cultural difference that Rayner et al. (2007) most clearly replicated from Chua, Boland et al. (2005), was that Chinese participants made shorter, more numerous fixations than Americans. Rayner et al. seem to view this as an effect of experience (perhaps language experience) rather than an effect of culture, but it is not clear to us how (or why) one would separate experience from culture. Unfortunately, the research described in Li et al. (this volume) and Rayner et al. was not designed to test cross-cultural theories of cognition. Their failure to replicate some of our findings is neutral with respect to Nisbett (2003)'s theory. Rather, the primary contribution of their very ambitious study is in providing novel insights concerning the stability of eye movements over various tasks. We see this as an important finding, especially given the cross-cultural sampling of their participants.

Open questions and related research

Of course, the Chua, Boland et al. (2005) study leaves many intriguing questions unanswered. What is it about Western and Eastern cultures that gives rise to the differences we observed? As noted at the outset, culture encompasses an amalgam of inter-related phenomena, and merely noting that there is a cross-cultural difference in some behavior is far from offering an explanation about why the differences arise, or how the differences might be generalized to other cultural groups.

One of us has written extensively about differences in eastern and western ways of thinking, and has proposed a general theory about why East Asians tend to behave more holistically in cross-cultural experiments, whereas Americans tend to be more analytic (e.g., Nisbett, Peng, Choi, & Norenzayan, 2001; Nisbett, 2003). The essence of the account is that East Asians depend, to a large degree, on social networks, and that attention to context is crucial for functioning effectively within these complex social structures (Markus & Kitayama, 1991). Westerners, on the other hand, function more independently, in less constraining social environments.

Nisbett's (2003) theory provides an account at a societal level, but it does not explain how a generic brain gets taught to exhibit the Chinese fixation pattern or the American fixation pattern. Our thoughts on this matter are quite speculative, but we do believe that the differences must arise from very early childhood experiences, prior to schooling. Childrearing practices are clearly influenced by societal differences, and reported differences in child-directed language could contribute to the fixation differences that Chua, Boland et al. (2005) observed. For example, Fernald and Morikawa (1993) found that American mothers tend to label objects for very young children, while Japanese mothers use more verbs, and use objects to engage very young children in social routines. Tardif, Gelman, and Xu (1999) found similar East/West differences when comparing English speaking mothers and Mandarin Chinese speaking mothers. Tardif and her colleagues also reported that the predominance of nouns in the early vocabularies of American children (and children from many other Western cultures) is not mirrored in the early vocabularies of Chinese children, which contain a larger proportion of predicates. Crucially, predicates often specify relations among objects. If Western children are encouraged from an early age to focus their attention narrowly on objects, while East Asian children are encouraged to understand the relations among different entities from an early age, this might be an important factor leading to the differences in orienting and sustaining visual attention that we observed in the eye movement study.

Finally, we confess to having done little since our paper was published to explore how the Chua, Boland et al. (2005) data generalize to eye movements for other cultural groups. (Though we have found that relatively interdependent Southern Italians group objects more thematically, and less categorically, than more independent Northern Italians (Knight & Nisbett, 2007). If our speculations above have any merit, then an analysis of child-directed speech might lead to clear predictions about which cultural groups should exhibit the American fixation pattern and which cultural groups should exhibit the Chinese pattern. More generally, one could predict that cultures that rely heavily on complex social networks should exhibit the Chinese pattern, and cultures with a more individualistic emphasis should exhibit the American pattern.

There is some support for the more general prediction: Bailey, Chuah, Siebold, LaBianca, and Bailey (2007) recently replicated our American pattern of eye movements with both American and Caribbean participants, and replicated our Chinese pattern with both Korean and Latin

American participants. As in our study, there was a single focal object against a richly featured background that comprised the majority of the image, e.g., a koala in a forest. And as in our study, Americans divided their time about equally between the focal object and the background regions during the three-second viewing interval. Thus, the Bailey et al. experiment provides an excellent testing ground for Nisbett's (2003) account of cross-cultural differences. The really interesting novel finding is that people from a Western culture (i.e., the Latin Americans) patterned like the Asian groups that have featured most prominently in Nisbett's account. Because Hispanic culture is often viewed as more wholistic than other American cultures (Hofstede, 1980; Hampden-Turner & Trompenaars, 1993; Triandis, 1995; Triandis, Marin, Betancourt, Lisansky, & Chang, 1984), these new results suggest that social and familial organization may be the most important factors driving the early experiences that lead to the cultural differences in how we allocate our visual attention.

In sum, there is growing evidence that cultural differences impact cognition in surprisingly deep ways. A clear implication of the Chua, Boland et al. (2005) finding, and related research by Bailey et al. (2007), is that differences in socialization, experience, or expertise can impact even highly automated, unconscious behaviors, such as eye movements, expanding the domain in which cultural variation is understood to impact cognition and perception.

References

Bailey, K. G. D., Chuah, M., Siebold, L. C., Labianca, Ø., & Bailey, R. N. (2007, May). *Cultural background affects eye movements during scene perception*. Poster presented at the 79th Annual Meeting of the Midwestern Psychological Association, Chicago, IL.

Baker, M. C. (2001). *The atoms of language: The mind's hidden rules of grammar*. New York: Basic Books.

Boroditsky, L. (2001). Does language shape thought? English and Mandarin speakers' conceptions of time. *Cognitive Psychology, 43*, 1-22.

Chomsky, N. (1965). *Aspects of the theory of syntax*. Cambridge, MA: MIT Press.

Chua, H. F., Boland, J. E., & Nisbett, R. E. (2005). Cultural variation in eye movements during scene perception. *Proceedings of the National Academy of Science, 102*, 12629-12633.

Fernald, A., & Morikawa, H. (1993). Common themes and cultural variations in Japanese and American mothers' speech to infants. *Child Development, 64,* 637-656.

Hampden-Turner, C., & Trompenaars, A. (1993). *The seven cultures of capitalism: Value systems for creating wealth in the United States, Japan, Germany, France, Britain, Sweden, and the Netherlands.* New York: Doubleday.

Henderson, J. H., & Hollingworth, A. (1999). High level scene perception. *Annual Review of Psychology, 50,* 243-271.

Hofstede, G. (1980). *Culture's consequences.* Beverly Hills, CA: Sage.

Intraub, H. (1997). The representation of visual scenes. *Trends in Cognitive Sciences, 1,* 217-222.

Kay, P., & Regier, T. (2006). Language, thought and color: Recent developments. *Trends in Cognitive Sciences, 10,* 51-54.

Kitayama, S., Duffy, S., Kawamura, T., & Larsen, J. T. (2003). Perceiving an object and its context in different cultures: A cultural new look. *Psychological Science, 14,* 201-206.

Knight, N., & Nisbett, R. E. (2007). Culture, class and cognition: Evidence from Italy. *Journal of Cognition and Culture, 7,* 283-291.

Li, X., Williams, C. C., Cave, K. R., Well, A. D., & Rayner, K. (this volume). Eye movements, individual differences, and cultural effects.

Lucy, J. (1992). *Grammatical categories and cognition: A case study of the linguistic relativity hypothesis.* Cambridge,UK: Cambridge University Press.

Majid, A., Bowerman, M., Kita, S., Haun, D. B. M., & Levinson, S. C. (2004). Can language restructure cognition? The case for space. *Trends in Cognitive Sciences, 8,* 108-114.

Markus, H. R., & Kitayama, S. (1991). Culture and the self: Implications for cognition, emotion, and motivation. *Psychological Review, 98,* 224-253.

Masuda, T., & Nisbett, R. E. (2001). Attending holistically versus analytically: Comparing the context sensitivity of Japanese and Americans. *Journal of Personality and Social Psychology, 81,* 922-934.

Masuda, T., & Nisbett, R. E. (2006). Culture and change blindness. *Cognitive Science, 30,* 381-389.

Morris, M. W., & Peng, K. (1994). Culture and cause: American and Chinese attributions for social and physical events. *Journal of Personality and Social Psychology, 67,* 949-971.

Miyamoto, Y., Nisbett, R. E., & Masuda, T. (2006). Culture and physical environment: Holistic versus analytic perceptual affordances. *Psy-*

chological Science, 17, 113-119.
Nisbett, R. E. (2003). *The geography of thought: How Asians and Westerners think differently... and why.* New York: The Free Press.
Nisbett, R. E., Peng, K., Choi, I., & Norenzayan, A. (2001). Culture and systems of thought: Holistic vs. analytic cognition. *Psychological Review, 108,* 291-310.
Potter, M. C. (1976). Short term conceptual memory for pictures. *Journal of Experimental Psychology: Human Learning, 2,* 509-522.
Potter, M. C., Staub, A., Rado, J., & O'Connor, D. H. (2002). Recognition memory for briefly presented pictures: The time course of rapid forgetting. *Journal of Experimental Psychology: Human Perception and Performance, 28,* 1163-1175.
Rayner, K., & Bertera, J. H. (1979). Reading without a fovea. *Science, 206,* 468-469.
Rayner, K., Li, X., Williams, C. C., Cave, K. R., & Well, A. D. (2007) Eye movements during information processing tasks: Individual differences and cultural effects. *Vision Research, 47,* 2714-2726.
Rensink, R. A. (2002). Change detection. *Annual Review of Psychology, 53,* 245-277.
Roberson, D., Davies, I., & Davidoff, J. (2000). Color categories are not universal: Replications and new evidence from a stone-age culture. *Journal of Experimental Psychology: General, 129,* 369-398.
Sera, M. D., Elieff, C., Forbes, J., Burch, M. C., Rodriguez, W., & Dubois, D. P. (2002). When language affects cognition and when it does not: an analysis of grammatical gender and classification. *Journal of Experimental Psychology: General, 131,* 377-397.
Simons, D. J., & Rensink, R. A. (2005). Change blindness: Past, present, and future. *Trends in Cognitive Sciences, 9,* 16-20.
Tardif, T., Gelman, S. A., & Xu, F.(1999). Putting the `noun bias ' in context: A comparison of English and Mandarin. *Child Development, 70,* 620-635.
Triandis, H. C. (1995). Individualism and Collectivism. Boulder, CO: Westview Press.
Triandis, H. C., Marin, G., Betancourt, H., & Chang, B. H. (1984). Simpatia as a cultural script of Hispanics. *Journal of Personality and Social Psychology, 47,* 1363-1375.

Chapter 19

Eye movements, individual differences, and cultural effects

Xingshan Li, Carrick C. Williams, Kyle R. Cave, Arnold D. Well, and Keith Rayner

In this chapter, we address two issues. First, how stable are eye movement measures (fixation duration and saccade length) across a number of different tasks? If a viewer's fixation durations and saccade lengths are long in one task, are they long in other tasks as well? Second, how does culture influence eye movements? Specifically, do Chinese and American participants differ across tasks in terms of their eye-movement behavior? The chapter is based on a large investigation we reported elsewhere (see Li, Rayner, Williams, Cave, & Well, 2007; Rayner, Li, Williams, Cave, & Well, 2007) in which American and Chinese participants engaged in the following tasks (as their eye movements were recorded): reading, scene perception, face perception, and visual search. We will first discuss the issue of stability of eye movements across tasks and then turn to the issue of cultural influences on eye movements.

Are eye movements stable across tasks?

Andrews and Coppolla (1999) reported the only prior study examining the stability of eye movements across tasks. The eye movements of fifteen viewers were examined in five different situations: (a) darkness, (b) viewing simple textured patterns (different combinations of dots, squares, and lines), (c) scene perception, (d) visual search, and (e) reading. In the darkness condition, viewers were instructed to keep their eyes open with their gaze straight ahead while they sat in a light-tight room. In the scene viewing task, five photographs of picturesque scenes were used; in the search task, five pages from the children's book *The Great Waldo Search* were used (and viewers had to locate Waldo). The reading material was taken from a number of sources.

Andrews and Coppola (1999) concluded (based on correlation and principal components analyses of their data) that the visual environment had a significant effect on eye movements, but that idiosyncrasies were also evident. For example, fixation duration and saccade size for scene viewing correlated with those same parameters when looking at visual patterns and also in the absence of visual stimulation. Conversely, eye-movement parameters during reading and visual search correlated with one another, but did not correlate with scene viewing, simple patterns, or in the dark. However, as we noted elsewhere (see Rayner et al., 2007), there are potential problems with the study. First, only a small number of stimuli were used in the scene perception, search, and simple pattern tasks, and the stimuli were used repeatedly. Thus, viewers may have been very familiar with each stimulus pattern and this could have easily influenced their eye movements. Second, the letters were rather large in the reading task. Third, although a considerable amount of data was obtained from each participant, given that correlation and principal component analyses were utilized, the number of participants was on the low side. In our study, we used more participants and more stimuli, as well as a wider range of information processing tasks, in an attempt to provide a more complete answer to the issue of how stable eye movements are across different tasks.

In our research, we compared the eye movements of participants as they (a) read English sentences, (b) examined faces in anticipation of a memory test, (c) examined scenes in anticipation of a memory test, (d) searched for a target in a standard visual search task, (e) counted the number of times a Chinese character occurred in a passage of text, or (f) searched for a Chinese character. In addition, all participants with knowledge of Chinese read the Chinese sentences. We used more tasks than Andrews and Coppola (1999) used in an attempt to obtain more reliable data. Furthermore, the tasks used are highly representative of those used in many eye-movement studies (Rayner, 1998).

The study included 74 participants who were divided into three groups (depending on their knowledge of and fluency with Chinese and English). The *native English* speaking group (who we will refer to as the *American* group) consisted of 24 participants; they attended school in the United States, and learned to read English in elementary school, but had no knowledge of Chinese. The *native Chinese* group consisted of 23 native speaking Chinese participants who attended school in China, learned to read Chinese in elementary school, studied English in middle school in China, and were fairly fluent in English. Though they could read Chinese and English, because they came to the United States after their college education, we call them native Chinese to distinguish them from the third group. The *bilingual* group[1] consisted of 27 participants. Thirteen of them had Chinese parents, but they were born in the United States or moved to the United States before the age of five, and they attended school and learned to read English in the United States. Seven other participants were Chinese who initially learned to read Chinese in elementary school in China, but moved to the United States to attend school before the age of 14. Finally, seven participants in this group were the same as native English readers except they learned to read and speak Chinese in college. Overall, the participants in the study differ in terms of their ability to read English and Chinese, and also in terms of their cultural background. All participants with knowledge of Chinese read Chinese sentences in addition to participating in the other six tasks.

The eye movements of all participants were recorded as they engaged in the various tasks (see Rayner et al., 2007 for further details regarding apparatus and stimuli). We used fixation duration and saccade size as primary indices of temporal and spatial processing in the tasks (see Rayner, 1998). Fixation duration is assumed to reflect the time needed to process the information around fixation and the time needed to plan the next saccade; saccade size is related to how much information can be processed on a fixation and how the next saccade target is selected.

Fixation durations and saccade sizes

Table 19.1 shows the average fixation durations and saccade sizes across the tasks for each group of participants. Across the different groups, visual search and Chinese character search yielded shorter fixation durations (210 ms and 199 ms, respectively) and longer saccades (5.66

1 The term "bilingual" is used for this group as a matter of convenience. All of the participants in the native Chinese group are clearly bilingual (in that they can read and speak both Chinese and English). Indeed, they are more fluent bilinguals than those in the group we have labeled "bilingual". The latter group does not speak or read Chinese nearly as well as they speak and read English.

degrees and 7.1 degrees, respectively) than the other tasks. The reading tasks yielded medium-size fixation durations (254 ms for English and 277 ms for Chinese) and the smallest saccade sizes (2.4 degrees for English and 2.6 degrees for Chinese). The Chinese count task yielded fixation durations (263 ms) that were similar to reading, but saccade size was somewhat larger (3.75 degrees). Face processing and scene perception yielded fairly long fixations (291 ms and 280 ms, respectively) and large saccades (3.86 degrees and 5.26 degrees) for all participant groups except the bilinguals, who had the longest fixation durations (330 ms) in the Chinese reading task (and also smaller saccades, 1.84 degrees). Most participants in this group acknowledged that their understanding of Chinese speech (which was generally good) exceeded their ability to read Chinese. Their long fixation durations and short saccade sizes are consistent with this fact.

Table 19.1 Mean fixation duration (ms) and saccade size (degrees) for the different groups of participants

Group	English reading	Face processing	Scene perception	Visual search	Chinese count	Chinese search	Chinese reading
			Fixation duration				
American (n=24)	247	296	289	209	277	204	-
Chinese (n=23)	268	275	264	206	238	193	230
Bilingual (n=27)	246	301	288	215	275	200	330
Total (n=74)	254	291	280	210	263	199	277
			Saccade size				
American (n=24)	2.31	3.96	5.18	5.64	2.97	6.38	-
Chinese (n=23)	2.19	3.73	5.21	5.45	4.29	7.41	3.26
Bilingual (n=27)	2.65	3.89	5.38	5.87	3.97	7.47	1.84
Total (n=74)	2.40	3.86	5.26	5.66	3.75	7.10	2.60

For the Chinese, fixation durations were similar for English reading (268 ms), face processing (275 ms), and scene perception (264 ms), and considerably shorter for visual search (206 ms) and Chinese search (193 ms). Fixation durations in the Chinese count task (238 ms) and Chinese reading (230) were similar and intermediate between the other two task categories. For the Americans and Bilinguals, in contrast, fixation durations were longer for face processing (296 ms and 301 ms) and scene perception (289 ms and 288 ms) than for English reading (247 ms and 246 ms). For the visual search task and the Chinese search task, there were no differences across the three groups. In contrast, the Chinese had shorter fixation durations in the Chinese count task (238 ms) than either the Americans (277 ms) or the Bilinguals (275 ms). Fixation durations were much shorter for the Chinese (230 ms) when reading Chinese than for the Bilinguals (330 ms) when reading Chinese, which is further evidence that the Bilingual group was not as comfortable with Chinese as the native Chinese. Finally, the Chinese fixations were shorter when reading Chinese (230 ms) than when reading English (268 ms).

The fixation duration results are generally quite consistent with what is known about fixation times in the various tasks (see Rayner, 1998). Most prior research has indicated that fixation times are longer for scene perception than reading, and that was again the case in the present study (see also Castelhano & Rayner, this volume). On the other hand, fixations were considerably shorter in the visual search tasks than for the reading task; Rayner (1998) reported just the opposite (collapsed across a number of studies). However, many recent studies have yielded fixation times in visual search tasks that, like the present study, are quite short (Greene & Rayner, 2000a, 2000b). In reality, there is probably a lot of variability in mean fixation duration in visual search tasks as a function of the exact nature of the task and stimuli.

In contrast to the fixation duration data, which showed some clear differences due to task and culture, there were fewer such differences in the saccade length data. There were obvious differences in saccade size due to task, with English reading yielding the shortest saccades (2.4 degrees) and the Chinese search task yielding the longest saccades (7.1 degrees). Scene perception and visual search both yielded average saccade sizes that were on the order of 5.5 degrees, and the face processing and Chinese count tasks yielded average saccade sizes that were on the order of 3.8 degrees. Across the three groups, saccade size tended to be quite similar for most of the tasks, with the main differences involving those where knowledge of Chinese led to longer saccades (in both the Chinese count and search tasks). Specifically, saccade size in the Chinese character count task (2.97 degrees) and the Chinese character search task (6.38 degrees) was smaller for the Americans than for the Chinese and Bilinguals. Finally, consistent with the view that the Bilinguals were not as skilled in reading Chinese, they made smaller saccades (1.84 degrees) than did the Chinese (3.26 degrees) while reading Chinese.

Correlations across tasks

To determine how stable the eye-movement data were across tasks, correlations were calculated to examine individual differences in the eye-movement measures. A strong positive correlation between two tasks for fixation duration, for example, would indicate that participants with longer fixation durations in one task also tended to have longer durations in the other. Table 19.2 shows the correlations collapsed across the participants. Obviously, the correlations involving Chinese reading could only be carried out with the participants who could read Chinese. The other correlations are based on the entire set of 74 participants. Although separate correlations were calculated for each of the three participant groups, we will not discuss those correlations in any detail here (see Rayner et al., 2007, for further details).

English reading was significantly correlated only with visual search and Chinese character search. This result is in agreement with the results reported previously by Andrews and Coppola (1999): They found that fixations durations in reading correlated significantly with fixation durations in visual search, but not in scene perception. Thus, participants who had long fixation durations in reading tended to have long fixation durations in search, but this relationship did not hold for scenes. While the correlation between English reading and scene perception was .18 (collapsed across all participants), there was a significant correlation for the Chinese group, but not for the American and Bilingual groups (see Rayner et al., 2007). However, it is interesting that Chinese reading was significantly correlated with only face processing and Chinese character count and that it did not correlate significantly with scene perception. Fixation durations in all of the other tasks were significantly correlated with each other, with the exception that there was no correlation between Chinese character count and visual search.

The correlations for saccade size yielded fewer significant correlations (see Table 19.2). Saccade size in English reading was significantly correlated with saccade size in scene perception, visual search, and Chi-

Table 19.2 Correlation coefficients for fixation duration (upper panel) and saccade size (bottom panel)

	English reading	Face processing	Scene perception	Visual search	Chinese count	Chinese search	Chinese reading
			Fixation duration				
English reading	-						
Face processing	0.23	-					
Scene perception	0.18	0.83**	-				
Visual search	0.27*	0.48**	0.44**	-			
Chinese count	0.09	0.53**	0.57**	0.18	-		
Chinese search	0.35**	0.53**	0.53**	0.53**	0.43**	-	
Chinese reading	-0.13	0.35*	0.22	0.26	0.56**	0.17	-
			Saccade size				
English reading	-						
Face processing	0.22	-					
Scene perception	0.39**	0.59**	-				
Visual search	0.33**	0.37**	0.27*	-			
Chinese count	0.20	-0.02	0.31**	0.19	-		
Chinese search	0.44**	0.09	0.36**	0.24*	0.54**	-	
Chinese reading	-0.13	0.07	0.10	-0.19	0.26	0.09	-

* p<0.05 **p<0.01

nese character search. Saccade size for face processing was correlated with saccade size in scene perception and visual search, while saccade size in scene perception was correlated with saccade size in all of the other tasks except Chinese reading. Saccade size for Chinese character search was correlated to all of the other tasks except face processing and Chinese reading. Interestingly, saccade size in Chinese reading was not significantly correlated with any other task.

In summary, we found that there was fairly good evidence that eye movements are quite stable across tasks. If participants had long fixations (or long saccades) in one task then they tended to likewise have long fixations (or saccades) in other tasks as well. There were some notable exceptions to this generalization as we have noted above.

How does culture influence eye movements?

In addition to examining the stability of eye movements across different tasks, we also examined the influence of culture on eye movements across the different tasks. Recently, Chua, Boland, and Nisbett (2005; see also Boland, Chua, & Nisbett, this volume) reported that native Chinese and native English speaking participants had different eye-movement patterns when looking at scenes. Specifically, they found that the Americans looked at the foreground objects in their study sooner and longer than the Chinese, and the Chinese were more likely to look at the background information in a scene (and to do so earlier in their looking sequence); they argued that cultural differences related to one's role in society were a causal factor in such an effect. We do not consider our study to be a direct replication of Chua et al.'s study because (a) the task we used (looking at the scene in preparation for a memory test) differed from their task (in which participants rated how much they liked each scene), and (b) our scenes were different from the scenes they used; however, our study did afford us the opportunity to examine this interesting issue.

The influence of language experience on reading and the Chinese related tasks

In order to examine the influence of language experience on reading, participants were categorized into different groups according to their experience with written English or Chinese. For English, Group E1 (n=44) consisted of all participants educated in the United States; Group

E2 (n=7) consisted of Chinese who started to read English in middle school in China, but then came to the United States and studied English in middle or high school for at least 3 years; and Group E3 (n=23) consisted of Chinese participants who started to read English in middle school in China but did not come to the United States until they started graduate school. For Chinese, Group C1 (n=29) consisted of native Chinese speakers who attended elementary school in China; Group C2 (n=7) were English speakers who started to study Chinese in middle or high school in the United States; and Group C3 (n=13) consisted of native English speakers who first started to study Chinese while attending college. In the reading tasks, fixation duration decreased and saccade size increased with increases in reading experience (see Table 19.3). This pattern was evident in both English and Chinese reading (see Rayner et al., 2007, for further details).

In the Chinese-character count and Chinese-character search tasks, fixation duration decreased and saccade size increased with increased knowledge of Chinese (see Table 19.3). Clearly, and not surprisingly, more experience with Chinese led to more efficient processing in the tasks that involved Chinese characters.

Eye movements, culture, and scene perception

To further examine how culture influences eye movements, we analyzed the eye movements in the scene perception task separately in an analysis which included three groups of participants: Native Chinese speakers, native English speakers, and Chinese who were born in the United States or came to the United States by the age of 5 (American-born Chinese, n=13). When looking at scenes, the Chinese had shorter fixation durations, but they also made more fixations than the other two groups[2] (see Table 19.4). Chua et al. (2005) also reported this same result.

Like Chua et al. (2005), we also examined the extent to which native Chinese were more likely to look at the background information and spend less time looking at important objects in the foreground of a scene in comparison to the Americans. We thus selected 18 scenes for which it was quite easy to discriminate the background from the foreground.

2 It is also interesting to note that in the face processing task, the Chinese made more fixations (27.2) than the Americans (25.7) and the Bilinguals (24.9). Thus, in both the face processing task and the scene perception task, the Chinese had shorter fixation durations, but made more fixations than the Americans and Bilinguals. The other task in which the Chinese had markedly shorter fixations than the American and Bilingual groups was the Chinese-character count task. Here, the Chinese actually made fewer fixations (132.5) than the Americans (160.1) or Bilinguals (154.1).

Table 19.3 Fixation duration and saccade size for reading, Chinese-character count and Chinese-character search tasks as a function of experience with written English and Chinese.

	English reading			
	Fixation duration (ms)		Saccade size (degree)	
English level	Mean	Std	Mean	Std
E1	243	5.1	2.5	0.1
E2	266	12.7	2.3	0.2
E3	268	7.0	2.2	0.1
Chinese level	**Chinese reading**			
C1	239	6.2	3.1	0.1
C2	343	14.9	1.8	0.3
C3	363	11.1	1.5	0.2
Chinese level	**Chinese count**			
C1	243	5.2	4.2	0.2
C2	253	11.5	3.9	0.4
C3	289	7.8	3.9	0.3
C4	278	5.5	3.1	0.2
Chinese level	**Chinese search**			
C1	194	3.2	7.5	0.2
C2	190	7.1	7.6	0.5
C3	199	4.8	7.2	0.3
C4	206	3.4	6.5	0.2

Table 19.4 Fixation duration, number of fixations, and saccade size in the scene perception task for different participant groups: Chinese (Chinese who attended school in China and came to the United States after their undergraduate education); Americans (Americans who attended school in the United States); ABChinese (American-born Chinese or Chinese who came to the United States before five years of age and attended school in the United States).

	Fixation duration (ms)		Number of fixations		Saccade size (degree)	
	Mean	Std	Mean	Std	Mean	Std
American	289	7.5	25.3	0.7	5.2	0.2
ABChinese	282	10.1	25.2	1.0	5.4	0.2
Chinese	264	7.6	27.6	0.7	5.2	0.2

The scenes used were both indoor and outdoor photographs that contained people or animals. We identified points of interest in the image and classified these points as foreground and the remainder as background. For example, one scene included three bears on a snowy mountainside. Each bear was selected as a foreground element, as was the mountaintop, and the remaining portions of the scene (e.g., the sky and ground) were identified as background. The number of foreground elements ranged from one to six. A region that encompassed each of these elements was defined as the smallest rectangle that could contain the element and was used for the analyses.

There was no difference between the Chinese and Americans in the mean amount of time spent viewing the background information. Actually, the Chinese (2489 ms) spent slightly less time viewing the background compared to the Americans (2565 ms). There was a nonsignificant tendency for the Chinese (6445 ms) to spend less time looking at the foreground elements than the Americans (6633 ms). Also, given that Chua et al. (2005) reported differences in the amount of time devoted to the background and foreground elements over time, we did a time-epoch analysis in which we examined the proportion of fixations devoted to the foreground elements and background elements for each ordinal fixation (up to the 16th fixation on the scene). However, we found no evidence for different eye-movement patterns over time in looking at the scenes (see Rayner et al., 2007 for further details).

One difference between our study and that of the Chua et al. (2005) study is that they used scenes in which they could clearly identify a single foreground object. Indeed, several of the scenes were originally background-type scenes with a central object added to the scene via photo-editing. This technique allowed Chua et al. to identify the number of objects present in any given scene. Our scenes on the other hand were selected to have multiple points of interest, including people, and the backgrounds were often large areas with no objects of interest. Given these differences, we selected six scenes which we thought were most like their stimuli (with one or two well-defined points of interest, or focal information). With these scenes, we did obtain results which were more consistent with Chua et al.'s findings (see Rayner et al., 2007, for full discussion). Thus, when given a limited number of points of interest in a scene, American and Chinese groups may differ. However, in our view, Chua et al.'s results become less interesting when we take into account the fact that viewers are confined to only a subset of possible scenes.

Discussion

We found that fixation durations tend to be fairly stable across different tasks. For the non-reading tasks, all of the correlations were positive and most were significant. As we noted earlier, saccade length did not correlate as well across tasks as did fixation duration, but when the reading tasks were eliminated, the correlations tended to be positive (and many were significant). Fixation durations in English reading tended to be significantly correlated with the visual search tasks, as reported by Andrews and Coppolla (1999). However, when the groups were considered separately, most of the correlations involving the non-reading tasks were significant, but fixation durations in reading tended to not correlate well with the other tasks, especially for the American and Bilingual groups (see Rayner et al., 2007).

We also found, not surprisingly, that the more experience participants had with either English or Chinese, the shorter the fixations and the longer the saccades. One might argue that this result is more of an effect of experience than of culture. With respect to cultural effects, we didn't find evidence consistent with the claims of Chua et al. (2005) that Chinese spend more time on the background information (and correspondingly less time on the foreground information) than Americans. We think the results reported by Chua et al. (see also the chapter by Boland et al. in this volume) are very intriguing, but we also suspect that they must be viewed with some caution given our results. Actually, as we noted earlier, our study is not a direct replication of Chua et al.'s study. In addition, the scenes differed across the studies and there were task differences (as we noted earlier). Also, Chua et al. used a cut and paste procedure to put a prominent object in the foreground of many scenes. Thus, one might want to argue that their materials may have been better controlled than ours in terms of defining foreground and background. On the other hand, our scenes were all very natural[3] and it was rather easy to differentiate background from foreground. Furthermore, one might argue that if the effect is highly robust then it should emerge in the scenes we used. Although we did not obtain the

3 In some of the scenes used by Chua et al. it appears obvious that a cut-and-paste procedure was used and they don't look fully natural. It is unclear to what extent this might influence their results.

same results as Chua et al. with our overall set of stimuli, we did obtain results that were somewhat similar to theirs when a selected subset of scenes was analyzed. As we noted previously, it isn't clear how interesting the results are if they are limited to certain types of scenes. However, we fully agree with Boland et al. that further research is needed to better elucidate the extent to which culture influences eye movements in scene perception.

We did find some cultural differences in eye movements in that our Chinese participants had systematically shorter fixations in the scene perception, face processing, and Chinese count tasks than the Americans. On the two search tasks, the fixation durations of the Chinese and Americans were quite similar. Naturally, the Americans had shorter fixations when reading English than did the Chinese, and the Chinese had shorter fixations when reading Chinese than English. The shorter fixation durations in the three tasks may provide evidence of a cultural effect. However, it is also important to note that the effect was due to the Chinese trading off number of fixations with fixation duration. In other words, while they made shorter fixations, they also made more fixations (see Figure 19.3). Interestingly, Chua et al. (2005) found similar results as their Chinese participants had shorter fixation durations (on both the foreground object and the background) and more fixations (particularly on the background) than the Americans. An examination of the fixation dispersion in our scenes indicated that there was no difference between the Chinese and Americans in terms of how much of the scene was covered by a fixation. Given the consistency between our results and Chua et al.'s results, shorter fixation durations in the scene and face processing tasks coupled with more fixations might be evidence of a strategy effect that is reflective of a cultural difference between Chinese and Americans. The exact nature of this cultural difference isn't fully clear at this point.

Finally, our Bilingual group participants were more variable overall in their eye-movement behavior than the other two groups, but they clearly were more like the Americans than the Chinese as is clear in Table 19.1. While their understanding and production of Chinese speech was reasonably good, their reading skill was not as good. Thus, they had some difficulty reading the Chinese sentences (their fixation durations were long and their saccade lengths were short), and their fixation durations in the Chinese count task were very similar to those of the Americans. However, as we have noted above, most of them indicated that English was their first language (even though some of them initially learned to speak Chinese).

In summary, our results yielded some important findings. First, there was consistency in eye-movement behavior across individuals over the different tasks. If fixation durations were long on one task, they tended to be long on other tasks; the same tended to be true for saccade size, though not as strongly. Second, eye movements in reading tended to not correlate particularly well with eye movements in the other tasks. Third, experience with a writing system had a large impact on eye movements. Fourth, there wasn't strong evidence overall that Chinese spend more time looking at the background information (and, conversely less time looking at the foreground) than the Americans (though we did find a hint of such an effect with a subset of scenes). Fifth, Chinese fixation durations tended to be systematically shorter than those of Americans in the face perception, scene perception, and Chinese count tasks, but this was largely because the Chinese traded off fixation durations with number of fixations. While eye-movement behavior tends to be fairly stable across tasks, there wasn't strong evidence in favor of the idea that culture systematically modulates eye movements except for the tradeoff we have noted between fixation duration and number of fixations in some of the tasks. Further research is needed to clarify the extent to which there might be cultural effects on eye movements.

Acknowledgments

This research was supported by Grant HD26765 from the National Institute of Health and a Grant from the Microsoft Corporation. We thank Barbara Juhasz for help in preparing the stimuli.

References

Andrews, T. J., & Coppola, D. M. (1999). Idiosyncratic characteristics of saccadic eye movements when viewing different visual environments. *Vision Research, 39*, 2947-2953.

Chua, H. F., Boland, J. E., & Nisbett, R. E. (2005). Cultural variation in eye movements during scene perception. *Proceedings of the National Academy of Sciences, 102*, 12629-12633.

Greene, H. H., & Rayner, K. (2001a). Eye movement control in direction-coded visual search. *Perception, 30,* 147-157.

Greene, H. H., & Rayner, K. (2001b). Eye movements and familiarity effects in visual search. *Vision Research, 41,* 3763-3773.

Li, X., Rayner, K., Williams, C. C., Cave, K. R., & Well, A. D. (2007). Eye movements and individual differences. *Visual Cognition, 15,* 105-108.

Rayner, K. (1998). Eye movements in reading and information processing: 20 years of research. *Psychological Bulletin, 124,* 372-422.

Rayner, K., Li, X., Williams, C. C., Cave, K. R., & Well, A. D. (2007). Eye movements during information processing tasks: Individual differences and cultural effects. *Vision Research, 47,* 2714-2726.

Chapter 20

Orthography and eye movements: The paraorthographic linkage hypothesis

Gary Feng

The past decade has witnessed spectacular success in understanding of eye movements during reading. Numerous computational models have been proposed to account for eye movements of skilled readers of English and related orthographies (Engbert, Nuthmann, Richter, & Kliegl, 2005, Feng, 2003, Legge, Klitz, & Tjan, 1997; Pollatsek, Reichle, & Rayner, this volume; Reichle, Pollatsek, Fisher, & Rayner, 1998; Reichle, Rayner, & Pollatsek, 2003; Reilly & O'Regan, 1998; Richter, Engbert, & Kliegl, 2006; Risse, Engbert, & Kliegl, this volume; Shillcock, Ellison, & Monaghan, 2000). This volume marks a significant new development as one of the most influential reading eye movement models, the E-Z Reader (Reichle, et al., 1998; Pollatsek et al., this volume), is extended to Chinese, a very different script from English (Rayner, Li, & Pollatsek, this volume; Rayner, Li, & Pollatsek, 2007). Amidst this great achievement and high expectations, it is perhaps time to reflect on the success of current theories and the prospect of a universal theory of reading.

The starting point of this chapter is what I shall call the *trinity of the word*, an often unstated assumption that the word is the basic unit of foveal (and parafoveal) word recognition, reading comprehension, and oculomotor planning. The notion of the word as a common unit linking sub-processes of reading is the common denominator of virtually all eye movement theories. This is obviously a problem for reading unspaced scripts such as Chinese, Japanese, and Latin before the introduction of spaces and punctuations.

This chapter advocates an alternative view that sees skilled reading processes as an optimal exploitation of the writing system in order to achieve maximal reading efficiency. Seen in this light, the *trinity of the word* is a convenient hypothesis, not a theoretical necessity. For linguistic and historical reasons, it works extremely well in English. But its utility ultimately depends on the nature of the *paraorthography*[1]—the use of punctuations and spaces—of a script. The history of paraorthography reveals an intriguing co-evolution between reading processes and paraorthogrphic conventions, where medieval readers struggled to adapt to the script but meanwhile constantly invented and adopted new paraorthographic symbols to facilitate oculomotor planning. Underneath seemingly haphazard historical changes the purpose is unambiguous—to embed clues in the script to optimize the coordination of reading processes.

We conclude the journey, which spans several millennia and disciplines, with the *Paraorthographic Linkage Hypothesis* (PoLH), a synthesis of psychological, linguistic, and historical observations on orthography and eye movements. The gist of the PoLH is that the mechanism of skilled reading is the product of an optimization process, not the other way around. To the extent all scripts provide useful statistical cues in the texts, readers will exploit the information in a way that maximizes reading efficiency, with or without the notion of words.

Words in reading eye movement models

Here is one way to appreciate the challenge of programming eye movements during reading: An average fixation lasts somewhere between 200 and 250 ms (Feng, 2003; McConkie, Kerr, & Dyre, 1994; Rayner, 1998), during which time the reader has to recognize written symbols in the fovea (and perhaps the parafovea), do syntactic and semantic analyses, and plan the next eye movement. According to Sereno and Rayner (2003), it takes approximately 60 ms for the retinal image to reach the vi-

1 Paraorthography is a term coined by the author; it refers to a set of graphical symbols and conventions that do not denote linguistic information themselves but help to highlight, disambiguate, or otherwise augment the main orthographical glyphs. In English, for example, paraorthographic symbols include spaces and punctuations, and paraorthographic conventions include capitalization, paragraph initial indentation, etc. The concept will be defined in the last section.

sual cortex, and another 100 ms or so for oculomotor planning. These physiological constraints leave very limited time for visual word recognition and language processing. Meanwhile, ERP evidence suggests that the earliest word frequency effects occur approximately 150 ms after the fixation onset and many syntactic and semantic effects show up much later, around 400 to 600 ms. Your assignment: Fit all these processes into a 200-250 ms fixation.

Obviously, a serial processing strategy will not work. The idea that the eyes randomly sample texts along a line—thus avoiding any linguistic constraints—has also been rejected long ago (Haber, 1976, Rayner, 1978; see also Rayner, 1998). A viable model needs to parallelize visual, oculomotor, and language processes in order to compress processing time. But these processes are naturally interlocked: One needs the output of another to proceed. The knack is to discover what elements can run in parallel and what cues can be used to coordinate these intricate actions.

Words appear to do the trick. Once words are recognized, sentence comprehension seems automatic—reminiscent of the Simple View of Reading (Hoover & Gough, 1990). It suggests that post-lexical processes could be excluded from the 200 ms limit, a major time saver. In addition, spaces between words make saccade programming easier (Juhasz, Inhoff, & Rayner, 2005; Pollatsek & Rayner, 1982). They are also important in foveal word recognition. Word recognition is most efficient at the *optimal viewing position* (OVP), which is generally at the center of the word (O'Regan, 1990; O'Regan & Jacobs, 1992). In continuous reading, McConkie and colleagues (McConkie, Kerr, Reddix, & Zola, 1988) showed that saccades are targeted at word centers, although oculomotor errors can skew the actual landing location (Rayner, 1979).

Theories of reading eye movement control

This review is not intended to be a comprehensive survey of models of reading eye movement control; rather, it illustrates how processing time could be squeezed into a 200 ms or so fixation by exploiting the notion of words in different ways.

A good starting point is the Morrison model. Morrison (1984) hypothesized that words are processed serially, and saccades are programmed to target the next word. In the case the next word is identified in parafoveal vision while waiting for oculomotor planning, the saccade target may be skipped. Fixation duration is determined by lexical processing time, plus the time to prepare the next saccade, and minus the benefit from parafoveal processing during the previous fixation. The

Morrison model achieved two parallel processes. By dropping post-lexical language processes out of the picture, Morrison implicitly assumed that they run in parallel with other processes. The hallmark of the Morrison theory is the parallelization of parafoveal previewing and oculomotor programming; foveal word recognition and saccade programming remain serial processes.

The E-Z Reader model (Pollatsek et al., this volume; Reichle et al., 1998, 2003) is the latest and most influential extension of the Morrison framework. A prominent change is the proposed L_1/L_2[2] stages in lexical processing. By allowing saccade programming to begin at the completion of L_1, as opposed to after L_2 (as in Morrison's model), E-Z Reader allows more overlapping between lexical access and saccade planning. The word is also the basis for saccade programming. The implementation of the OVP effect (the eccentricity variable), for example, awards fixations landed near OVP with addition savings in recognition time. It does inherit from Morrison (1984) the strict serial foveal and parafoveal processing—the covert attention is only moved to the next word in the parafovea when the foveal word recognition is completed.

SWIFT (Engbert et al., 2005; Risse et al., this volume; Richter et al., 2006) introduced two types of parallel processes. First, all words within the perceptual span are activated in parallel. This affords a lot of flexibility to account for potential interactions among words: for example, the parafoveal-on-foveal effect (Kennedy & Pynte, 2005; White, Rayner, & Liversedge, 2005). The other parallelization disengages saccade preparation from saccade target selection. In SWIFT, the preparation of a saccade happens at the end of L_1, but the target of the saccade is probabilistically determined at the time of saccade execution, based on word activation levels. Fixation duration is largely determined by a random process, but is also under the stochastic influence of the foveal processing ("foveal inhibition"). Overall, SWIFT allows the highest degree of parallelization among current models, based—implicitly or explicitly—on the notion of words.

The Strategy-tactics theory (O'Regan, 1990; Reilly & O'Regan, 1998) also relies heavily on words. The main feature of the model is the division between inter-word saccades and intra-word saccades. The former targets word centers (McConkie et al., 1988) whereas the latter are refixations that try to compensate for eccentric landing locations. Further

2 L_1 was originally called the "Familiarity Check (fc) stage" in Reichle et al. (1998) and L_2 the "Lexical Completion" stage. They have been referred to as simply L_1 and L_2 since Reichle et al. (2003).

reading efficiency is achieved by strategically selecting inter-word saccade targets, e.g., skipping short words and/or fixating long words (Reilly & O'Regan, 1998).

The "ideal observer" approach focuses on the identification of constraints of the problem space and search for optimal solutions. In this tradition, the challenge of eye movement programming is often recast as how to determine the optimal saccade target position in order to maximize the efficiency of lexical identification. Mr. Chips, a model which aspires to account for reading with retinal defects (Legge, et al., 1997; Legge, Hooven, Klitz, Mansfield, & Tjan, 2002), meticulously calculates the landing position in order to minimize the ambiguity in word recognition. Similarly, the recent *Split-fovea* model (Shillcock, et al., 2000; McDonald, Carpenter, & Shillcock, 2005) also focuses on optimizing landing position to ensure equal distribution of lexical information between the two hemispheres. The suggestion from these ideal observer models is clear: pre-position the landing location of the next fixation to facilitate foveal word recognition. In the presence of oculomotor noise, this optimal theoretical solution can be well approximated by the heuristics of always targeting word centers (Legge et al., 1997).

Troubles with spaces

Every aforementioned model requires texts to be pre-segmented into words. Removing spaces will disrupt saccade programming, slow down word recognition (and perhaps disable parafoveal previewing), and greatly increase ambiguities in sentence processing. Reading will be disorganized and deficient, if not downright impossible, according to these models.

There are, however, writing systems that do not visually mark word boundaries in any way. Chinese, Japanese, and Thai are contemporary examples. And until the 12th century or so Latin, Greek, and other European languages were typically written unsegmented. Together, these comprise most of the human written history and a large portion of readers in the world today.

From the perspective of a word-based theory, the lack of word marking presents a challenge because the perceptual unit (letters, characters, or other glyphs) that serves as the basis for saccade programming is disconnected from the unit of language processing, i.e., words. In other words, oculomotor and linguistic processes run on different tracks, complicating the coordination of reading sub-processes. Some difficult choices have to be made in adapting a word-based theory to unsegmented orthographies. Saccade programming could be based on perceptual units (e.g., Yang & McConkie, 1994), but this would lead to random landing positions and thus impede word recognition. Alternatively, one could salvage the word-based hypothesis by assuming that word segmentation occurs inconspicuously in the parafovea. This, however, is a potentially risky assumption. Word parsing in Chinese is notoriously difficult even for linguists (e.g., Duanmu, 1998). It is unlikely that Chinese readers can accomplish this linguistic feat, with only limited preview of upcoming characters, without adding time to the fixation duration. Either way, suboptimal reading performance is predicted for reading unsegmented scripts. This contradicts empirical observations that skilled readers of Chinese and English show remarkable similarities and few differences in eye movement parameters (see Feng, 2006 for a summary).

A potential solution is proposed by Tsai (2002), who suggested instead of identifying the "true" word (in the linguistic sense), saccade planning could be based on a proxy of words. Tsai specifically recommended a statistics based on the co-occurrence of characters, but presumably other shortcuts can work as well to drastically reduce the overhead of word parsing in real time. It is also tempting to justify the current word-centric approach by saying that orthographic words are a proxy to linguistic words.

Although this may appear to be an issue of modeling technique, I argue it represents a significant breach from the word-based tradition. It effectively rejects the often unstated axiom that oculomotor programming is based on the linguistic unit *word*. Instead, it replaces it with a much softer assumption that saccade planning is based on perceptual units (e.g., Chinese characters) in a way that is linked to linguistic processing. The divorce between oculomotor planning and linguistic processes has far reaching consequences. Regarding reading unspaced scripts, it directs research attention to the statistical information in the orthography and connects different processes in reading. Furthermore, it raises questions about the status of the word in reading spaced orthographies such as English. What is a word? Is it conceptually necessary for a theory of reading? Or perhaps it is a marriage of convenience between the oculomotor and linguistic processes?

The illusion of words

What is special about the word that makes it the preferred unit of analysis in eye movement modeling? The justification—at least to English speakers—seems straightforward: Words are the fundamental linguistic unit and, as it happens, they are conveniently individualized in print. This, however, may be a happy linguistic coincidence. In the context of reading, words are not necessarily the most basic, natural, or critical level of linguistic processing. In fact, they are nothing more than what are flanked between spaces.

The elusive word

Despite strong intuitions of (literary) speakers, the word is notoriously hard to define in linguistics (e.g., Coulmas, 2003; Spencer, 1991; Crystal, 1997). A number of criteria have been proposed. For example, an influential definition by the prominent American linguist Leonard Bloomfield referred to *minimal free forms*, i.e., the smallest units of speech that can meaningfully stand on their own. Nonetheless, this leaves out functional words, such as English *the* and *to* or French *de*, which are conventionally written as words but can never stand alone in speech. The criterion of *indivisibility*—that no extra words may be inserted within a word—is intuitive, but it leads to the awkward conclusion that "*kick the bucket*" is a word but "*fantastic*" is not, because Robin Williams once exclaimed "*fan-bloody-tastic*" in the movie *Mrs. Doubtfire*. Individually or together, these criteria do not amount to an accurate, coherent definition of *word* that applies to all human languages and all levels of linguistic analyses (Spencer, 1991; Coulmas, 2003).

A practical solution is to define *word* within each domain of study. For example, *phonological words* can be identified by stress patterns in English or by vowel harmony in Finnish. *Lexical words*, also called the *lemmata or citation forms* (as in dictionary entries), often come to mind as the prototype of words. But what goes into a dictionary is conventional and language-dependent. English happens to allow uninflected root morphemes (e.g., verb infinitives or singular nouns) to stand freely. Latin dictionaries customarily list the first-person singular present tense form of verbs. Modern Arabic, which has no infinitives, uses the third-person singular of the past tense as the citation form of verbs.

The *orthographic word* is arguably the closest to the notion of *word* in reading theories. Orthographic words are "the unit bounded by spaces in the written language" (Crystal, 1997, p. 420), although there are many other conventions to demarcate words (e.g., in Devanagari, letters are grouped by a horizontal head stroke that breaks at word boundaries; Daniels & Bright, 1996). Notions such as "word center", "landing position", and "word length" in the reading literature are clearly based on orthographic words.

Words identified at different levels of linguistic analyses do not necessarily correspond to one another. Some orthographic words (e.g., *a*, *of* and *to*) do not qualify as phonological words. Likewise, phrasal verbs such as "*put up with*" or "*take advantage of*" are effectively units of semantic analyses but are nonetheless orthographically divided. The distinction between compound words and phrases has always been subtle in English, and now instant messaging has made the fine line between *chat-room* and *bathroom* even thinner. Finally, the linguistic notion of words may not be universal. Yuen Ren Chao, the prominent Chinese linguist, concluded, "Not every language has a kind of unit which behaves in most (not to speak all) respects as does the unit called 'word' ... It is therefore a matter of fiat and not a question of fact whether to apply the word 'word' to a type of subunit in the Chinese sentence (1968, p. 136)."

Words are composed of morphemes, the smallest meaningful unit of a language. Words often take on various *grammatical forms* when used in a sentence, and inflections and other morphological changes can dramatically transform the root word. Languages vary greatly in the degree of morphological complexity. At one extreme, *isolating* languages such as Chinese and Vietnamese make little use of inflectional or derivational morphology (e.g., no prefixes or suffixes); *words* are either bare root morphemes or simple compounds of them. At the other end, the entire sentence in a *polysynthetic* language may simply be an inflection of the root morpheme. English has a fairly impoverished inflection system (Booij, 2005; Crystal, 1997). English inflectional morphology is a largely *fusional*, where a single morpheme simultaneously represents a number of morphosyntactic properties.[3] In contrast, *agglutinative* languages such as Turkish and Finnish tend to attach numerous suffixes, each with their own meanings, to the root morpheme (Crystal, 1997; Niemi, Laine, & Tuominen, 1995). This results in a larger number of

3 E.g., the suffix "-s" in walks represents PRESENT-TENSE, THIRD-PERSON, and SINGULAR at the same time.

morphemes per word and thus a longer word on average. It is estimated that Turkish, a language closely related to Finnish, has four times more morphemes per word than English has (Johanson & Csató, 1998).

Implications for reading

No linguistic theory is based on orthographic words. The argument that (orthographic) words are the basic unit of linguistic processing has at least two problems.

Even in English, orthographic words do not correspond to the basic elements in syntactic or semantic analysis. The English-style word marking provides only limited help to the syntactic parser because it does not signal phrasal boundaries at all. In fact, the English orthography disrespects the syntactic boundary between phrases and compound words and frequently breaks compound words into morphemic components (e.g., the *White House*, rather than the *Whitehouse*). On the other hand, English orthographic words are hardly the basic semantic unit either. Although English words tend to be short, it does not mean they are morphologically simple, thanks to its fusional inflection system. English rarely marks morpheme boundaries (e.g., no **cran-berry* or **dis-please-d*; Booij, 2005). This suggests that some words may have to be parsed into morphemes before they are recognized. While most models of visual word recognition (for reviews see Coltheart, Rastle, Perry, Langdon, & Ziegler, 2001; Seidenberg, 2005) do not include morphological analysis, psycholinguistic evidence for morphological analysis in word recognition is paramount (see Reichle & Perfetti, 2003). English readers' gaze duration on a compound word is a function of the frequency of the whole word as well as that of its morphological components (Andrews, Miller, & Rayner, 2004), suggesting a competition between direct access and morphological decomposition (Caramazza, Laudanna, & Romani, 1988; Reichle & Perfetti, 2003).

Across languages, differences in orthographic conventions may entail different processes. When presented with long compound words, Finnish readers' first fixation duration was influenced only by the frequency of the first morpheme but not the second constituent, indicating serial morphological processing in Finnish (Hyönä, Bertram, & Pollatsek, 2004). Reflecting differences in morphology, English compound words in the Andrews et al. study were typically 8-10 letters, whereas the Finnish compound words in the Hyönä et al. study were much longer, approximately 12-18 letters. While the majority of the English compounds received a single fixation, over 90% of the long Finnish compounds were refixated, often for multiple times. When shorter Finnish compound words were used (7-9 letters; Bertram & Hyönä, 2003), Finnish readers switched to an English-like pattern. But given the prevalence of long, morphologically complex words in agglutinative languages, word-based models of eye movement control have to be outfitted with additional mechanisms to deal with within-word eye movement programming.

To summarize, the notion of *words* in reading refers to orthographic words. Orthographic words provide the natural targets for saccade programming by virtue of being separated by spaces. Beyond this, however, they may or may not map onto any meaningful linguistic units, across languages or even within a language. They are, after all, defined by the convention of writing.

Paraorthographical marking and eye-movement planning

The reader may object at this point: Orthographic words may be what are flanked between spaces, but isn't the case that where we put spaces is based on our linguistic intuitions about words? My answer is "no," at least not historically. There is little evidence that a clear sense of the *word*—not as a vague idea but an operational concept—predates the widespread practice of orthographic word segmentation. Moreover, evidence suggests the interesting possibility that our intuition about the word may be an unintended side-effect of the development of conventions to facilitate visual and oculomotor processing.

I will begin this section by turning the clock back 2,000 years. We need to broaden the scope of investigation to include punctuations, because the earliest segmental signs were not spaces. The first obstacle we encounter, though, is notational: Because there is no word for the union of spaces, punctuations, capitalization, and other symbols or conventions that visually parse texts, we need to invent one.

What is paraorthography?

Paraorthography, a neologism, refers to a set of graphic symbols and conventions of a writing system that does not directly transcribe linguistic information but exists to ensure faithful transmission of the written message. "*Para-*" is a Greek prefix meaning *alongside of* or *beyond,* and by extension a *role ancillary* or *subsidiary to a role with higher status.* "*Orthography,*" also of Greek origin, literally means *correct writing.* Just like spoken language, which is aided by *paralinguistic* elements such as body language, pauses, and intonations, written languages exploit a rich set of visual symbols and conventions—punctuations, spaces, capitalization and font variations, page layout, etc.—to ensure and enrich the communication. The prefix "*para-*" is accurate in both historical and functional senses: Paraorthographic systems evolved alongside of writing, and their primary role in writing is to assist and complement the work of the primary orthographic symbols—letters and other glyphs.

While many contemporary definitions of orthography include punctuations and capitalization rules (e.g., Crystal, 1997), these elements receive only sporadic scholastic attention (but see Nunberg, Briscoe, & Huddleston, 2001) and are often left to the hands of prescriptive language pundits (Truss, 2004). The proposal here is to separate the domains of orthography—which concerns itself with transcribing linguistic messages—and paraorthography, the convention (and often an art) of parsing and annotating written messages.

A brief history

Elements of paraorthography are as old as writing itself. For example, a conventional direction of writing—essential for planning eye movements in reading—was present in the Cuneiform writing some 6,000 years ago. Indentation and letter size (*litterae notabiliores*, the large and decorative initial letter of a chapter) were used by 2nd-century B.C. scribes to indicate the beginning of important discourse units such as chapters or paragraphs (Parkes, 2003, p. 10).

However, separation of linguistic elements within major divisions of texts (i.e., paragraphs or arguments) was rare in Latin until the 6th century C.E. Although words in 1st-century Latin monuments and manuscripts were sometimes separated by small points (the *interpunct*; see Parkes, 2003, p. 263), by the end of the 1st century the practice was replaced by the Greek style *scriptio continua*, i.e., writing without any indication of word boundaries or places for pauses. The likely motivation for *scriptio continua* was to present the reader with a neutral text free of interpretations by the scribe: Authoring at the time meant dictating to scribes, who would mechanically write down the sounds without processing (or even understanding) the message. Any markings on surviving manuscripts from this period were likely supplied by later readers rather than the oringinal authors.

The lack of visual segmentation of the text took tolls on the reader as he read the text aloud—the standard practice then. When asked to read an unfamiliar text, the 2nd-century writer, Aulus Gellius, exclaimed,

"How can I read what I do not understand? What I shall read will be confused and not properly phrased" (Parkes, 2003, p. 11). The 4th-century grammarian Servius recorded one of the earliest cases of misparsing by his colleague because of the lack of word spacing: *collectam exilio pubem* ("a people gathered for exile") was mistaken as *collectam ex Ilio pubem* ("a people gathered from Troy") (Parkes, 2003, p. 11). Silent reading was a stunt, far from the norm (Saenger, 1997).

In the 2nd century, systematic punctuations were used chiefly by teachers to help pupils' literacy acquisition. The marks, which would include today's equivalent of spaces, commas, periods, hyphens, stress markers, paragraph markers, etc., were punctuated by the teacher or by students themselves, not authors. By the 5th century, the demand for pre-punctuated texts surged as literacy spread to individuals not familiar with classical literary traditions. The usefulness of punctuations became widely recognized. Conventions of punctuations had emerged by the 5th and the 6th century (Parkes, 2003, p. 13), although individual idiosyncrasies abounded.

Two significant changes occurred during this period. The first is a shift of the function of punctuations. The primary concern for readers before the 5th century was to find sensible places to pause and breathe. For example, large comma-like signs drawn at different heights were used to mark pauses of various lengths. As silent reading became prevalent and as the need for accurate interpretation of Christian Scriptures became paramount, authors began to consciously put in punctuations to guide readers. Punctuation marks now took on a new role as indicators of text structure. For example, the *diple*, a long vertical bar on the margin, was used in the 6th century to indicate direct quotations from the Bible (Parkes, 2003, p. 17).

Another important change is the introduction of spaces between "words," a practice pioneered by Irish scribes at the end of the 7th century to compensate for their lack of familiarity with Latin (Parkes, 2003, p. 23). Slowly this practice spread to Anglo-Saxons scribes, to France, and eventually to most European countries by around the 12th century (Saenger, 1997). Historically, spaces were not always word-bound, though. Saenger (1997, p. 32) documented "aerated scripts," frequently used in the early Middle Ages, where spaces were sparsely used to segment long lines into letter strings approximately 20 letters long. Sometimes minor spaces further divided the text into smaller blocks. The resulting units, though, often did not correspond to meaningful linguistic units or rhetorical pauses. The purpose of the aerated scripts was to assist saccade planning. Saenger maintains that

> *While the reader of aerated script cannot identify a word by its Bouma shape [the outline] or regularly rely on parafoveal vision to glean preliminary information about word meaning, aeration helped the reader to reduce ocular regressions by providing points of reference for orientation of the eye movements within a line of text as the reader grouped letters to form syllables and words. ... Thus, aeration made it possible for the reader to begin the cultivation of cognitive skills that had not been exploited by either the ancient Greeks or Romans. [p. 33]*

It appears highly unlikely that medieval readers had an acute sense of word boundaries but simply refrained themselves from applying that knowledge. The struggle to invent a text segment system supports the alternative hypothesis, where readers of *scriptio continua* did not have a clear intuition of what words were, and the sense of words is a by-product of inserting spaces in texts.

The next defining moment in the evolution of paraorthography was the introduction of printing technologies, which began to standardize shapes and conventions of punctuation marks. This process lasted several centuries after the first moveable type print shops were set up in the late 15th and early 16th centuries (Parkes, 2003, p. 51). A number of other paraorthographic conventions were also established: capitalization of the sentence initial letter, use of line spaces and indentation to indicate paragraphs, use of italic and bold type faces for various marking purposes, etc.

The establishment of paraorthographic conventions has forever changed the reading habit. Paraorthography has become a hard addiction to break. "Lord Timothy" Dexter, the 19th century American eccentric, published his memoir *A Pickle for the Knowing Ones, or Plain Truths in a Homespun Dress* with no punctuations (and plenty of idiosyncratic spelling). In response to the publisher's demands for punctuations, he offered a full page of them in his 2nd edition, along with a note:

> *fouder mister printer the Nowing ones complane of my book the fust edition had no stops I put in A Nuf here and thay may peper and solt it as they plese [Dexter, 1838/2004, p. 36]*

Paraorthographic variations

There are important cross-linguistic differences in paraorthographic conventions. Even within European languages, systematic differences in paraorthography abound. For example, English uses commas to bracket relative clauses, but only for the unrestricted type; in German all relative clauses require commas. German also keeps the tradition to capitalize all major nouns, a practice once popular in English publications but that has been replaced by the current style of only capitalizing sentence initial and proper nouns. The rules for spaces also differ from language to language. English uses spaces liberally, often dividing compound nouns such as "high school" as if they were phrases. Formal distinctions between compounds and phrases, e.g., the differences in stress between "blackbird" and "black bird", escape most native speakers. German, on the other hand, keeps all noun-noun compounds spelled together. Recent spelling reforms attempt to separate other types of compound words, but the reforms are under heated debate and the fate of German compounds is remains to be seen (Johnson, 2005).

While most writing systems today use spaces to some extent, the linguistic units they mark can be quite different. Spaces often mark linguistic units smaller than words. Written Chinese clearly demarcates individual characters, which are always monosyllabic and usually correspond to a single morpheme; words, in the phonological or grammatical sense, are not marked in any way in writing. Japanese, under the influence of Classic Chinese, also leaves no extra spaces between words; its Kana and Kanji characters represent different linguistic units. Kanji (Chinese) characters typically correspond to lexical and phonological words, whereas the kanas correspond to syllables (or moras; Coulmas, 2003). Derived from Devanagari, Thai is a well-known non-spaced, alphabetic orthography. The Thai language is a tonal, uninflected, and predominantly monosyllabic language (Coulmas, 2003). There are polysyllabic loan words, but word boundaries are not indicated with additional spaces. Thai does not use Western punctuation; in fact, it rarely uses any punctuation at all, other than the extra space at the end of a sentence. The Korean Hangul is an alphabetic writing system that also features syllables as visual units. It differs from the above languages in that it puts additional spaces between words, a recent adaptation from the West (Sohn, 2001).

Functions of paraorthographic marking

The oldest function of punctuation goes back to its origin two millennia ago, i.e., as transcriptions of paralinguistic features such as pauses, intonation, stress, etc. (Crystal, 1997; Lawler, 2006). The Spanish inverted question mark (¿) alerts the reader of an upcoming question, because a statement may be syntactically indistinguishable from a question except for the intonation. A subtle case in English is the comma, which often represents a *mid-low-high-mid* sequence (Lawler, 2006). Thus the use of commas in counting "fifty-one, fifty-two, fifty-three, ..." gives an "authorial voice."

More relevant to reading eye movement planning are two relatively new functions of paraorthographic symbols. The first is to provide a hierarchical segmentation of a written text. It is evident from the evolution of punctuation that paraorthographic conventions distinguish four levels of linguistic objects: (a) paragraphs or major sections of texts, which are discourse level objects that are among the earliest to be marked; (b) sentences, or major pauses, are marked not only with periods (or "!" or "?") but also with capitalization of the initial letter; (c) the clause and/or phrasal level, or minor pauses, often marked with commas; and (d) words, flanked by spaces and occasionally with hyphens. The paraorthographic system not only segments the text with a rich set of explicit markers but also visualizes the hierarchical structure. This is a great advantage over spoken language and is exploited in eye movement programming.

Another role of punctuations is to indicate status of a constituent, what Nunberg called the "text grammar," a set of rules that determine syntactic relations among elements of written texts (Lawler, 2006; Nunberg, 1990; Nunberg, et al., 2001). For example, the following example (Nunberg, et al., 2001, p. 1736) is invalid because it requires a matching comma to the left of "in fact" in order to signal that the parenthetical phrase is not at the same level as the main sentence.

Jill was in fact, keeping her opinions open.

By using punctuations and other paraorthographic conventions, the author embeds a series of visual clues in the text, with the intention of illuminating the hierarchical structure of the text and guiding readers through potential parsing hazards. No paralinguistic system in spoken language provides as much systematic scaffolding, despite the inherent idiosyncrasy and inconsistency in the everyday usage of paraorthographic symbols. This is necessitated by the nature of written communications—one-way, asynchronous, solitary, and without paralinguistic support. And history shows that its evolution was driven primarily by the readers. What are the paybacks to the readers, then?

Paraorthography and eye movements

Paraorthography is designed for eye movement guidance. This is a hypothesis entertained by medievalists Parkes (2003) and Saenger (1997). In addition to the historical evidence they have amassed, some eye movement data also support the conjecture.

First, there is a history of extraordinary difficulties in parsing unsegmented text into meaningful linguistic units, words or otherwise. Whatever eye-movement strategies *scriptio continua* required, it could not have been efficient for word recognition. There are a handful of studies on reading English without spaces. Epelbiom and colleagues (Epelboim, Booth, & Steinman, 1994; see also Epelboim, Booth, Ashkenazy, Taleghani, & Steinman, 1997) found that native and second language readers of English can read *scriptio continua* (albeit with punctuations), but 30% slower. Rayner and colleagues estimated an approximately 50% decrease in reading rate (Morris, Rayner, & Pollatsek, 1990; Rayner et al., 1996; Pollatsek & Rayner, 1982). While readers are able to comprehend unspaced text fairly well, just like readers 2,000 years ago, their reading efficiency suffers.

Second, paraorthography is designed to group orthographic symbols linguistically as well as visually. Indeed, what could visually segment a letter string better than blank spaces, or blank spaces with minuscule dots? Were it just for linguistic segmentation, less visually salient symbols would suffice. Spaces around words reduce lateral inhibition at word borders and therefore make the initial and final letters much more perceivable. Johnson, Perea, and Rayner (2007) showed that extreme letters contribute more to the parafoveal preview benefits than word-medial letters. Most importantly, orthographic words now stand out as individual visual objects, allowing them to be recognized as perceptual wholes. Its significance can only be appreciated when one considers how reading was done before this point. Saenger (1997, p.85) wrote that "word separation ... provided shortcuts for achieving the reading skills that an elite among the ancients had mastered only through a prolonged and arduous grammatical apprenticeship."

The final observation, perhaps more of a conjecture, is that segmental punctuation marks are evolved to guide parafoveal saccade programming. Evidence comes from historical changes in the shapes of many punctuation marks and word delimiters: The general trend is a reduction in their spatial frequency, either through simplifying strokes or by widening the symbols. In other words, punctuation becomes more like blank space. Until 11th century letter *h* and the diacritic *dasia*, silent letters in Medieval Latin, were sometimes used as word separators (Saenger, 1997, p. 84). The Irish scribes used a '7'-like sign for pauses, and the letter *K* (for *kaput*, or 'head' in the argument) to introduce a new periodus (Parkes, 2003, p. 12). Eventually all these symbols were replaced by ones visually distinctive from letters. This would be a welcome change for the oculomotor system. Punctuated texts appear in the peripheral as separated objects of variable lengths. Our oculomotor system knows how to deal with this kind of visual input (Findlay & Walker, 1999).

The evolution of paraorthography was a history of pluralism and idiosyncrasy. But what emerged from the chaos was a set of symbols and conventions that segment texts linguistically as well as visually. Compare our reading experience with Quintilian's description in the 1st century: Reading requires "dividing the attention so that the eyes are occupied in one way and the voice another" (*dividenda intentio animi ut aliud voce aliud oculis agatur*; Parkes, 2003, p. 10). The co-evolution between eye movement planning and the paraorthographic system has changed the nature of reading.

The paraorthographic linkage hypothesis

This chapter began by examining a common assumption among current theories of reading eye movements, i.e., that the concept of the word links visual word identification, post-lexical linguistic processes, and saccade planning together as an optimal system. I argued the *word* is not a unit of linguistic analysis but a result of writing conventions. The last section took a historical look at the emergence of paraorthogrphic conventions and suggested that paraorthography was developed, at least in part, to ease all three aspects of reading. We now come to the natural conclusion: Paraorthographic symbols, not *words*, enable optimal coordination of sub-processes in reading.

Unlike the word, which is presumably a unit of language, paraorthographic symbols result from intentional human actions. They are the breadcrumbs[1] the author left to lead the readers to the correct interpretation of the message. Paraorthography also provides optimal (or near optimal) solutions to the time-compression challenge in reading, by virtue of trial-and-error over millennia. By this account, the reason word-based theories enjoy extraordinary success in English reading is because they capture the essence of what the English paraorthographic system set out to do. By the same token, a key to understanding eye movement control in a different language is to know what paraortho-

1 In the Brothers Grimm fairytale *Hansel and Gretel*, the two boys left breadcrumbs along the trail in order to find home.

graphic aids readers and writers of the language have already established.

The Paraorthographic Linkage Hypothesis (PoLH) is an attempt to formalize these insights. It starts with the assumption that at the initial stage the three main components of reading—foveal and parafoveal object (word) identification, language comprehension, and saccade planning—are independent and not well coordinated. Their coordination will improve with reading experience, but optimality is often achieved with the guidance of the paraorthography. Specifically, PoLH involves three principles:

Loose coupling

A basic premise of the PoLH is that saccade planning, visual recognition, and language comprehension are three separate modules prior to the emergence of reading and writing. They are loosely connected in the initial stage. In other words, proficient reading processes originate from a set of ineffective, poorly coordinated sub-systems.

The disassociation among the three sub-systems is self-evident. We move our eyes when we are not reading. Our linguistic faculty exists long before we can read or write. Foveal processing can also be divorced from saccade planning. Word recognition can be accomplished without moving the eyes. In fact, classic RSVP (Rapid Serial Visual Presentation) studies have shown that reading speed can be temporarily raised to 1200 words per minute if words are flashed in succession at the fovea (Juola, Ward, & McNamara, 1982, but see Masson, 1983, on effects on comprehension). Conversely, we also appear to have no trouble making reading-like eye movements without any linguistic processing. A number of studies asked readers to "read" nonsense letter strings that resemble print, i.e., with comparable paraorthographic marking such as paragraphs, punctuations, and "word" spaces (Vitu, O'Regan, Inhoff, & Topolski, 1995). At the surface level eye movements in scanning nonsense strings share some important similarities with those in reading.

A reasonable but obviously ineffective strategy, one that may be initially adopted by beginning readers, is to plan the next saccade only after foveal word recognition is completed. This would leave approximately 100 milliseconds per fixation in idle while waiting for oculomotor programming and execution. Improvement over this strategy relies on two additional factors—our intrinsic capacity to learn and optimize and the paraorthographic clues authors left.

Paraorthographic linkage

Spaces, punctuations, capitalizations, and the like are intentional cues left by the author. Paraorthography not only prevents readers from wandering astray but also enables seamless integration of the reading processes. This hypothesis follows from the functions of paraorthographic symbols—they visually parse written symbols into meaningful linguistic units, and they signal syntactic and semantic relations among linguistic entities.

The disambiguating function of interword spaces is discussed in the previous section. Much less discussed in the eye-movement literature is the role of paraorthography in signaling relations among linguistic constituents (Nunberg, 1990). As the current sentence shows, even with words clearly identifiable note this gives the reader a huge advantage over first century monks comprehension is still impaired to a point of pain. The use of punctuation releases us from constant struggles with syntactic ambiguities during reading. Ironically, the ubiquity of punctuation in today's texts gives rise to models of reading eye movements that ignore their presence.

Spaces or other word separators reduce the difficulty of foveal processing in a number of ways. First, having spaces eliminates the need for parsing letter strings into linguistic units for recognition. Furthermore, the initial and final letters of a word are more salient and identifiable with spaces. Last, paraorthographic symbols enable consistent representations of individual orthographic words, as opposed to words embedded in unpredictable letter sequences. This should amplify perceptual learning during repeated print exposure and further speed up foveal—and potentially parafoveal—word recognition. Similarly, parafoveal processing also benefits from paraorthography. For example, readers use the length of the upcoming word to plan the next eye movement (see Rayner 1998). In addition, by reducing lateral inhibition, spaces also allow at least partial identification of the extreme letters of parafoveal words (Johnson et al., 2007).

Compared to *scriptio continua*, separated and punctuated texts afford more efficient reading strategies (McConkie et al., 1988): Programming the eye to go to the OVP of a parafoveal word, which minimizes foveal processing time, leaves more time for parafoveal processing; this in turn allows more judicious choice of the next saccade target. In addition, with most of the potential syntactic and discourse parsing ambiguities taken care of by punctuation, foveal word identification becomes the primary constraint in eye movement programming. This confirms one of the assumptions of current eye movement models.

The optimal strategy for reading English may not necessarily be adaptive for reading other languages. When orthographic words are long and morphologically complex, multiple fixations may be required for word identification. It would not be advisable to target the center of a long word in the parafovea; instead, shooting for somewhere left of the center is more likely to provide the morphological parser with useful information.

The optimal reading strategy is neither hardwired nor explicitly taught. The only way to achieve efficiency is through unsupervised learning from experiences. And reading provides a plethora of opportunities to do so.

Optimality

The third principle is concerned with the acquisition of proficient reading strategies. An optimal strategy is defined here as one that maximizes system performances in the long haul. One way to characterize reading performance is the speed of reading at a certain level of comprehension (Carver, 1990). In other words, the goal of optimization is to achieve the most efficient reading while maintaining comprehension. A computational model of the optimization process is presented elsewhere (Feng, 2007). Here I will focus on evidence for the optimization process and the facilitative role of paraorthography.

Evidence of developmental changes in reading is overwhelming. By 5th grade, an avid reader is exposed to over 4 million words per year, and even the average 5th grader reads over a half million words each year (Anderson, Wilson, & Fielding, 1988). The sheer amount of practice dwarfs any other complex cognitive skills that are not part of our biological endowment. The impact of these exercises is profound. From first grade to college, children's reading speed increases more than threefold, from approximately 80 wpm to 300 wpm (Taylor, 1965; Carver, 1990). The average fixation duration decreases over time and saccade length increases, along with other changes toward a more adult-like pattern (see Rayner, 1998). Children's ability to consciously control saccade programming also improves with age (Fischer, Biscaldi, & Gezeck, 1997).

Paraorthography contributes to the optimization of reading processes in two ways. New paraorthographic conventions changed the nature of the text and the task of reading. In addition to these "hard" changes in the text and processing, paraorthography also introduces more subtle or "soft" cues that are no less important. Specifically, spaces and punctuations allow readers to further improve reading performance based on probabilistic regularities.

For example, additional time could be saved if the foveal word recognition time were known before hand. In this case the timing of oculomotor planning would be adjusted to minimize the "idle" time, i.e., the time between the completion of foveal word processing and the initiation of the next saccade. Such information can potentially be calculated by a learning algorithm. With a sample size in the millions, the estimates are potentially very informative for eye movement programming.

Clearly, these statistics are unimaginable in *scriptio continua*. Foveal processing would be preoccupied by lexical parsing and other processes. Parafoveal information such as word length was also unattainable. First century Latin readers must have optimized their reading processes in some ways, but the range of information provided by the paraorthography was extremely impoverished by today's standard. This reiterates the point that the reading process, as we know it, down to the split-second decisions readers make, is ultimately the creation of the paraorthographic system. Understanding the co-evolution of the two may shed new light on current debates in the literature.

Conclusions

At the onset of the chapter I contrasted the trinity of the word with a view that rejects the notion of the word as the conceptual basis for reading eye movement control. I argued that words—more precisely the orthographic words—bear no direct relationship with levels of linguistic analyses. As the foundation of a theory of reading eye movements, the concept of the word is convenient, intuitive, but ultimately illusive.

As an alternative, the Paraorthographic Linkage Hypothesis (PoLH) argues that, historically and cross-linguistically, reading processes are strongly constrained by paraorthography, which are embedded cues to help readers to reach intended interpretation of the author's message. To the extent paraorthography differs across language, the optimal reading processes should also differ accordingly.

The proposal here, however, is not one of linguistic relativism (e.g., Hoosain, 1991). Quite the contrary: The moral of the story is that readers constantly adapt and optimize their reading behaviors. It is this ability to adapt and to optimize that forms the basis for the universal theory of reading, not any of its end products.

Lastly, the PoLH has direct implications for reading Chinese, Japanese, and other non-spaced languages. From the point of view of current eye movement models, which are almost invariantly word-based, eye movement programming in these orthographies is paradoxical: how do you move the eyes to the next word if you don't know where the word is? The advice from PoLH is: Forget words, look for other cues. According to the PoLH, proficient readers in these languages are well-adapted to their own writing systems. Thus the paradox has always been in the researcher's mind, never the reader's. The starting point of an eye movement model for a new language should be to investigate constraints of the language and writing system, with the assurance that readers will always find the best solution, provided that they, well, read.

References

Anderson, R. C.,Wilson, P. T.,& Fielding, L. G. (1988). Growth in reading and how children spend their time outside of school. *Reading Research Quarterly, 23,* 285-303.

Andrews, S., Miller, B., & Rayner, K. (2004). Eye movements and morphological segmentation of compound words: There is a mouse in mousetrap. *European Journal of Cognitive Psychology, 16,* 285-311.

Booij, G. (2005). *The grammar of words: An introduction to linguistic morphology*. Oxford University Press, USA.

Bertram, R., & Hyönä, J. (2003). The length of a complex word modifies the role of morphological structure: Evidence from eye movements when reading short and long Finnish compounds. *Journal of Memory and Language, 48,* 615-634.

Caramazza, A., Laudanna, A., & Romani, C. (1988). Lexical access and inflectional morphology. *Cognition, 28,* 297-332.

Carver, R. P. (1990). *Reading rate: A review of research and theory.* NY: Academic Press.

Coulmas, F. (2003). *Writing systems: An introduction to their linguistic analysis.* Cambridge University Press.

Chao, Y. R. (1968). *A grammar of spoken Chinese.* Berkeley: University of California Press.

Coltheart, M., Rastle, K., Perry, C., Langdon, R., & Ziegler, J. (2001). DRC: A dual route cascaded model of visual word recognition and reading aloud. *Psychological Review, 108,* 204-256.

Crystal, D. (1997). *The Cambridge encyclopedia of language.* Cambridge University Press.

Daniels, P. T., & Bright, W. (1996). *The world's writing systems*. Oxford University Press, USA.

Dexter, T. (1838). *A pickle for the knowing ones, or, plain truths in a homespun dress*. Boston: Otis, Broaders and Co. Reprinted (2004) by Whitefish, MT: Kessinger Publishing.

Duanmu, S., (1998). Wordhood in Chinese. In J. Packard (Ed.), *New approaches to Chinese word formation: Morphology, phonology and the lexicon in modern and ancient Chinese* (pp.135-196). Berlin: Mouton de Gruyter.

Engbert, R., Nuthmann, A., Richter, E., & Kliegl, R. (2005). SWIFT: A dynamical model of saccade generation during reading. *Psychological Review, 112*, 777-813.

Epelboim, J., Booth, J. R., & Steinman, R. M. (1994). Reading unspaced text: Implication for theories of reading eye movements. *Vision Research, 34*, 1735-1766.

Epelboim, J., Booth, J. R., Ashkenazy, R., Taleghani, A., & Steinman, R.M. (1997). Fillers and spaces in text: The importance of word recognition during reading. *Vision Research, 37*, 2899-2914.

Feng, G. (2003). From eye movement to cognition: Toward a general framework of inference. Comment on Liechty et al., 2003. *Psychometrika, 68*, 551-556.

Feng, G. (2006). Eye movements in Chinese reading. In P. Li, L. Tan, E. Bates, & O. J. L. Tzeng (Eds.), *Handbook for east Asian psycholinguistics: Vol. 1*. London: Cambridge.

Feng, G. (2007). *Eye movement planning as stochastic optimization: Reinforcement learning in SHARE*. Paper presented at the 14th European Conference on Eye Movement.

Findlay, J. M., & Walker, R. (1999). A model of saccade generation based on parallel processing and competitive inhibition. *Behavioral & Brain Sciences, 22*, 661-721.

Fischer, B., Biscaldi, M., & Gezeck, S. (1997). On the development of voluntary and reflexive components in human saccade generation. *Brain Research, 754*, 285-297.

Haber, R. N. (1976). Control of eye movements during reading. In R. A. Monty, & J. W. Senders (Eds.), *Eye movements and psychological processes* (pp. 443-454). Hillsdale, NJ: Lawrence Erlbaum.

Hoosain, R. (1991). *Psycholinguistic implications for linguistic relativity: A case study of Chinese*. Hong Kong: Lawrence Erlbaum Assoc.

Hoover, W. A., & Gough, P. (1990). The simple view of reading. *Reading and Writing: An Interdisciplinary Journal, 2*, 127-160.

Hyönä, J., Bertram, R., & Pollatsek, A. (2004). Are long compound words identified serially via their constituents? Evidence from an eye-movement-contingent display change study. *Memory & Cognition, 32*, 523-532.

Johanson, L., & Csató, É. (1998). *The Turkic languages*. Routledge.

Johnson, R. L., Perea, M., & Rayner, K. (2007). Transposed-letter effects in reading: Evidence from eye movements and parafoveal preview. *Journal of Experimental Psychology: Human Perception and Performance, 33*(1), 209-229.

Johnson, S. A. (2005). *Spelling trouble? Language, ideology and the reform of German orthography*. Multilingual Matters Limited.

Juhasz, B. J., Inhoff, A. W., & Rayner, K. (2005). The role of interword spaces in the processing of English compound words. *Language and Cognitive Processes, 20*, 291-316.

Juola, J. F., Ward, N. J., & McNamara, T. (1982). Visual search and reading of rapid serial presentations of letter strings, words, and text. *Journal of Experimental Psychology: General, 111*, 208-227.

Kennedy, A., & Pynte, J. (2005). Parafoveal-on-foveal effects in normal reading. *Vision Research, 45*, 153-168.

Lawler, J. (2006). Punctuations. In K. Brown (Ed.), *Encyclopedia of language and linguistics*, 2ed. Elsevier.

Legge, G. E., Hooven, T. A., Klitz, T. S., Mansfield, S. J., & Tjan, B. S. (2002). Mr. Chips: New insights from an ideal-observer model of reading. *Vision Research, 42*, 2219-2234.

Legge, G. E., Klitz, T. S., & Tjan, B. S. (1997). Mr. Chips: An ideal-observer model of reading. *Psychological Review, 104*, 1524-1553.

Masson, M. E. J. (1983). Conceptual processing of text during skimming and rapid sequential reading. *Memory & Cognition, 11*, 262-274.

McConkie, G. W., Kerr, P. W., & Dyre, B. P. (1994). What are "normal" eye movements during reading: Toward a mathematical description. In J. Ygge, & G. Lennerstrand (Eds.), *Eye movements in reading* (pp. 315-327). Tarrytown, NY: Pergamon.

McConkie, G. W., Kerr, P. W., Reddix, M. D., & Zola, D. (1988). Eye movement control during reading: I. The location of initial eye fixations on words. *Vision Research, 28*, 1107-1118.

McDonald, S. A., Carpenter, R. H. S., & Shillcock, R. C. (2005). An anatomically constrained, stochastic model of eye movement control in reading. *Psychological Review, 112*, 814-840.

Morris, R., Rayner, K., & Pollatsek, A. (1990). Eye movement guidance in reading: The role of parafoveal letter and space information. *Journal of Experimental Psychology: Human Perception and Performance, 16*, 268-281.

Morrison, R. E. (1984). Manipulation of stimulus onset delay in reading: Evidence for parallel programming of saccades. *Journal of Experimental Psychology: Human Perception and Performance, 10*, 667-682.

Niemi, J., Laine, M., & Tuominen, J. (1995). Cognitive morphology in Finnish: Foundations of a new model. *Language and Cognitive Processes, 9*, 423-446.

Nunberg, G. (1990). *The linguistics of punctuation*. Center for the Study of Language and Information.

Nunberg, G., Briscoe, T., & Huddleston, R. (2001). Punctuation. In G. Pullum, & R. Huddleston (Eds.), *The Cambridge grammar of the English language* (pp.1723-1764). Cambridge University Press.

O'Regan, J. K. (1990). Eye-movements and reading. In E. Kowler (Ed.), *Eye movements and their tole in visual and cognitive processes* (pp. 395-453). Amsterdam: Elsevier.

O'Regan, J. K., & Jacobs, A. M. (1992). Optimal viewing position effect in word recognition: A challenge to current theory. *Journal of Experimental Psychology: Human Perception* and *Performance, 18*, 185-197.

Parkes, M. (2003). *Scribes, scripts and readers: Studies in the communication, presentation and dissemination of medieval texts*. Hambledon & London.

Pollatsek, A., & Rayner, K. (1982). Eye movement control in reading: The role of word boundaries. *Journal of Experimental Psychology: Human Perception and Performance, 8*, 817-833.

Rayner, K. (1978). Eye movements in reading and information processing. *Psychological Bulletin, 85*, 618-660

Rayner, K. (1979). Eye guidance in reading: Fixation locations within words. *Perception, 8*, 21-30.

Rayner, K. (1998). Eye movements in reading and information processing: 20 years of research. *Psychological Bulletin, 124*, 372-422.

Rayner, K., Li, X., & Polllatsek, A. (2007). Extending the E-Z Reader model of eye movement control to Chinese readers. *Cognitive Science, 31*, 1021-1034.

Reichle, E. D., & Perfetti, C. A. (2003). Morphology in word identification: A word-experience model that accounts for morpheme frequency effects. *Scientific Studies of Reading, 7*, 219-237.

Reichle, E. D., Pollatsek, A., Fisher, D. L., & Rayner, K. (1998). Toward a model of eye movement control in reading. *Psychological Review, 105*, 125-157.

Reichle, E. D., Rayner, K., & Pollatsek, A. (2003). The E-Z Reader model of eye-movement control in reading: Comparisons to other models. *Behavioral and Brain Sciences, 26*, 445-476.

Reilly, R. G., & O'Regan, J. K. (1998). Eye movement control during reading: A simulation of some word-targeting strategies. *Vision Research, 38*, 303-317.

Richter, E. M., Engbert, R., & Kliegl, R. (2006). Current advances in

SWIFT. *Cognitive Systems Research, 7*, 23-33.

Saenger, P.H. (1997). *Space between words: The origins of silent reading.* Stanford, Calif: Stanford University Press.

Seidenberg, M. (2005). Connectionist models of word reading. *Current Directions in Psychological Science, 14*, 238-242.

Sereno, S. C., & Rayner, K. (2003). Measuring word recognition in reading: Eye movements and event-related potentials. *Trends in Cognitive Sciences, 7*, 489-493.

Shillcock, R., Ellison, T., & Monaghan, P. (2000). Eye-fixation behavior, lexical storage, and visual word recognition in a split processing model. *Psychological Review, 107*, 824-851.

Sohn, H. (2001). *The Korean Language*. Cambridge University Press.

Spencer, A. (1991). *Morphological theory : An introduction to word structure in generative grammar* . Oxford: Basil Blackwell.

Taylor, S. E. (1965). Eye movements while reading: Facts and fallacies. *American Educational Research Journal, 2*, 187-202.

Truss, L. (2004). *Eats, shoots & leave : The zero tolerance approach to punctuation*. Gotham Books.

Tsai, C. H. (2002). *Word identification and eye movements in reading Chinese: A modeling approach.* Unpublished Ph. D. dissertation, U Illinois at Urbana-Champaign.

Vitu, F., O'Regan, J. K., Inhoff, A.W., & Topolski, R. (1995). Mindless reading: Eye-movement characteristics are similar in scanning letter strings and reading texts. *Perception & Psychophysics, 57*, 352-364.

White, S., Rayner, K., & Liversedge, S. (2005). Eye movements and the modulation of parafoveal processing by foveal processing difficulty: A reexamination. *Psychonomic Bulletin & Review, 12*, 891-896.

Yang, H. M., & McConkie, G. W. (1994). Eye movement control in Chinese reading. *Bulletin of the National TaiNan Teacher's College, 29*, 193-229.

Author index

Subject index

A.

B.

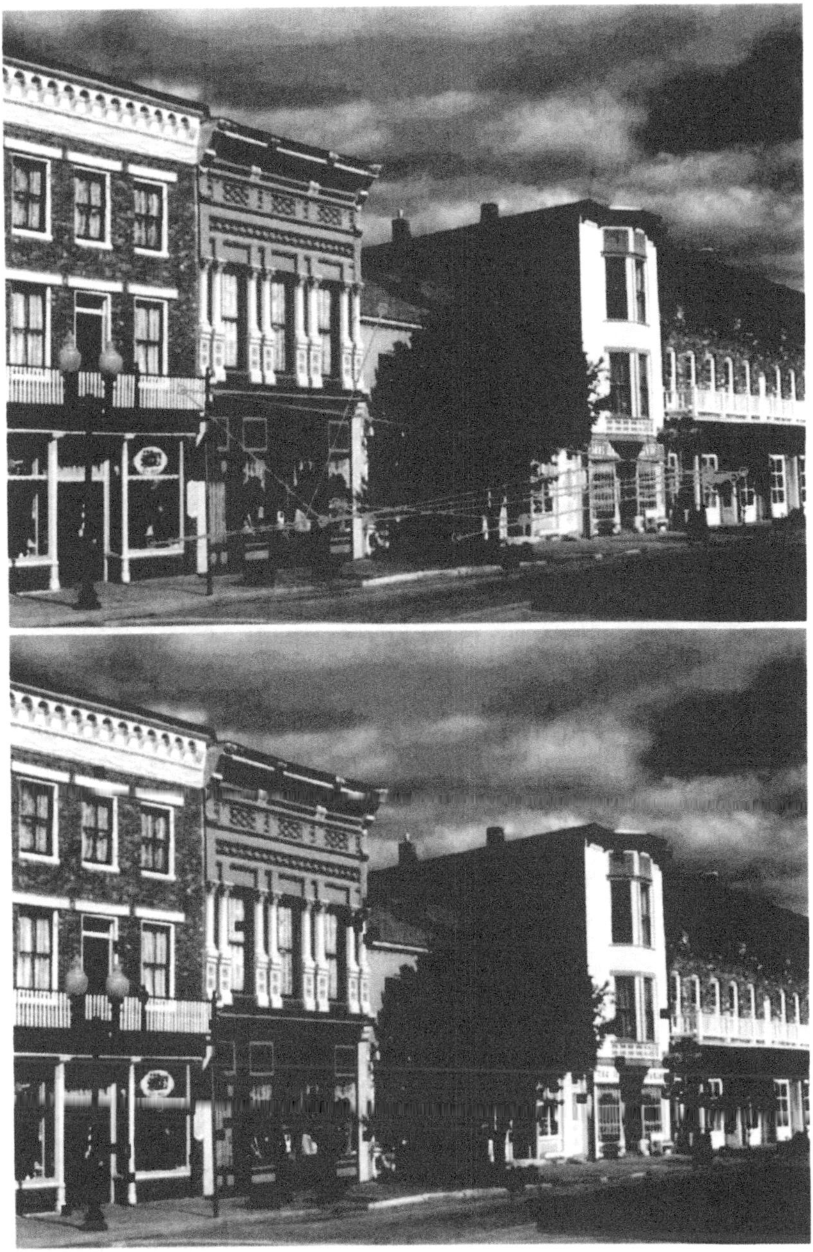

Plate 1 Examples of where viewers look in scenes. The top portion of the figure shows where one viewer fixates in the scene (the dots represent fixation points and the lines represent the sequence). The bottom portion shows where a number of different viewers fixate (with the dots representing fixation locations across a number of viewers). (*See Figure 1.3, Chapter 1, p. 16.*)

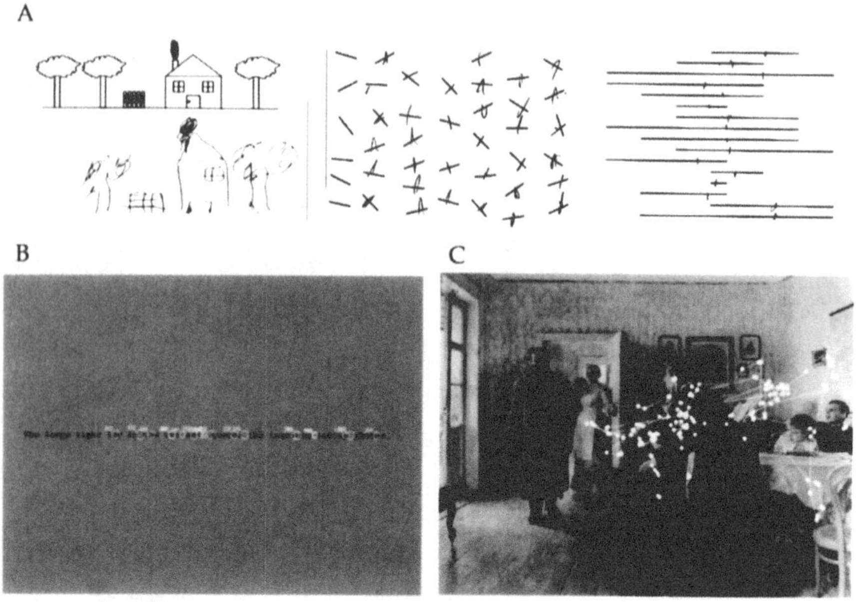

Plate 2 (A) screening data for MB for a cancellation task, a line bi-section task and a scene copying task, (B) the number, location and duration of fixations that were made by MB when reading a single sentence, and (C) the scanpath made by MB as he inspected the 'Repin' picture under free viewing conditions. (The Repin picture was downloaded from http://www.abcgallery.com/R/repin/repin46.JPG). (*See Figure 6.3, Chapter 6, p. 131.*)

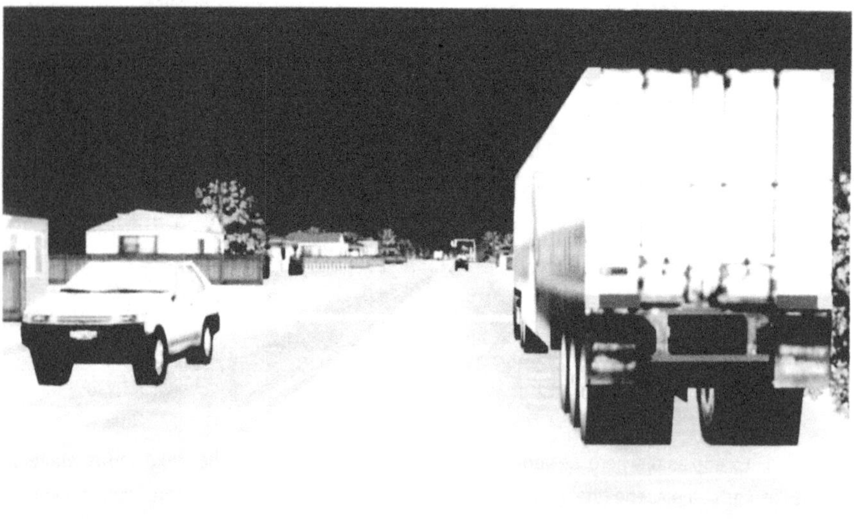

Plate 3 Perspective view in driving simulator: truck crosswalk scenario (*See Figure 8.2, Chapter 8, p. 160.*)

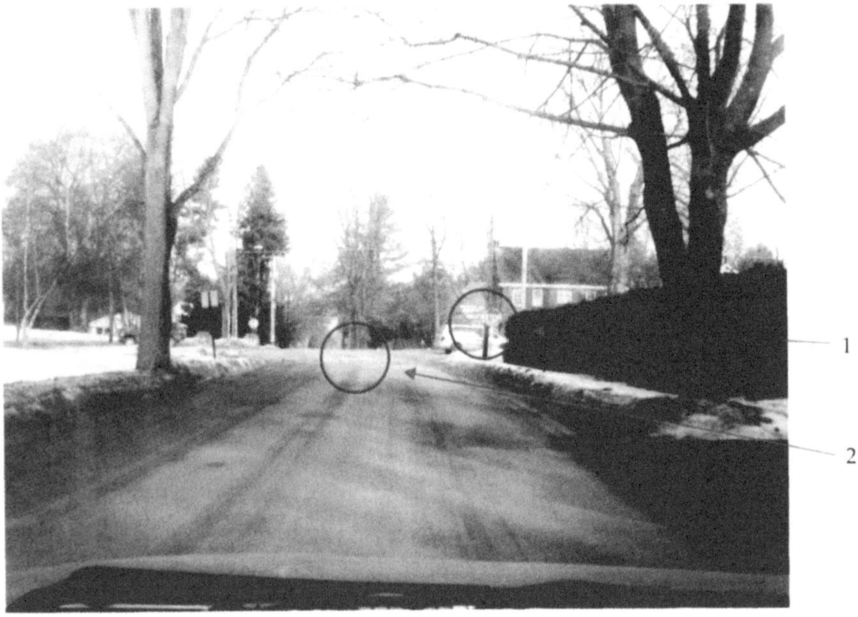

Plate 4 Still photograph used In PC-based training (*See Figure 8.3, Chapter 8, p. 163.*)

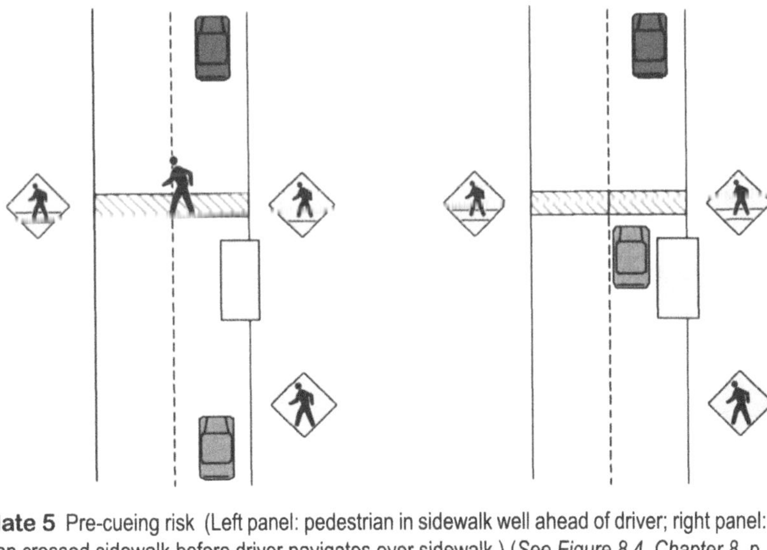

Plate 5 Pre-cueing risk (Left panel: pedestrian in sidewalk well ahead of driver; right panel: pedestrian crossed sidewalk before driver navigates over sidewalk.) (*See Figure 8.4, Chapter 8, p. 167.*)

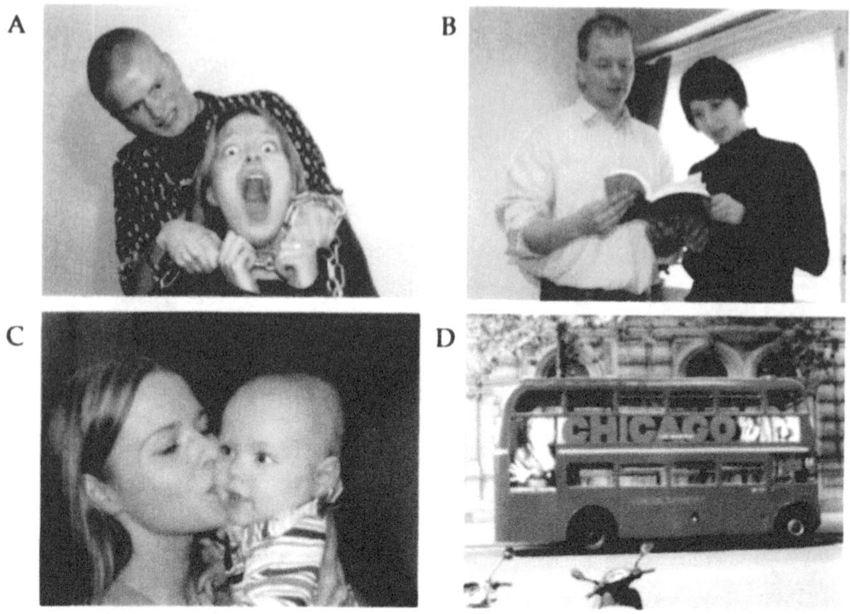

Plate 6 Illustration of unpleasant (A), neutral (B), pleasant (C), and control (D) stimuli used in the studies. Note that these example pictures were not among the experimental stimuli. (*See Figure 9.1, Chapter 9, p. 180.*)

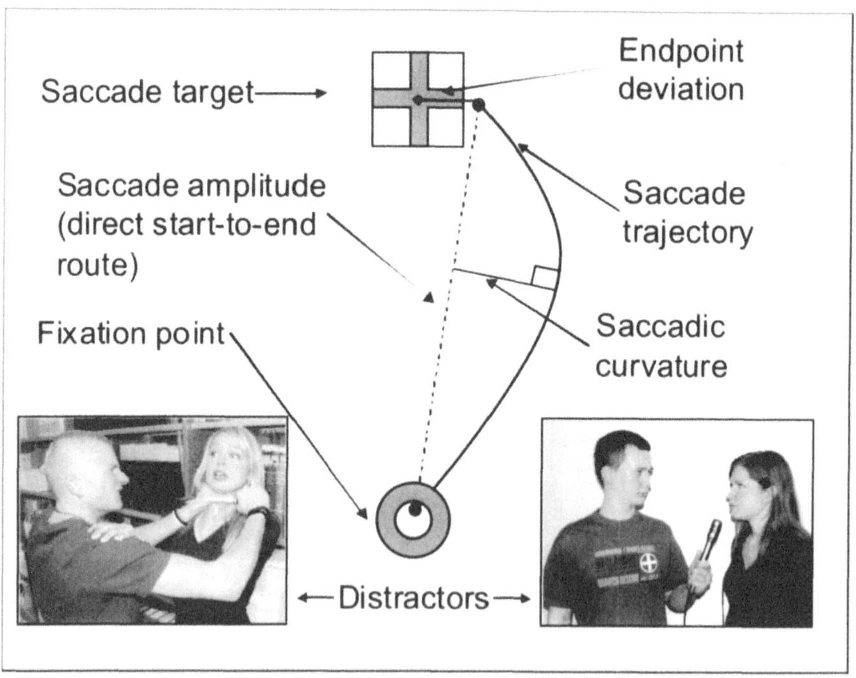

Plate 7 An illustration of the measure of saccadic curvature and saccade endpoint deviation. An emotional distracter appears on the left and a neutral distracter on the right. (*See Figure 9.3, Chapter 9, p. 185.*)

Plate 8 Examples of the three types of stimuli use: gun, IED and plain rectangle. The gun and the IED shown here comprise a target pair for dual-target search. (*See Figure 10.3, Chapter 10, p. 202.*)

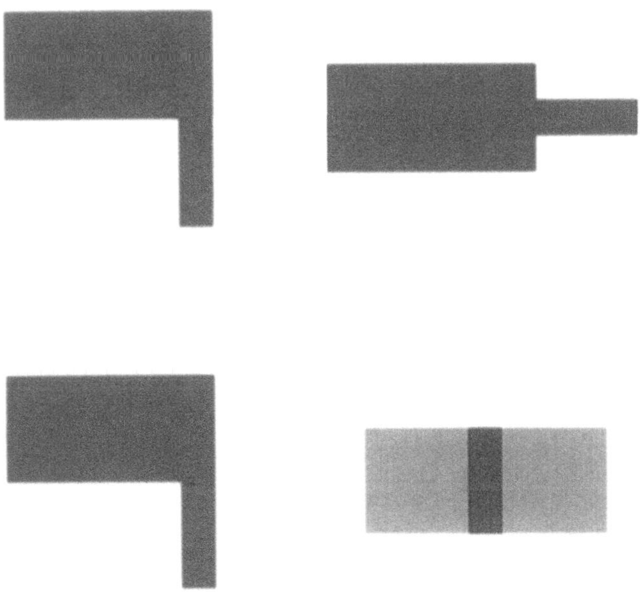

Plate 9 Example pairs of targets. Upper panel: same-color gun and knife targets. Lower panel: different-color gun and IED targets. (*See Figure 10.4, Chapter 10, p. 203.*)

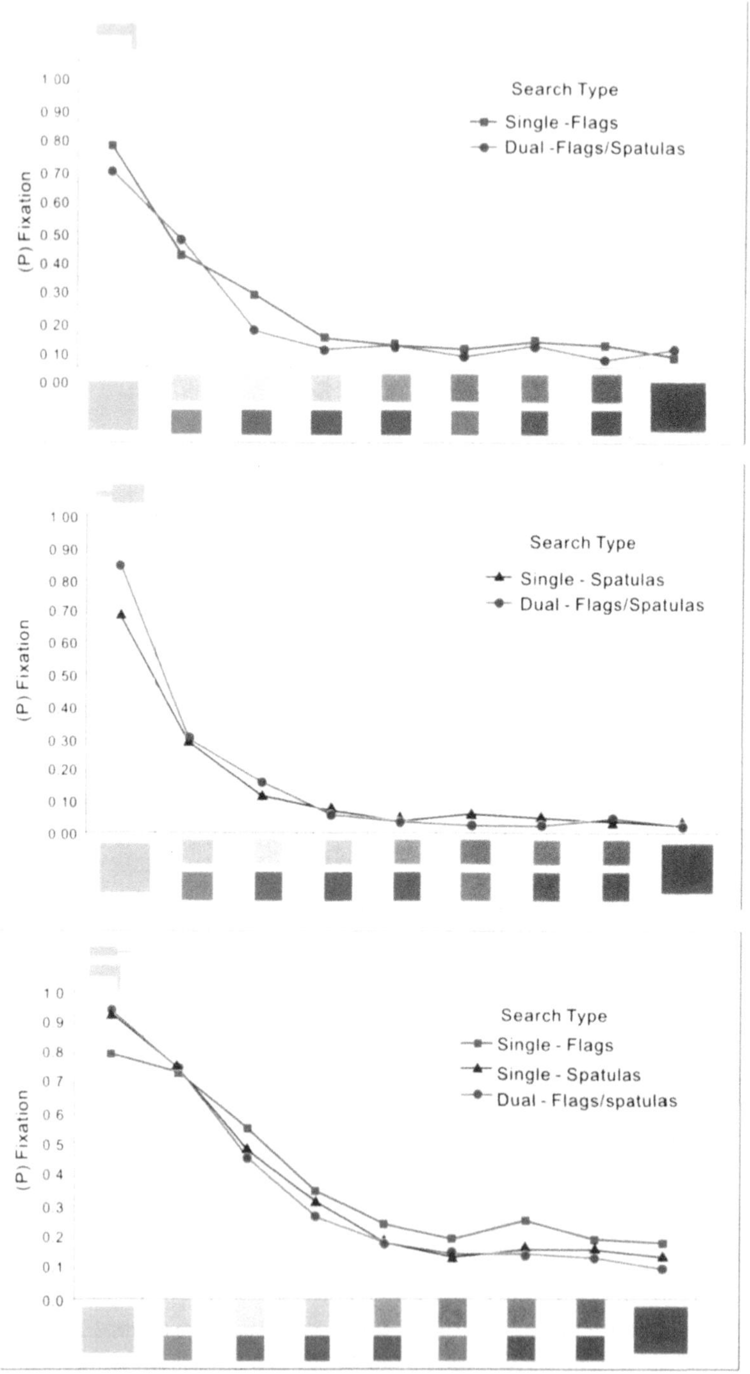

Plate 10 Probability of fixating a target of a given color when targets share the same color on gun present trials, knife present trials and absent trials. (*See Figure 10.5, Chapter 10, p. 205.*)

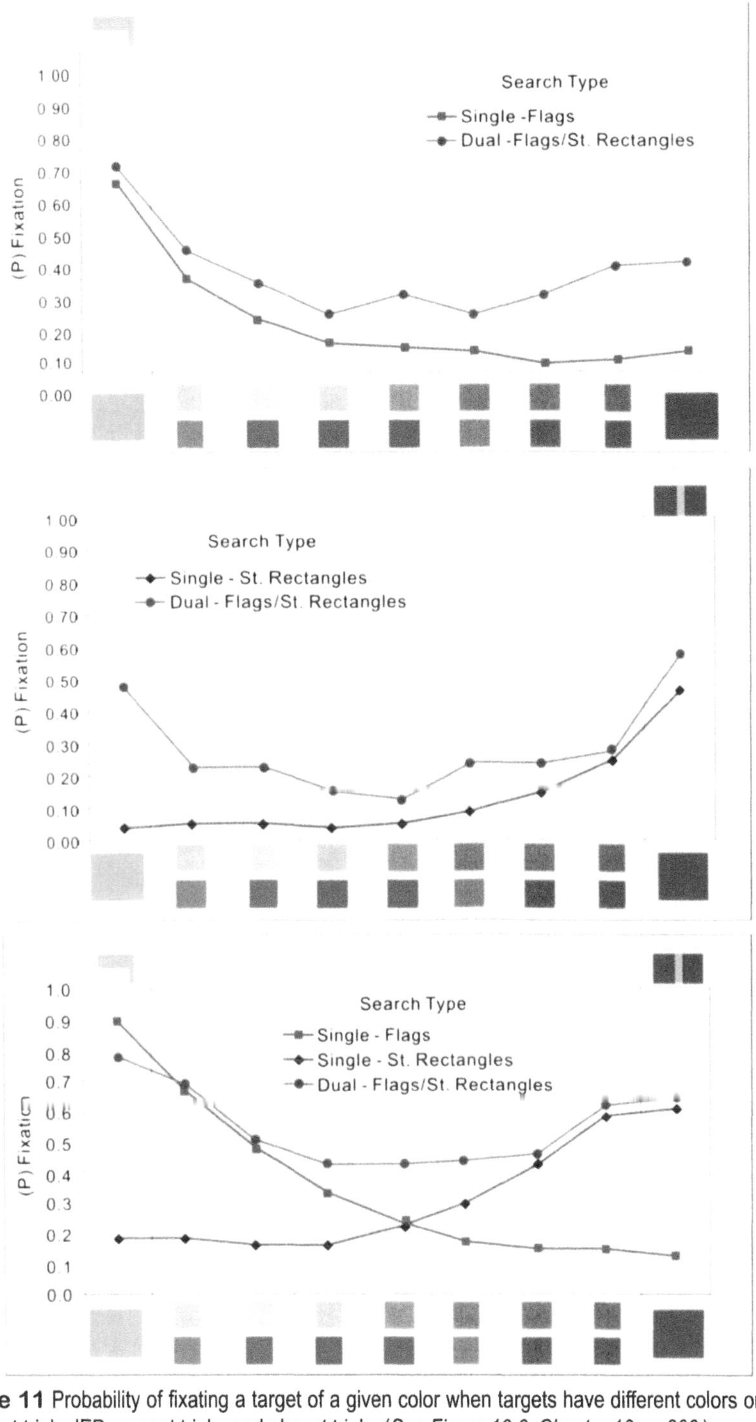

Plate 11 Probability of fixating a target of a given color when targets have different colors on gun present trials, IED present trials, and absent trials. (*See Figure 10.6, Chapter 10, p. 206.*)

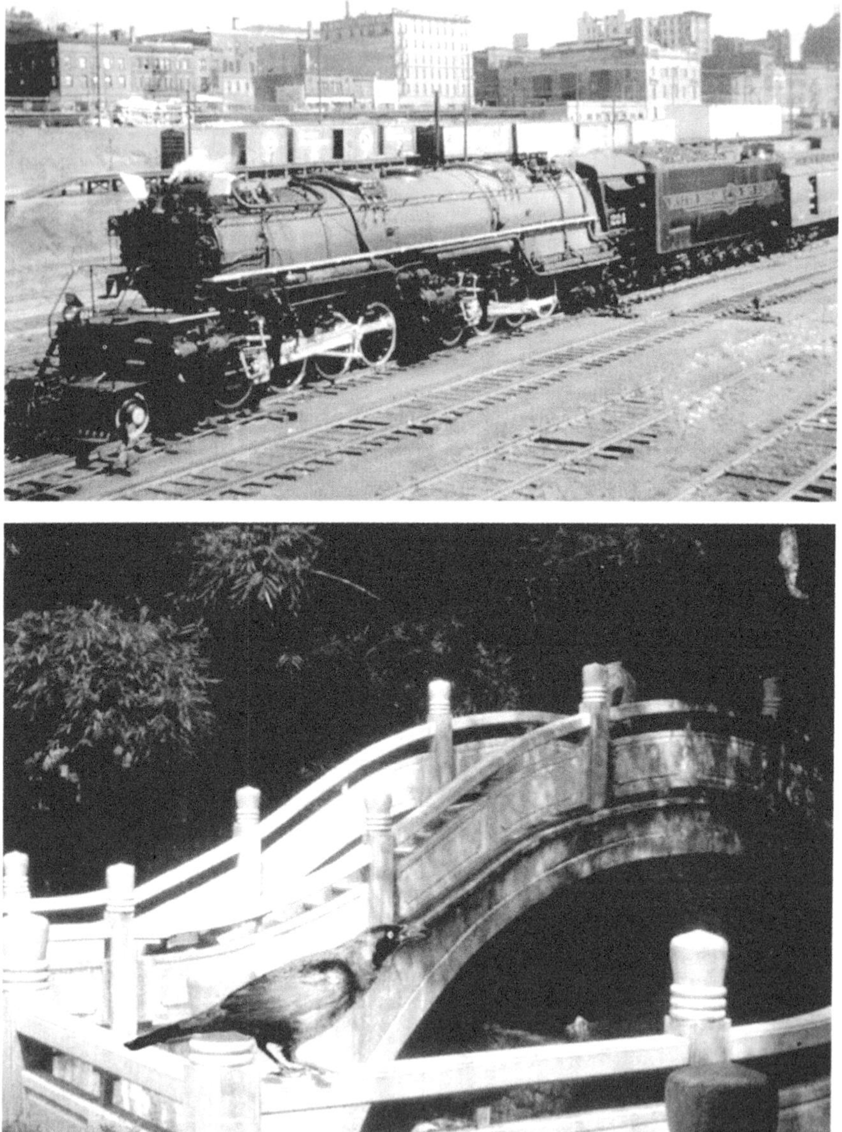

Plate 12 Two example scenes from Chua, Boland, and Nisbett (2005) illustrate the range in size and placement of our focal objects and the salience of the background objects. In the train yard picture, the train in the foreground was considered the focal object. In the bird/bridge picture, only the bird was considered the focal object. (*See Figure 18.1, Chapter 18, p. 368.*)